Atlas of Differential Diagnosis in
DERMATOLOGY

Atlas of Differential Diagnosis in
DERMATOLOGY

Klaus F. Helm, M.D.
Associate Professor
Division of Dermatology
Departments of Medicine and Pathology
Pennsylvania State University College of Medicine
Hershey, Pennsylvania

James G. Marks, Jr., M.D.
Professor
Division of Dermatology
Department of Medicine
Pennsylvania State University College of Medicine
Hershey, Pennsylvania

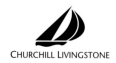

CHURCHILL LIVINGSTONE

New York, Edinburgh, London, Madrid, Melbourne, San Francisco, Tokyo

CHURCHILL LIVINGSTONE
Medical Division of Pearson Professional Limited

Distributed in the United States of America by Churchill Livingstone Inc., 650 Avenue of the Americas, New York, N.Y. 10011, and by associated companies, branches and representatives throughout the world.

First published 1998

ISBN 0 443 05605 6

British Library of Cataloguing in Publication Data
A catalogue record for this book is available from the British Library.

Library of Congress Cataloging in Publication Data
A catalog record for this book is available from the Library of Congress.

Acquisitions Editor: *Sheila Khullar*
Production Editor: *Dave Terry*
Production Supervisor: *Sharon Tuder*
Desktop Coordinator: *Kathy Jo Dunayer*
Cover Design: *Jeannette Jacobs*

Printed in Hong Kong

To Jan and Joyce

Preface

This book presents both common and uncommon dermatologic differential diagnoses in a problem-oriented manner. Unlike other atlases that catalog diseases, this book stresses the viewpoint of the clinician. A repeatable and discerning approach to evaluating skin diseases is the unifying theme. Algorithms, clinical photographs, and tables that compare diseases present specific points important in arriving at the correct diagnosis.

To facilitate accurate diagnoses, several different approaches have been used. The reader who knows the differential diagnosis in question can go directly to the appropriate table or discussion by using the index. If the diagnosis is unclear, possible diagnoses can be obtained by using the following algorithm in conjunction with the algorithm found at the beginning of each chapter. Finally, in each chapter, tables of differential diagnoses for different types of eruptions or neoplasms are included with accompanying illustrative photographs. The etiology, important clinical features, and therapy for each disease is succinctly presented in the last section of each chapter.

Klaus F. Helm, M.D.
James G. Marks, Jr., M.D.

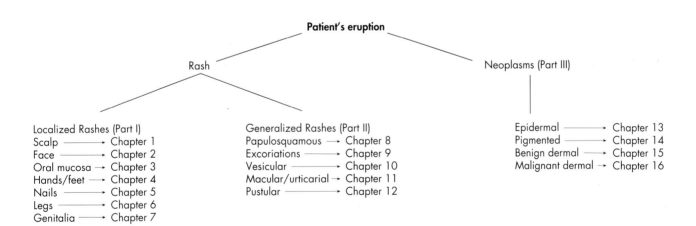

Acknowledgments

We thank Dr. Thomas Helm for proofreading the manuscript, and acknowledge Dr. Frederick Helm and the staff and dermatology residents at the Pennsylvania State University College of Medicine for providing some of the photographs. We also thank Dianne Safford for typing portions of the manuscript.

Contents

I

Localized Rashes

1 Scalp

ALGORITHM FOR INFLAMMATORY DISEASES OF THE SCALP

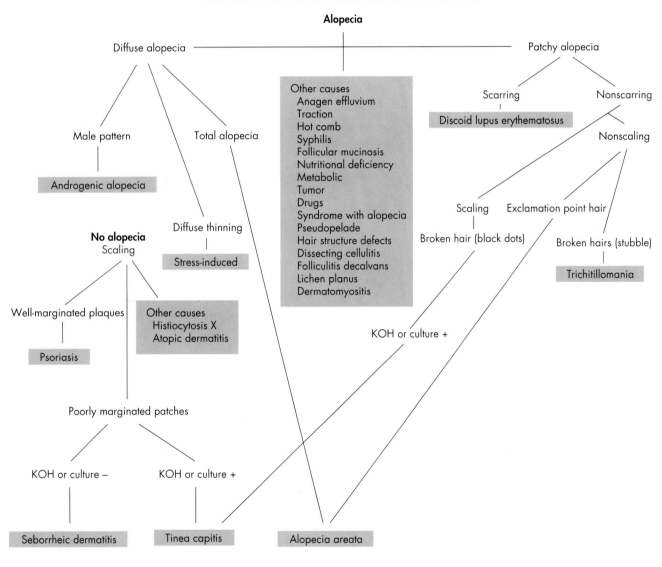

Introduction

The average scalp contains more than 100,000 hairs in a mixture of different growth phases. Eighty-five percent are in an active growing phase (anagen), 5% are in a transitional phase (catagen), and 10% are in a resting phase (telogen). The average number of hairs shed daily is approximately 100. The hair grows approximately 1 cm each month. In the adult, there are two types of hair: *vellus* (fine, usually light colored, fuzzy hair) and *terminal* (coarse, thick, usually pigmented hair).

Disorders of the hair and scalp are fairly frequent presenting complaints. The physical examination is often the most critical component in the evaluation of these patients. However, a detailed history and, on occasion, laboratory tests or a biopsy may also be required to establish a definitive diagnosis. Initially, the examination should determine whether there is hair loss. Diseases such as psoriasis, seborrheic dermatitis, and diffuse tinea capitis present as inflammatory conditions of the scalp without associated hair loss. When alopecia (hair loss) is present, it is helpful to observe the pattern—diffuse or patchy. *Diffuse alopecia* may occur in a typical distribution involving the frontal and vertex regions of the scalp, characteristic of androgenic or male pattern baldness. Diffuse, thinning, or total alopecia can be seen in alopecia areata, following physically or mentally stressful events (telogen effluvium), or secondary to a metabolic disorder, drug reactions, or a dietary deficiency. In patients with *patchy alopecia*, the presence or absence of scarring is important in the differential diagnosis. Discoid lupus erythematosus is the prototype of the scarring form of alopecia. Nonscarring patchy alopecia can be seen in alopecia areata, trichotillomania, and tinea capitis. Additionally, scarring is an important prognostic sign, since destruction of the hair follicle results in permanent loss of hair, whereas nonscarring alopecia may be a temporary phenomenon.

1. TINEA CAPITIS
VERSUS
ALOPECIA AREATA

Features in common: Nonscarring patches of hair loss.

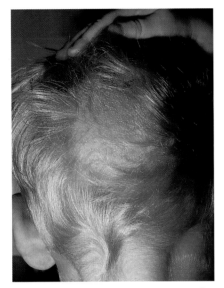

Figure 1.1.1 Tinea capitis.

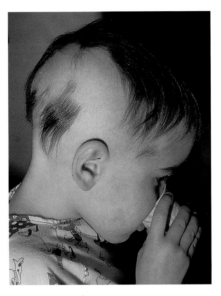

Figure 1.1.2 Alopecia areata.

Distinguishing features

	TINEA CAPITIS	ALOPECIA AREATA
Physical examination		
Morphology	Scaling	No scaling
	Inflammation	No or slight inflammation
	Kerion—boggy, crusted, purulent plaque	No kerion
	Broken hair—black dot	No broken hair
	No exclamation point hairs	Exclamation point hairs
Distribution	Scaling patches scattered on face, trunk, extremities	Alopecia elsewhere on face, trunk, extremities
History		
Symptoms	Family member or friend with tinea	Family history positive
	Pet with tinea	
Exacerbating factors	None	None
Associated findings	Cervical lymphadenopathy	No lymphadenopathy
	Nail dystrophy	Nail pits and dystrophy
	No autoimmune disease	Vitiligo, thyroiditis, anemia

Continues

Distinguishing features (Continued)

	TINEA CAPITIS	ALOPECIA AREATA
Epidemiology	Epidemic among inner-city school children	Sporadic
Biopsy	Usually not done Fungal structures	Usually not necessary Dystrophic hair with lymphocytic infiltrate around hair bulb
Laboratory	No blood work KOH and/or culture positive	Complete blood count Thyroid-stimulating hormone KOH and/or culture negative
Treatment	Oral antifungals	Steroids
Outcome	Curable	Variable and unpredictable

Abbreviation: KOH, potassium hydroxide.

Differential diagnosis of patchy alopecia

Nonscarring
    Trichotillomania
    Secondary syphilis
    Bacterial infection
Scarring
    Discoid lupus erythematosus
    Lichen planus
    Malignant tumor

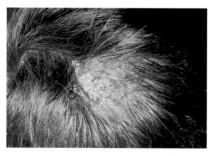

Figure 1.1.3 Tinea capitis. *Clue to diagnosis:* Boggy, crusted, scaling plaque with alopecia (kerion).

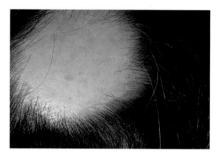

Figure 1.1.4 Alopecia areata. *Clue to diagnosis:* Smooth patch of alopecia with exclamation point hairs in the periphery.

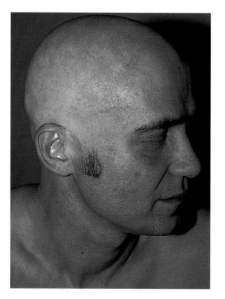

Figure 1.1.5 Alopecia areata. Almost total loss of scalp hair is termed *alopecia totalis*.

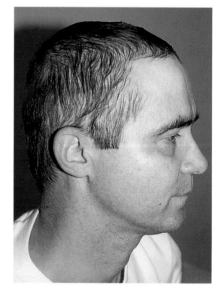

Figure 1.1.6 Alopecia areata showing regrowth of hair after treatment.

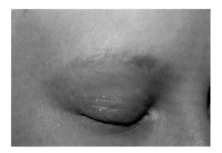

Figure 1.1.7 Alopecia areata with loss of eyebrow and eyelashes.

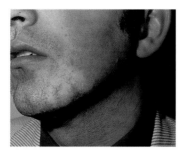

Figure 1.1.8 Alopecia areata with patches of alopecia in beard.

2. SEBORRHEIC DERMATITIS
VERSUS
TINEA CAPITIS

Features in common: Scaling patches *without* hair loss.

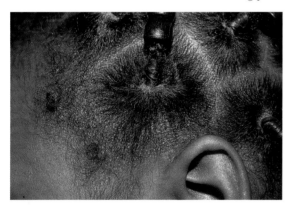

Figure 1.2.1 Seborrheic dermatitis.

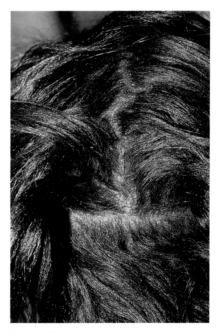

Figure 1.2.2 Tinea capitis.

Distinguishing features

	SEBORRHEIC DERMATITIS	TINEA CAPITIS
Physical examination		
Morphology	Yellow or white scaling	White scaling
	No hair loss	No hair loss or possible hair loss
	No broken hair	Broken hair—black dot
Distribution	Eyebrows, eyelids, nasolabial folds, ears, chest	Scaling patches scattered on face, trunk, extremities

Continues

Distinguishing features (Continued)

	SEBORRHEIC DERMATITIS	TINEA CAPITIS
History Symptoms	Mild itching No one else affected	Mild itching Family member or friend with tinea Pet with tinea
Exacerbating factors	Poor hygiene	None
Associated findings	AIDS, Parkinson's disease	Cervical lymphadenopathy
Epidemiology	5% of healthy adults affected 33% of AIDS patients affected	Epidemic among inner-city school children
Biopsy	Not done Nonspecific dermatitis No fungal structures	Usually not done Fungal structures
Laboratory	KOH and/or culture negative HIV testing in severe or treatment-resistant cases	KOH and/or culture positive No HIV testing
Treatment	Antidandruff shampoos	Oral antifungals
Outcome	Chronic	Curable

Abbreviations: AIDS, acquired immunodeficiency syndrome; KOH, potassium hydroxide; HIV, human immunodeficiency virus.

Differential diagnosis of nonscarring, scaling scalp patches without hair loss

Psoriasis   Histiocytosis X   Atopic dermatitis

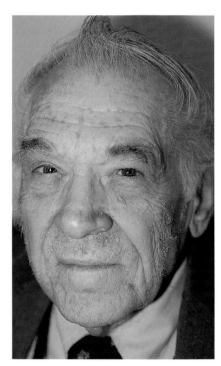

Figure 1.2.3 Seborrheic dermatitis. *Clue to diagnosis:* Scaling patches involving eyebrows and nasolabial fold.

3. TRICHOTILLOMANIA
VERSUS
TINEA CAPITIS

Features in common: Patchy alopecia with broken hairs.

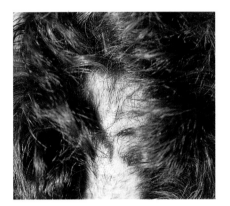

Figure 1.3.1 Trichotillomania.

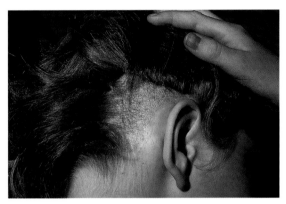

Figure 1.3.2 Tinea capitis with a patch of alopecia, broken hairs, and scaling scalp.

Distinguishing features

	TRICHOTILLOMANIA	TINEA CAPITIS
Physical examination		
Morphology	No scaling No inflammation Hairs unequal lengths—stubble No kerion	Scaling Inflammation Broken hair—black dot Kerion

Distribution	"Friar Tuck" sign—rim of normal
	  hair in periphery of scalp
	Loss of eyebrows and eyelashes—plucked
		Scaling patches elsewhere on face,
		  trunk, extremities
		No loss of eyebrows or eyelashes

History		
Symptoms	No itching Emotional distress No one else affected	Mild itching Family member or friend with tinea Pet with tinea
Exacerbating factors	Stress	None
Associated findings	No cervical lymphadenopathy Psychiatric or emotional problems	Cervical lymphadenopathy No emotional problems
Epidemiology	Sporadic Children and female adults	Epidemic among inner-city school children

Continues

Distinguishing features (Continued)

	TRICHOTILLOMANIA	TINEA CAPITIS
Biopsy	Often not required No fungal structures Empty hair shafts	Usually not done Fungal structures No empty hair shafts
Laboratory	KOH and/or culture negative	KOH and/or culture positive
Treatment	Supportive	Oral antifungals
Outcome	Chronic Children—usually self limited Adults—resistant to psychotherapy	Curable

Abbreviation: KOH, potassium hydroxide.

Differential diagnosis of patchy alopecia without scarring

Alopecia areata

Secondary syphilis

4. ALOPECIA AREATA
VERSUS
TRICHOTILLOMANIA

Features in common: Patchy alopecia without scarring.

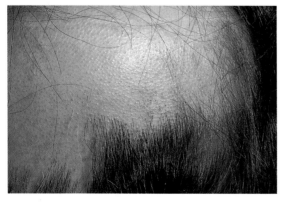

Figure 1.4.1 Alopecia areata.

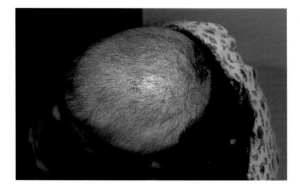

Figure 1.4.2 Trichotillomania with a rim of normal hair (the "Friar Tuck" sign).

Distinguishing features

	TRICHOTILLOMANIA	**ALOPECIA AREATA**
Physical examination Morphology	No inflammation No exclamation point hairs Hairs unequal lengths—stubble	No or slight inflammation Exclamation point hairs Hair same length

Distribution	"Friar Tuck" sign—rim of normal hair
	  in periphery of scalp
	Loss of eyebrows and eyelashes—plucked
		Alopecia elsewhere on face, trunk,
		  extremities

History Symptoms	Family history negative	Family history positive
Exacerbating factors	Stress	None
Associated findings	No nail pits or dystrophy No autoimmune diseases Psychiatric or emotional problems	Nail pits and dystrophy Vitiligo, thyroiditis, anemia No psychiatric problems
Epidemiology	Sporadic Children and female adults	Sporadic All ages
Biopsy	Often not required Empty hair shafts	Usually not necessary Dystrophic hair with lymphocytic infiltrate around hair bulb
Laboratory	None	Complete blood count Thyroid-stimulating hormone
Treatment	Supportive	Steroids
Outcome	Chronic Children—usually self-limited Adults—resistant to psychotherapy	Variable and unpredictable

Differential diagnosis of patchy alopecia without scarring

Tinea capitis
Secondary syphilis

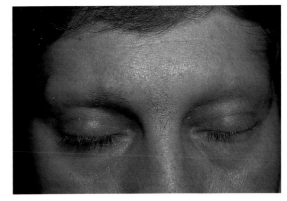

***Figure* 1.4.3** Alopecia areata. *Clue to diagnosis:* Loss of eyebrows and eyelashes. Examination of scalp confirms the diagnosis.

5. DISCOID LUPUS ERYTHEMATOSUS
VERSUS
ALOPECIA AREATA

Features in common: Patchy alopecia.

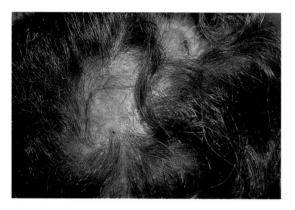

Figure 1.5.1 Discoid lupus erythematosus.

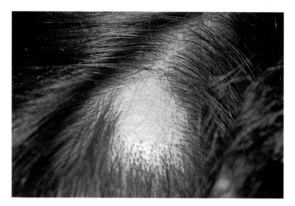

Figure 1.5.2 Alopecia areata.

Distinguishing features

	DISCOID LUPUS ERYTHEMATOSUS	ALOPECIA AREATA
Physical examination		
Morphology	Scarring	Nonscarring
	Inflammation	No or slight inflammation
	Scaling	No scaling
	No exclamation point hairs	Exclamation point hairs
Distribution	Sun-exposed areas	Not in sun-exposed areas
History		
Symptoms	May itch	No itching
	Family history negative	Family history positive
Exacerbating factors	Sunlight may cause flare-up	None
Associated findings	No nail changes	Nail pits and dystrophy
	Systemic lupus erythematosus in 5% to 10%	Vitiligo, thyroiditis, anemia
Epidemiology	Sporadic	Sporadic
Biopsy	Yes—hyperkeratosis with follicular plugging, vacuolar degeneration of basal cell layer, perivascular and perifollicular inflammation	Usually not necessary. Dystrophic hair with lymphocytic infiltrate around hair bulb

Continues

Distinguishing features *(Continued)*

	DISCOID LUPUS ERYTHEMATOSUS	ALOPECIA AREATA
Laboratory	Complete blood count Platelet count Urinalysis Antinuclear antibody testing	Complete blood count Thyroid-stimulating hormone
Treatment	Steroids, antimalarials	Steroids
Outcome	Chronic—spontaneous remission in 50%	Variable and unpredictable

Differential diagnosis of patchy alopecia

Nonscarring
    Trichotillomania
    Secondary syphilis
    Tinea capitis
    Alopecia areata

Scarring
    Lichen planus
    Malignant tumor
    Folliculitis decalvans
    Dissecting cellulitis
    Discoid lupus erythematosus

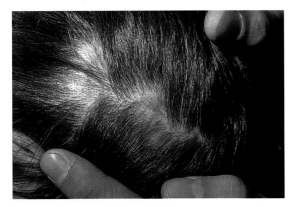

Figure 1.5.3 Discoid lupus erythematosus. *Clue to diagnosis:* Scarring discoid plaques.

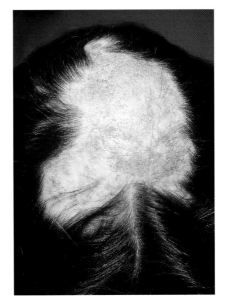

Figure 1.5.4 Old burned-out discoid lupus erythematosus.

6. STRESS-INDUCED ALOPECIA (TELOGEN EFFLUVIUM) VERSUS
ANDROGENIC ALOPECIA

Features in common: Nonscarring diffuse alopecia.

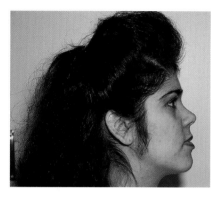

Figure 1.6.1 Stress-induced alopecia.

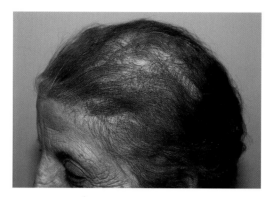

Figure 1.6.2 Androgenic alopecia in a female showing diffuse thinning of top of scalp without frontal regression.

Distinguishing features

	STRESS-INDUCED ALOPECIA (TELOGEN EFFLUVIUM)	ANDROGENIC ALOPECIA
Physical examination		
Morphology	No obvious alopecia	Obvious alopecia
Distribution	Diffuse	Frontotemporal and vertex—males No frontal recession—females
History		
Symptoms	Acute onset Hair comes out by "handfuls" after shampooing, combing	Gradual onset Asymptomatic No stressful event
Exacerbating factors	Stressful event No androgens, progesterones	Androgens, progesterones
Associated findings	Drug-induced—heparin, coumadin, retinoids, β-blockers	Females with androgen excess—acne, hirsutism, clitoromegaly
Epidemiology	Sporadic	Family history positive
Biopsy	Not done	Not done

Continues

Distinguishing features (*Continued*)

	STRESS-INDUCED ALOPECIA (TELOGEN EFFLUVIUM)	ANDROGENIC ALOPECIA
Laboratory	None	Usually none In females suspected to have androgen excess—free and total testosterone, dehydroepiandrosterone sulfate testing
	Hair pull—greater than 5 hairs	Hair pull—1–2 hairs
Treatment	Reassurance	Minoxidil, surgery
Outcome	Resolves	Chronic

Differential diagnosis of nonscarring diffuse hair loss

Alopecia areata

Systemic lupus erythematosus

Metabolic (thyroid) disorders

Drug induced disorders

Nutritional deficiency

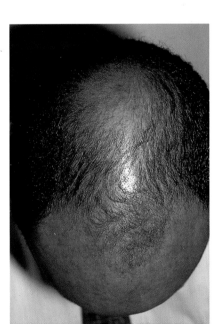

Figure 1.6.3 Androgenic alopecia. *Clue to diagnosis:* Frontal and vertex regression (in men).

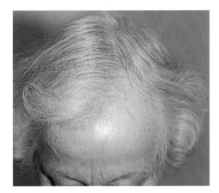

Figure 1.6.4 Androgenic alopecia in a woman with recent onset of frontal regression. She had a testosterone-producing ovarian tumor.

7. PSORIASIS
VERSUS
SEBORRHEIC DERMATITIS

Features in common: Scaling patches *without* alopecia.

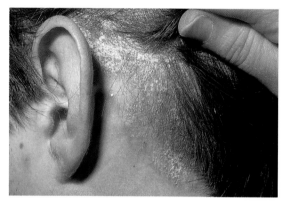

Figure 1.7.1 Psoriasis.

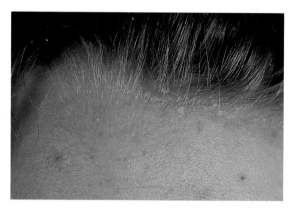

Figure 1.7.2 Seborrheic dermatitis.

Distinguishing features

	PSORIASIS	SEBORRHEIC DERMATITIS
Physical examination		
Morphology	Well-demarcated patches/plaques Silvery scaling	Poorly demarcated patches Yellow or white scaling
Distribution	Elbows, knees, nails, elsewhere	Eyebrows, eyelids, nasolabial folds, ears, chest
History		
Symptoms	Moderate itching	Mild itching
Exacerbating factors	Trauma Physical or emotional stress/illness Medications—β-blockers, lithium	No trauma Poor hygiene
Associated findings	Arthritis Nail dystrophy	No arthritis AIDS Parkinson's disease No nail changes
Epidemiology	Positive family history	No family history 5% of healthy adults affected 33% of AIDS patients affected
Biopsy	Not done Hyperkeratosis, acanthosis, neutrophils in epidermis, dermal capillary proliferation, perivascular inflammation	Not done Nonspecific dermatitis

Continues

Distinguishing features *(Continued)*

	PSORIASIS	SEBORRHEIC DERMATITIS
Laboratory	None	HIV testing in severe or treatment-resistant cases
Treatment	Topical steroids, tar shampoos	Antidandruff shampoos
Outcome	Chronic	Chronic

Abbreviations: AIDS, acquired immunodeficiency syndrome; HIV, human immunodeficiency virus.

Differential diagnosis of scaling scalp patches without alopecia

Tinea capitis   Histiocytosis X   Atopic dermatitis

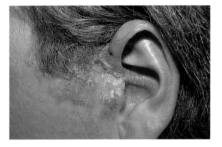

Figure 1.7.3 Psoriasis. *Clue to diagnosis:* Well-marginated, inflamed, scaling plaque.

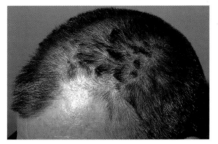

Figure 1.7.4 Psoriasis. *Clue to diagnosis:* Hair clumps together in tentlike configuration ("tent sign").

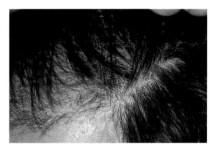

Figure 1.7.5 Seborrheic dermatitis. *Clue to diagnosis:* Poorly marginated patches.

Discussion

ANDROGENIC ALOPECIA

Definition and etiology: Androgenic alopecia, or common baldness, is the nonscarring replacement of dark terminal hairs by vellus hairs and atrophic follicles. This hair loss is androgen-dependent and involves the vertex and frontotemporal regions of the scalp of genetically predisposed males and females.

Clinical features: Common baldness is an androgen-dependent inherited condition that begins in late adolescence or early adulthood. The onset and progression are gradual and highly variable. It affects almost 100% of whites, whereas in other ethnic groups, such as Native Americans and Asians, it is uncommon.

Initially, the young male or female may notice increased hair shedding after washing or combing with subsequent thinning of the hair in the frontotemporal and vertex regions of the scalp. The coarse dark terminal hairs are replaced by finer depigmented vellus hairs. These vel-

lus hairs then become atrophic, leaving a smooth shiny scalp with few or no follicular orifices. Characteristically, the posterior and lateral margins of the scalp are spared. In males, there is bitemporal hair recession and balding of the vertex, which can progress to complete baldness. In females, the frontal hairline remains intact, but there is mild to moderate diffuse thinning over the top of the scalp. This rarely results in total baldness. Although thinning continues throughout life, it is most prominent between the ages of 30 and 50 years.

The diagnosis is usually straightforward and made without difficulty in men. In women, a hormonal abnormality should be considered if frontal recession develop together with other signs of androgen excess such as acne, hirsutism, or menstrual irregularities. A skin biopsy is rarely done. In females in whom androgen excess is suspected, serum-free and total testosterone and dehydroepiandrosterone sulfate tests are ordered to screen for pituitary, adrenal, or ovarian disorders.

Therapy: A 2% solution of minoxidil (Rogaine) applied twice a day is somewhat effective in growing hair in areas that were previously bald. Men are more responsive than women. Additionally, minoxidil may stop or retard the progression of baldness, but it must be used continuously to preserve growth. The use of antiandrogens such as finasteride is being investigated. Surgical treatment involving hair transplants, scalp reduction, and flaps remains an important therapeutic option. Baldness can also be covered with a hairpiece or wig.

ALOPECIA AREATA

Definition and etiology: Alopecia areata is an idiopathic disorder that causes round or oval patches of nonscarring alopecia.

Clinical features: Alopecia areata affects both children and adults but most often occurs in early adulthood. Both sexes are affected equally. The emotional stress that accompanies alopecia areata appears to be reactive rather than causative. Although the pathogenesis of alopecia areata is poorly understood, an immunologic process is probable. Occasionally, autoimmune disease such as Hashimoto's thyroiditis and pernicious anemia have been associated with alopecia areata. In approximately 25% of patients, a family history of the disorder is found.

The clinical findings include round or oval patches of complete hair loss. The underlying skin is smooth without any evidence of scarring. Closer inspection may reveal the presence or absence of follicular orifices. In the absence of orifices, regrowth of the hair will not occur. In the periphery of the patches of alopecia, "exclamation point" hairs occur. These are so named because of their resemblance to this punctuation mark—the diameter of the distal hair is greater than that of the proximal segment. In some cases the hair loss can involve the entire scalp; this is referred to as *alopecia totalis*. If it occurs over the entire body, it is referred to as *alopecia universalis*. Erythema and slight tenderness may be present early in the course of the disease. Subsequently, the scalp may become slightly depressed. Fine stippling and pitting of the nails are infrequent associated findings.

The differential diagnosis of nonscarring forms of alopecia includes trichotillomania, secondary syphilis, and tinea capitis. Although a skin biopsy is not usually necessary, biopsy findings will reveal small dystrophic hair structures with an infiltrate of lymphocytes surrounding the hair bulbs of anagen hairs like a swarm of bees. For extensive alopecia areata, a complete blood count and thyroid-stimulating hormone assay are done to rule out associated autoimmune diseases.

Therapy: A variety of treatments have been tried, but topical, intralesional, and oral corticosteroids are used most often. Other therapeutic modalities include topical anthralin, topical minoxidil, topical retinoic acid, immunotherapy with contact irritants and allergens, psoralens plus

ultraviolet light (PUVA), and immunomodulating agents such as thymopentin, azathioprine, and inosiplex. None of these treatments is uniformly successful, and many have significant side effects. The majority of patients with alopecia areata will experience a spontaneous recovery and therefore need no treatment. Relapses, however, are not uncommon. Extensive hair loss and disease duration of more than 1 year are poor prognostic signs. The patient needs to be aware that alopecia areata has a variable and often unpredictable course.

DISCOID LUPUS ERYTHEMATOSUS

Definition and etiology: Discoid lupus erythematosus is an autoimmune disorder that causes scarring alopecia of the scalp.

Clinical features: Discoid lupus erythematosus causes scarring plaques on the scalp, head, trunk, and extremities. The preferential distribution is in sun-exposed areas. Five to ten percent of patients with discoid lupus erythematosus also have systemic disease.

The examination reveals oval scarring patches of alopecia, with an active erythematous border and white atrophic center. Within the plaques, prominent keratin-filled hair follicles and telangiectasia are present.

The differential diagnosis of scarring alopecia includes lichen planus and malignant tumor. It should be fairly easy to differentiate discoid lupus erythematosus from nonscarring types of alopecia, such as alopecia areata. Biopsy findings, usually diagnostic for discoid lupus erythematosus, reveal an atrophic epidermis and dystrophic hair follicles without hair shafts. A lymphocytic infiltrate characteristically occurs at the dermal/epidermal junction, where hydropic degeneration of the basal cells occurs. The infiltrate is also distributed in a patchy manner around dermal vessels and hair follicles. In addition to general history and physical examination, a complete blood count, platelet count, urinalysis, and antinuclear antibody testing are done to rule out systemic lupus erythematosus.

Therapy: The initial treatment of discoid lupus erythematosus is application of a potent topical or intralesional corticosteroid. When this fails to control the inflammatory process, the use of antimalarials such as hydroxychloroquine is indicated.

PSORIASIS

Definition and etiology: Psoriasis is an inflammatory disease characterized by increased proliferation of the epidermis. The cause of psoriasis is unknown, but abnormal epidermal kinetics as well as activation of the immune system within the skin must be taken into account.

Clinical features: Approximately one-third of patients have a family history positive for psoriasis. This is a relatively common skin disease affecting approximately 2% of the population of the United States. The most common time of onset is in the third decade of life, but it can present at any time. The major precipitating or aggravating factors include streptococcal pharyngitis, trauma to the skin, emotional stress, and use of drugs such as β-blocking agents and lithium.

The examination reveals sharply demarcated, erythematous, silvery, scaling plaques without associated alopecia. The extensor surfaces of the elbows and knees are typically involved, and dystrophic nail changes occur as well.

The differential diagnosis of psoriasis of the scalp includes seborrheic dermatitis, tinea capitis, histiocytosis X, and atopic dermatitis. Usually, a skin biopsy is not necessary. If a biopsy is done, however, characteristic findings will include hyperkeratosis, parakeratosis, acanthotic epidermis, inflammatory infiltrate in the dermis, and neutrophils migrating into the epidermis, forming microabscesses.

Therapy: Psoriasis of the scalp is more difficult to treat than it is elsewhere because delivery of the therapeutic agent is more difficult. Treatment modalities include topical preparations containing steroids, tars, and anthralin. For thick, scaling plaques, phenol and sodium chloride (P & S) liquid or mineral oil is used to remove the scale.

SEBORRHEIC DERMATITIS

Definition and etiology: Seborrheic dermatitis is a common chronic eczematous process predominantly affecting the scalp, eyebrows, face, and, to a lesser extent, other hairy regions of the body. The cause is thought to be an inflammatory reaction to the lipid-loving yeast, *Pityrosporum ovale.*

Clinical features: Seborrheic dermatitis has a waxing and waning course with a variable amount of pruritus. It occurs in infancy and after puberty when the sebaceous glands secrete sebum, which encourages the growth of *Pityrosporum ovale.* Seborrheic dermatitis has been associated with Parkinson's disease and acquired immunodeficiency syndrome (AIDS). Rarely, seborrheic dermatitis can be generalized, resulting in exfoliative dermatitis.

Physical examination demonstrates the predilection of seborrheic dermatitis for the hairy, sebaceous-gland-rich regions of the body. Characteristically, the scalp, eyebrows, eyelids, nasolabial creases, ears, and chest are involved. This distribution is distinctive and helps to differentiate this disease from other scaling or eczematous eruptions. Patches of seborrheic dermatitis are characterized by ill-marginated borders, mild to moderate erythema, and yellow or white, greasy, fine scaling. Alopecia does not occur. The most mild form of seborrheic dermatitis without inflammation is the fine, white scaling of dandruff.

The differential diagnosis of seborrheic dermatitis of the scalp includes psoriasis, tinea capitis, histiocytosis X, and atopic dermatitis. Usually, the ill-marginated patches and disease distribution (involving the face) make the diagnosis of seborrheic dermatitis straightforward. Biopsy is rarely performed because it reveals only nonspecific dermatitis.

Use of an antiseborrheic shampoo containing zinc pyrithione, selenium sulfide, or ketoconazole is the treatment of choice. For patients with a form of disease that is more inflammatory and more pruritic, a topical steroid is added.

STRESS-INDUCED ALOPECIA (TELOGEN EFFLUVIUM)

Definition and etiology: An alteration in the normal hair cycle that results in excessive loss of telogen (resting) hairs is characteristic of stress-induced alopecia. It is also referred to as *telogen effluvium.* This alteration of the hair cycle is precipitated by marked emotional or physiologic stress.

Clinical features: The onset of stress-induced alopecia occurs 2 to 3 months after the causative stressful event, which may be high fever, childbirth, major surgery, or a severe emotional disorder. The growing anagen hairs are prematurely converted to resting telogen hairs, which are then shed. These patients are distressed because their hair is coming out by the "handful" after shampooing and combing.

Close physical examination reveals diffuse mild thinning of the hair that may not be readily apparent. The scalp is normal without inflammation or scaling. A hair pull test, which is accomplished by gently pulling 2 to 3 dozen hairs, will result in the loss of more than five hairs, when normally only 1 or 2 hairs pull out. A loss of 400 to 500 hairs daily is not uncommon. (Fewer than 100 is normal.)

The differential diagnosis of stress-induced alopecia includes alopecia areata, systemic lupus erythematosus, abnormal thyroid function, drug-induced disease, androgenic alopecia, and nutritional deficiencies involving essential fatty acids, biotin, or zinc. Although a biopsy is usually not done, biopsy findings will show that more than 25% of the hairs are telogenic. Appropriate laboratory studies and history taking will rule out other causes of diffuse alopecia.

Therapy: For most patients with stress-induced alopecia, the stressful event is short-lived, and reassurance is all that is required.

TINEA CAPITIS

Definition and etiology: Tinea capitis is a superficial fungal infection of the scalp caused by dermatophytes—usually *Trichophyton tonsurans* and *Microsporum canis*. *Trichophyton tonsurans* is the most common cause of tinea capitis in the United States, particularly in urban black children. *Microsporum canis* is the most common causative organism worldwide.

Clinical features: Human to human spread of *Trichophyton tonsurans* results in epidemics of tinea capitis among urban black children. The fungus can be cultured from hairs and scales found on combs, hats, and brushes. *Microsporum canis* is spread from cats and dogs to humans and is sporadic in occurrence.

The clinical appearance of tinea capitis varies. Sometimes it may appear as a mild to moderate, diffuse, scaling, seborrheic-like dermatitis with minimal inflammation. At other times, there may be inflamed, scaling patches of alopecia containing broken hair shafts (black dots) and indurated, boggy, purulent plaques of alopecia referred to as *kerion*. Prominent cervical adenopathy is commonly associated with inflammatory tinea capitis.

The differential diagnosis of tinea capitis includes seborrheic dermatitis, alopecia areata, trichotillomania, psoriasis, and bacterial scalp infection. Results of a potassium hydroxide (KOH) preparation or fungal culture confirm the diagnosis of tinea capitis.

Therapy: Effective treatment of tinea capitis requires oral antifungal agents. Topical preparations are inadequate. For children, microsized griseofulvin, 10 mg/kg daily for 6 to 8 weeks, is usually effective, but larger doses in the range of 20 to 25 mg/kg daily may be required for cure. Additionally, shampooing with ketoconazole, selenium sulfide, and povidone-iodine several times a week is helpful in reducing the number of viable fungal spores. Alternative oral medications include ketoconazole, itraconazole, fluconazole, and terbinafine. In some instances, asymptomatic family members should also be treated because they may be carriers of *T. tonsurans*. Household pets should also be examined for the presence of a dermatophyte infection.

TRICHOTILLOMANIA

Definition and etiology: Trichotillomania is a self-induced traumatic alopecia that results from pulling, plucking, and breaking one's own hair.

Clinical features: Trichotillomania affects children and adults, predominantly female, who have emotional or psychiatric problems. In children, sibling rivalry, mental retardation, hospitalization, or discord at home or in school can trigger trichotillomania. In adults, it is usually a sign of a personality disorder, sometime severe.

Coarse-feeling broken hairs or stubble are characteristic of trichotillomania. The scalp is normal without inflammation or scarring. Ill-marginated, irregularly shaped patches of alopecia are the most common presentation. In some individuals, however, almost all the scalp hair has been pulled, plucked, or broken, resulting in a rim of normal hair in the periphery referred to as the "Friar Tuck" sign. The eyebrows and eyelashes may also be plucked.

The differential diagnosis includes tinea capitis, alopecia areata, and secondary syphilis. The clinical examination is usually enough to establish the diagnosis, but occasionally a biopsy is required. Examination reveals normally growing hairs, empty hair follicles in a noninflamed dermis, and traumatized follicles with broken or no hair and perifollicular hemorrhage.

Therapy: Treatment is generally supportive. Insight into the self-induced nature of the disorder should be provided. In children, the condition is usually self-limited. In adults, however, trichotillomania may be a sign of a severe emotional or mental disturbance requiring a psychiatric referral. Clomipramine, a tricyclic antidepressant, appears to have a role in the short-term treatment of this obsessive-compulsive disorder.

Suggested Readings

ALOPECIA AREATA
Chanco Turner ML. Guidelines of care for alopecia areata. J Am Acad Dermatol 1992;26:247–50.
Fiedler VC. Alopecia areata. A review of therapy, efficacy, safety, and mechanism. Arch Dermatol 1992;128:1519–29.

ANDROGENIC ALOPECIA
DeVillez RL, Jacobs JP, Szpunar CA, Warner ML. Androgenetic alopecia in the female. Treatment with 2% topical minoxidil solution. Arch Dermatol 1994;130:303–7.
Olsen EA, Weiner MS, Amara IA, DeLong ER. Five-year follow-up of men with androgenetic alopecia treated with topical minoxidil. J Am Acad Dermatol 1990;22:643–46.
Venning VA, Dawber RPR. Patterned androgenic alopecia in women. J Am Acad Dermatol 1988;18:1073–77.

DISCOID LUPUS ERYTHEMATOSUS
Tuffanelli DL, Dubois EL. Cutaneous manifestations of systemic lupus erythematosus. Arch Dermatol 1964;90:377–85.

PSORIASIS
Drake LA, Ceilley RI, Cornelison RL et al. Guidelines of care for psoriasis. J Am Acad Dermatol 1993;28:632–37.

Cram DL. Psoriasis: current advances in etiology and treatment. J Am Acad Dermatol 1981;4:1–14.

Griffiths CEM. Cutaneous leukocyte trafficking and psoriasis. Arch Dermatol 1994;130:494–99.

SEBORRHEIC DERMATITIS

Danby FW, Maddin WS, Margesson LJ, Rosenthal D. A randomized, double-blind, placebo-controlled trial of ketoconazole 2% shampoo versus selenium sulfide 2.5% shampoo in the treatment of moderate to severe dandruff. J Am Acad Dermatol 1993;29:1008–12.

Peter RU, Richarz-Barthauer U. Successful treatment and prophylaxis of scalp seborrhoeic dermatitis and dandruff with 2% ketoconazole shampoo: results of a multicentre, double-blind, placebo-controlled trial. Br J Dermatol 1995;132:441–45.

Van Cutsem J, Van Gerven F, Fransen J et al. The in vitro antifungal activity of ketoconazole, zinc, pyrithione, and selenium sulfide against *Pityrosporum* and their efficacy as a shampoo in the treatment of experimental pityrosporosis in guinea pigs. J Am Acad Dermatol 1990;22:993–98.

STRESS-INDUCED ALOPECIA

Headington JT. Telogen effluvium. Arch Dermatol 1993;129:356–63.

TINEA CAPITIS

Babel DE, Baughman SA. Evaluation of the adult carrier state in juvenile tinea capitis caused by *Trichophyton tonsurans.* J Am Acad Dermatol 1989;21:1209–12.

Drake LA, Dinehart SM, Farmer ER et al. Guidelines of care for superficial mycotic infections of the skin: tinea capitis and a tinea barbae. J Am Acad Dermatol 1996;34:290–94.

Elewski BE, Weil ML. Dermatophytes and superficial fungi. In Sams MW, Lynch PJ (eds): Principles and Practice of Dermatology, 2nd Ed. pp. 149–58. Churchill Livingstone, New York, 1996.

Herbert A. Tinea capitis. Current concepts. Arch Dermatol 1988;124:1554–57.

TRICHOTILLOMANIA

Muller SA. Trichotillomania: a histopathologic study in sixty-six patients. J Am Acad Dermatol 1990;23:56–62.

Oranje AP, Peereboom-Wynia JDR, De Raeymaecker DMJ. Trichotillomania in childhood. J Am Acad Dermatol 1986;15:614–19.

Swedo SE, Leonard HL, Rapoport JL et al. A double-blind comparison of clomipramine and desipramine in the treatment of trichotillomania (hair pulling). N Engl J Med 1989;321:497–501.

ALGORITHM FOR FACIAL RASHES

Papulopustular

Central face — Perioral

Comedones — No comedones

Photodistributed

No pustules
Vesicular papules — Telangiectasias

Onset in spring

Dermatitic appearing — Ingrown hairs

Other causes
  Adenoma sebaceum
  Drugs (halogenodermas)
  Granuloma faciale
  Lymphocytic infiltrate of Jessner
  Pyoderma faciale
  Sarcoidosis
  Sycosis barbae
  Trichoepitheliomas

| Acne vulgaris | Polymorphous light eruption | Acne rosacea | Perioral dermatitis | Pseudofolliculitis barbae |

Erythema/scaling

No scarring — Scarring

Accentuation of nasolabial area
Scalp involvement

Photodistributed

Patient healthy

Patient complaining
of malaise

Pruritic/contactant

Telangiectasia
Papules

Onset in spring
Improves over summer

Other causes
  Actinic reticuloid
  Atopic dermatitis
  Erysipelas
  Keratosis pilaris atrophicans
  Leishmaniasis
  Leprosy
  Lupus pernio
  Pemphigus foliaceus
  Psoriasis
  Tuberculosis

| Seborrheic dermatitis | Contact dermatitis | Acne rosacea | Polymorphous light eruption | Cutaneous lupus erythematosus |

Vesicles/bullae

Grouped — Not grouped

Tzanck prep +

Urticarial lesions

Golden-colored crust
Localized rash
Primarily erosions

Contactant present

Other causes
  Acrodermatitis enteropathica
  Actinic prurigo
  Bullous pemphigoid
  Erythema multiforme
  Hydroa vacciniforme
  Photocontact dermatitis
  Phototoxic drug eruption

| Herpes simplex (herpes zoster) | Contact dermatitis | Impetigo contagiosum |

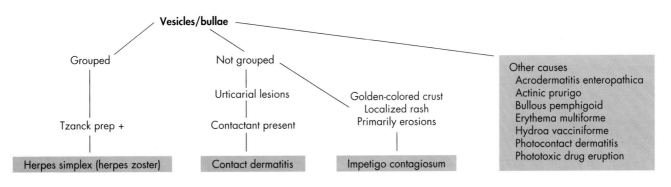

Introduction

Of the many locations affected by dermatologic diseases, from a patient's and a cosmetic perspective, facial rashes are most important. Patients frequently ignore or are content not to treat inconspicuous cosmetic rashes like tinea pedis, but may be distressed by even a single pimple on the face. The face is involved in many different dermatologic diseases because it contains numerous sebaceous glands and is constantly exposed to the environment. Diseases involving the follicular-sebaceous gland apparatus include seborrheic dermatitis, acne vulgaris, pseudofolliculitis barbae, and acne rosacea. Exposure to sunlight can result in photodistributed rashes such as polymorphous light eruption, photocontact dermatitis, and lupus erythematosus. Exposure to chemicals found in cosmetics and other products can produce contact dermatitis.

1. ACNE VULGARIS
VERSUS
ACNE ROSACEA

Features in common: Erythematous papules and pustules.

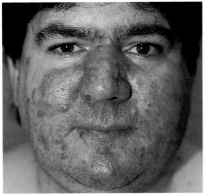

Figure 2.1.1 Acne vulgaris.

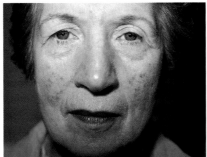

Figure 2.1.2 Acne rosacea.

Distinguishing features

	ACNE VULGARIS	**ACNE ROSACEA**
Physical examination	Primary lesion is comedo	Comedones rarely found
Morphology	Telangiectasias not prominent Nodular-cystic lesions may be present Lesions always present No background erythema No rhinophyma	Telangiectasias often prominent No cystic lesions Early on, no circumscribed lesions Mainly erythema and easy blushing Rhinophyma in advanced cases
Distribution	Involves face, back, chest	Affects face, eyelids, rarely axilla
History Symptoms	No history of easy blushing	Occasionally history of easy blushing

Exacerbating factors	Cosmetics and chemicals
	Medications: androgens, lithium,
	  corticosteroids
		Sunlight, spicy foods, heat, cold,
		  steroid creams

Associated findings	None, occasionally signs of androgen excess: hirsutism, oily skin	Conjunctivitis

Epidemiology	Primarily affects teenagers and
	  young adults
	Family history of acne may be present
		Primarily affects adults
		Frequently found in fair-skinned
		  patients of Celtic origin

Continues

Distinguishing features (Continued)

	ACNE VULGARIS	ACNE ROSACEA
Biopsy	Follicular plugging	Perivascular and perifollicular mixed inflammatory infiltrate, telangiectatic blood vessels
Laboratory	None In case of suspected androgen excess: testosterone, free testosterone, dehydroepiandrosterone testing	None
Treatment	If mild: topical benzoyl peroxide, retinoids, azelaic acid, sulfacetamide, antibiotics If severe: systemic antibiotics, rarely systemic retinoids	Avoid sunlight, alcohol, spicy foods Topical sulfur or metronidazole preparations Laser surgery for erythema or rhinophyma
Outcome	Chronic; end result of severe acne may be depressed icepick-like scars	Chronic; end result of severe rosacea is rhinophyma

Differential diagnosis of acneiform eruption

Common causes
  Acne rosacea
  Acne vulgaris
  Drug-induced acne
    Androgens
    Corticosteroids
    Dilantin
    Halogenoderma
    Lithium
  Perioral dermatitis
  Pseudofolliculitis barbae
  Tinea faciei

Rarer causes
  Adenoma sebaceum (tuberous sclerosis)
  Androgen excess (due to tumors or genetic factors)
  Favre-Racouchot's disease (actinic comedones)
  Haber's syndrome
  Lupus miliaris disseminatums faciei (may be variant of rosacea)
  Nevus comedonicus
  Pyoderma faciale
  Sycosis barbae
  Trichoepitheliomas

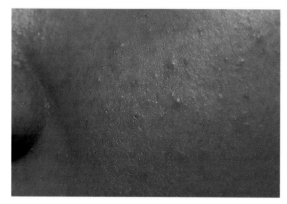

Figure 2.1.3 Acne vulgaris. *Clue to diagnosis:* Comedones.

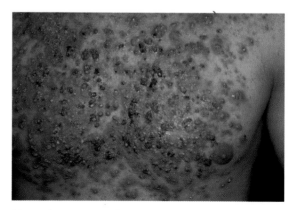

Figure 2.1.4 Acne vulgaris. *Clue to Diagnosis:* Numerous cysts on chest.

2. ACNE ROSACEA
VERSUS
SYSTEMIC LUPUS ERYTHEMATOSUS

Features in common: Malar erythema.

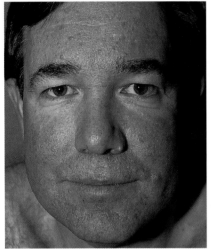

Figure 2.2.1 Acne rosacea.

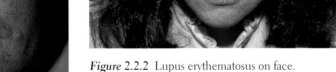

Figure 2.2.2 Lupus erythematosus on face.

Distinguishing features

	ACNE ROSACEA	SYSTEMIC LUPUS ERYTHEMATOSUS
Physical examination		
Morphology	Papules and pustules on erythematous base	No papules or pustules
	Rhinophyma in severe cases	No rhinophyma
	No discoid lesions seen	Occasionally discoid lesions present
Distribution	Face, chest, back	Central face, sun-exposed skin
History		
Symptoms	Patient asymptomatic; occasionally discomfort from papular-cystic lesions	Generalized malaise
Exacerbating factors	Sunlight, food, alcohol, heat, cold	Sunlight
	Also exacerbated by topical steroids	Occasionally drug-induced: hydralazine, procainamide
Associated findings	Conjunctivitis	Arthritis, pleurisy, renal insufficiency, anemia, central nervous system disorders, cardiac disorders

Continues

Distinguishing features (Continued)

	ACNE ROSACEA	SYSTEMIC LUPUS ERYTHEMATOSUS
Epidemiology	Adults; predilection for males	Adults; much more common in women

Biopsy	No
	Perivascular and periappendiceal
	  mixed inflammatory infiltrate
	Telangiectatic blood vessels
		Occasionally
		Epidermal atrophy, hydropic changes,
		  follicular plugging, superficial and
		  deep lymphocytic infiltrate

Laboratory	None	Testing for antinuclear antibodies,
		  anti-ds DNA, anti-Sm antibody,
		  RO and LA antigens, and complement
		  levels; complete blood count,
		  platelet count, urinalysis

Treatment	Avoid sunlight, topical steroids,
	  alcohol, spicy foods, hot drinks
	Topical sulfur and metronidazole creams
	Laser therapy for rhinophyma or erythema
		Avoid sunlight
		
		Topical or systemic steroids if systemic
		  symptoms present
		Immunosuppressive agents
		Antimalarial agents

Outcome	Chronic	Chronic relapsing disease; in acute
		  lupus erythematosus, lesions heal
		  without scarring

Differential diagnosis of
macular facial rashes

Common causes
  Acne rosacea
  Contact dermatitis
  Photocontact dermatitis
  Phototoxic drug eruption
  Polymorphous light eruption
  Lupus erythematosus
  Seborrheic dermatitis
  Tinea faciei

Rarer causes
  Actinic reticuloid
  Dermatomyositis
  Erysipelas
  Herpes zoster
  Keratosis pilaris atrophicans
  Leprosy
  Leishmaniasis
  Lupus pernio (sarcoidosis)
  Lymphoma
  Pemphigus foliaceus/erythematosus

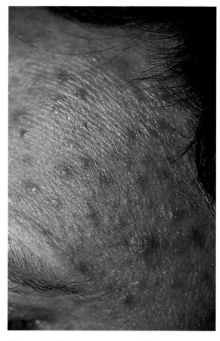

Figure 2.2.3 Acne rosacea. *Clue to diagnosis:* Papules and pustules, but no comedones on face.

3. ACNE VULGARIS VERSUS PSEUDOFOLLICULITIS

Features in common: Follicular-based papules and pustules on the face.

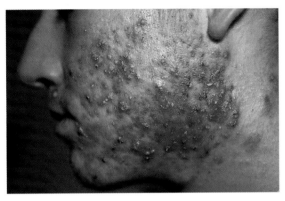

Figure 2.3.1 Acne vulgaris.

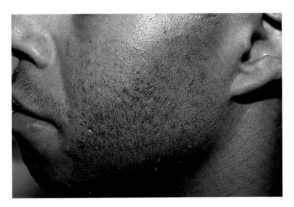

Figure 2.3.2 Pseudofolliculitis barbae.

Distinguishing features

	ACNE VULGARIS	PSEUDOFOLLICULITIS
Physical examination Morphology	Comedones present Nodular-cystic lesions may be present No ingrown hairs	No comedones No nodular-cystic lesions Ingrown hairs present
Distribution	Face, back, chest Neck rarely involved	Beard area and cheeks Neck area usually involved
History Symptoms	None	None
Exacerbating factors	Exacerbated by some cosmetics, chemicals, occlusion Drugs: androgens, lithium	Exacerbated by shaving
Associated findings	Occasionally signs of androgen excess: hirsutism, oily skin Curly hairs (if present) coincidence	No androgen excess Majority of patients have curly hairs
Epidemiology	Primarily affects teenagers and young adults Genetic predisposition in many patients	Most common in black men Genetic predisposition may be present
Biopsy	No Follicular plugging with surrounding inflammation	No Hairs penetrating skin or hair shaft

Continues

Distinguishing features (*Continued*)

	ACNE VULGARIS	PSEUDOFOLLICULITIS
Laboratory	None In case of suspected androgen excess: testosterone, free testosterone, dehydroepiandrosterone testing	None
Treatment	Oral or systemic antibiotics, topical retinoids, azelaic acid, benzoyl peroxide Rarely oral *cis*-retinoic acid	Avoid shaving too close or long Topical antibiotics, retinoids, low-potency corticosteroids for irritation Glycolic acid preparations to soften hair; use of specially designed electric razors
Outcome	Chronic; end result of severe acne is icepick-like scars	Chronic; may result in scars

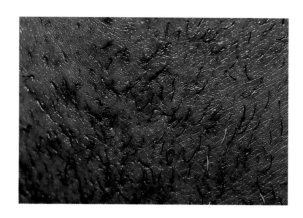

Figure 2.3.3 Pseudofolliculitis barbae.
Clue to diagnosis: Ingrown hairs.

4. SEBORRHEIC DERMATITIS
VERSUS
CONTACT DERMATITIS

Features in common: Erythema and scaling.

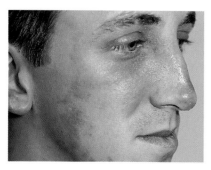

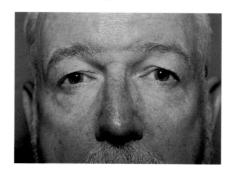

Figure 2.4.1 Contact dermatitis.

Figure 2.4.2 Seborrheic dermatitis.

Distinguishing features

	SEBORRHEIC DERMATITIS	CONTACT DERMATITIS
Physical examination Morphology	Erythematous scaling patches Occasionally follicular papules No oozing or weeping No vesicles seen Yellow- to white-colored scale	Red patches with vesicles and erythematous plaques Oozing or weeping of serous fluid in established cases Vesicles may be present White-colored scale
Distribution	Involves areas with increased oil production (seborrhea): nasolabial areas, cheeks, eyebrows, scalp, axilla, anterior chest, groin	Can affect any cutaneous surface
History Symptoms	Asymptomatic or mildly pruritic	Usually very pruritic
Exacerbating factors	Infrequent washing, poor hygiene	Contact with irritant or allergen
Associated findings	Underlying diseases may be present such as human immunodeficiency virus infection, cardiac disease or Parkinson's disease	No associated disease
Epidemiology	Generally affects neonates, middle-aged, or older patients	Affects any age group
Biopsy	Epidermal spongiosis, parakeratotic mounds around follicular infundibuli	Epidermal spongiosis, parakeratotic mounds, superficial inflammatory infiltrate with few eosinophils
Laboratory	None	Patch testing
Treatment	Topical ketoconazole, sulfur preparations, and low-potency corticosteroid creams; benzoyl peroxide, selenium sulfide, zinc pyrithione cleansers	Avoid allergens Topical or systemic corticosteroids
Outcome	Chronic; no scarring; good response to therapy	Self-limited once exposure to irritant or allergen halted

Differential diagnosis of erythematous and scaly seborrheic dermatitis-like eruptions

Common causes
  Contact dermatitis
  Lupus erythematosus
  Rosacea
  Photodermatitis
  Psoriasis (sebopsoriasis)
  Seborrheic dermatitis
  Tinea faciei

Rarer causes
  Histiocytosis X
  Leishmaniasis
  Leprosy
  Pellagra
  Pemphigus foliaceus/erythematosus
  Riboflavin, biotin, or pyridoxine deficiency
  Tuberculosis

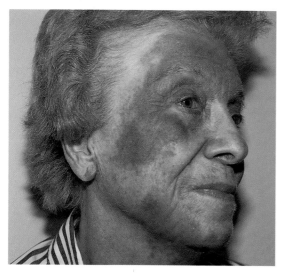

Figure 2.4.3 Contact dermatitis. *Clue to diagnosis:* Geometric sharply demarcated urticarial plaques (in contact dermatitis due to fragrance).

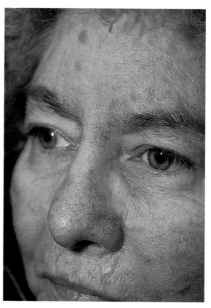

Figure 2.4.4 Seborrheic dermatitis. *Clue to diagnosis:* Scaling in eyebrows (or nasolabial folds).

5. IMPETIGO CONTAGIOSA
VERSUS
HERPES SIMPLEX

Features in common: Vesicles.

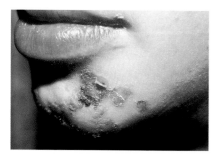

Figure 2.5.1 Impetigo.

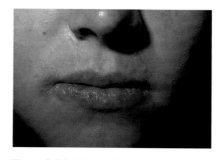

Figure 2.5.2 Herpes simplex.

Distinguishing features

	IMPETIGO CONTAGIOSA	HERPES SIMPLEX
Physical examination		
Morphology	Bullae may be present Blisters contain pus Blisters not grouped Blisters not umbilicated No scalloped borders Golden-orange-colored crust	No bullae No pus unless secondarily infected Blisters grouped Umbilicated blisters Scalloped borders Crust red-colored
Distribution	Any glabrous portion, frequently on face	Any skin surface, most frequently on lip
History		
Symptoms	No prodromal symptoms Not associated with fever	Prodromal tingling or burning sensation in most cases Primary lesions may be associated with fever and malaise
Exacerbating factors	Usually not recurrent Immunosuppression	May be recurrent Immunosuppression
Associated findings	None	Occasionally lymphadenopathy
Epidemiology	Most common in children	Common in children and adults
Biopsy	No Subcorneal pustule containing gram-positive organisms	No Ballooning necrosis of keratinocytes with mulinucleated giant cells
Laboratory	Bacterial culture	Viral culture Tzanck preparation
Treatment	Topical mupirocin Systemic: penicillin derivatives or erythromycin	Antiviral therapy effective if given first 1–2 days: oral acyclovir, valacyclovir, famciclovir, or pencyclovir cream
Outcome	Excellent; heals without scarring	Good; no scarring, but may be recurrent

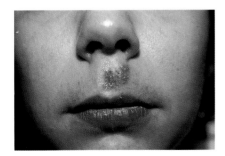

Figure 2.5.3 Herpes simplex. *Clue to diagnosis:* Grouped vesicles.

6. POLYMORPHOUS LIGHT ERUPTION
VERSUS
LUPUS ERYTHEMATOSUS

Features in common: Erythematous papules and plaques in
sun-exposed skin that are exacerbated by sunlight. Polymorphous light
eruption can clinically be confused with both discoid lupus erythematosus
and systemic lupus erythematosus.

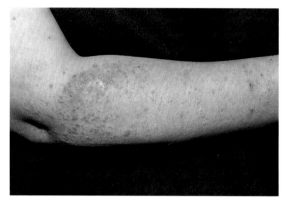

Figure 2.6.1 Polymorphous light eruption.

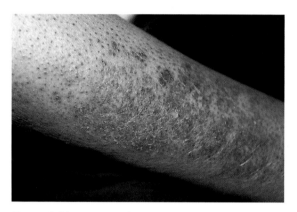

Figure 2.6.2 Lupus erythematosus.

Distinguishing features

	POLYMORPHOUS LIGHTS ERUPTION	LUPUS ERYTHEMATOSUS
Physical examination Morphology	Urticarial papules, vesicular eczematous plaques	Round, "discoid" plaques
	No atrophy, telangiectasias, or follicular plugging	Atrophy, follicular plugging telangiectasias present
	No pigmentary changes	Hyper- and hypopigmentation frequently present
	Note: Lesions of subacute lupus erythematosus indistinguishable from lesions of PMLE	
Distribution	Sun-exposed sites	Sun-exposed and also protected sites
History	Eruption starts in spring	Eruption may start any time of year
Symptoms .	Symptoms vary from burning to pruritus	Arthralgias, malaise if associated with systemic lupus erythematosus
Exacerbating factors	Sunlight	Sunlight Medications
Associated findings	None	Arthritis, hair loss, mouth ulcers, renal disease
Epidemiology	Children and young adults; more common in females	Young adults; more common in females

Continues

Distinguishing features *(Continued)*

	POLYMORPHOUS LIGHTS ERUPTION	LUPUS ERYTHEMATOSUS
Biopsy	No Superficial and deep lymphocytic infiltrate with edema in papillary dermis	Occasionally Superficial and deep lymphocytic infiltrate Epidermal atrophy, follicular plugging, hydropic changes
Laboratory	Antinuclear antibody, SSA (Ro), SSB (LA) antigen tests negative; lesions sometimes reproduced by phototesting	Antinuclear antibody testing positive; frequently SSA (Ro) and SSB (La) antigen testing positive; low white blood cell and hemoglobin levels; platelets, urinalysis
Treatment	Sunscreens Topical steroids, antimalarials	Sunscreens Topical steroids, antimalarials, oral gold
Outcome	Chronic; nonscarring disease; tends to worsen with age	Chronic scarring disease

Abbreviation: PMLE, polymorphous light eruption.

Differential diagnosis of photodistributed rashes

Common causes
  Lupus erythematosus
  Photocontact dermatitis
  Phototoxic drug eruption
  Phytophotodermatitis
  Polymorphous light eruption

Rarer causes
  Actinic reticuloid
  Actinic prurigo
  Dermatomyositis
  Hydroa vacciniforme
  Porphyria
  Photodistributed psoriasis
  Pellagra

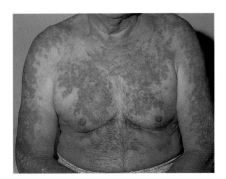

Figure 2.6.3 Lupus erythematosus.
Clue to diagnosis: Photodistributed rash.

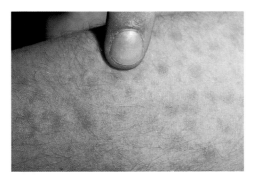

Figure 2.6.4 Polymorphous light eruption.
Clue to diagnosis: Urticarial-appearing papules.

7. SEBORRHEIC DERMATITIS
VERSUS
LUPUS ERYTHEMATOSUS

Features in common: Red, scaly rash in malar distribution.

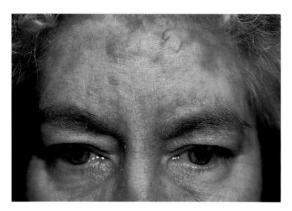

Figure 2.7.1 Seborrheic dermatitis with erythema and scale on eyebrows.

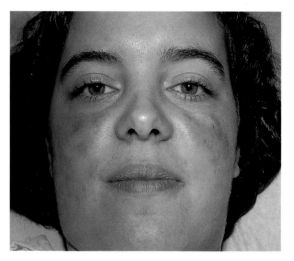

Figure 2.7.2 Systemic lupus erythematosus with erythema in a malar distribution.

Distinguishing features

	SEBORRHEIC DERMATITIS	LUPUS ERYTHEMATOSUS
Physical examination		
Morphology	Persistent erythema	**Acute cutaneous LE:** transient erythema in malar area, minimal scaling
	Yellow- to white-colored, greasy-appearing scale	**Chronic discoid LE:** atrophy, telangiectasias, follicular plugging in round scaly plaques
	Telangiectasias due to sun damage	Telangiectasias in lesions
	Scaling and erythema most prominent in nasolabial fold	Nasolabial area usually spared
Distribution	Scalp, eyebrows, anterior chest, nasolabial area, occasionally axilla and groin	Sun-exposed sites and occasionally nonexposed sites
History		
Symptoms	Asymptomatic	If systemic disease: malaise, arthritis, pleurisy, fatigue
Exacerbating factors	Infrequent washing No medications	Sunlight Medications: procainamide, hydralazine

Continues

Distinguishing features (*Continued*)

	SEBORRHEIC DERMATITIS	LUPUS ERYTHEMATOSUS
Associated findings	Parkinson's disease, human immunodeficiency virus infection, cardiac disease No associated physical findings	Arthritis, renal disease, anemia, pleurisy Diffuse or patchy hair loss Periungual telangiectasias Oral ulcers
Epidemiology	Older adults	Young adults, female predominance
Biopsy	No Superficial perivascular dermatitis with parakeratotic mounds around follicular orifices	Yes Superficial and deep perivascular and periappendiceal lymphocytic infiltrate Epidermal atrophy, telangiectasia, follicular plugging in DLE
Laboratory	None	Antinuclear antibody, anti-DS DNA, SS-A and SS-B antigen testing, complete blood count with differential; urinalysis
Treatment	Topical ketoconazole, sulfur preparations, low-potency corticosteroid creams; benzoyl peroxide, selenium sulfide or zinc pyrithione cleansers	Sun avoidance Topical steroids Antimalarials, oral gold Occasionally systemic steroids
Outcome	Chronic but nonscarring; good response to therapy	Chronic; may leave scars; fair response to therapy

Abbreviation: DLE, discoid lupus erythematosus.

Differential diagnosis: See p. 28.

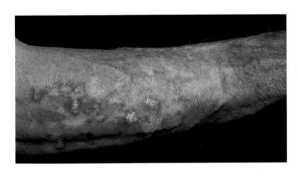

Figure 2.7.3 Discoid lupus erythematosus. *Clue to diagnosis:* Atrophic scarring hyperpigmented plaques.

8. PERIORAL DERMATITIS
VERSUS
CONTACT DERMATITIS

Features in common: Red, scaly patches and plaques on face.

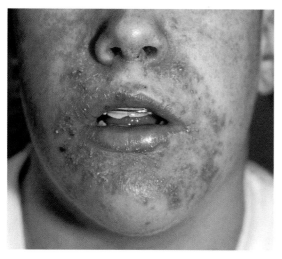

Figure 2.8.1 Contact dermatitis with sharply demar-cated erythema.

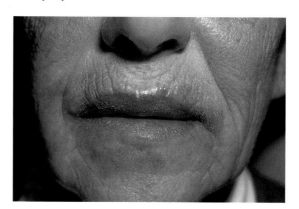

Figure 2.8.2 Perioral dermatitis with erythema and scaling in a perioral distribution.

Distinguishing features

	PERIORAL DERMATITIS	CONTACT DERMATITIS
Physical examination		
Morphology	Erythema, scaling, and papules distributed around the mouth Pustules No geometric shape	Erythema, scaling, and vesicles in area of contact No pustules Eruption may have sharp borders or geometric shape
Distribution	Rim of normal skin surrounding mouth Perioral, rarely periocular	No area of sparing No particular distribution
History		
Symptoms	Little or no pruritus	Severe pruritus frequent
Exacerbating factors	Topical steroids	Fragrances and preservatives in cosmetics or toiletries are most common culprits
Associated findings	None	None
Epidemiology	Adult females	Any age or sex
Biopsy	No Spongiotic dermatitis with granulomatous folliculitis	No Spongiotic dermatitis

Continues

Distinguishing features (*Continued*)

	PERIORAL DERMATITIS	CONTACT DERMATITIS
Laboratory	None	Patch testing
Treatment	Low-dose tetracycline and topical moisturizers; taper off corticosteroid preparations	Avoid allergen Topical or parenteral corticosteroids
Outcome	Chronic Resolves over several months with therapy	Curable Rapid improvement over 1 to 2 weeks with therapy and avoidance of contactant

Possible causes of contact dermatitis of the face based on location

Entire face: Cosmetics and topical pharmaceuticals
Eyelids: Nail cosmetics, adhesives for artificial nails, eyedrops, mascara
Nose: Eyeglasses, handkerchiefs, nasal medications
Forehead: Hair care products
Lips, perioral area: Lipstick, oral medications, foods
Chin, beard area: Shaving products, chin straps

Discussion

ACNE VULGARIS

Definition and etiology: Acne is a follicular disease that is a result of blockage of pilosebaceous units by keratinous material and sebum. This forms a comedo, the primary lesion in acne. Subsequent inflammation results in papules, pustules, nodules, and cysts.

Clinical features: The blocked pore in acne becomes enlarged and produces a clinically visible comedo. If the opening of the pore is visible, the comedo clinically appears to be filled with black-colored debris known as a blackhead. If the pore opening is not visible, the comedo looks like a small white- to yellow-colored papule, the whitehead. The inflammatory response to colonization of the comedo by *Propionibacterium acnes* produces papular and pustular lesions. Rupture of the blocked pore produces nodular-cystic lesions. In an individual patient, the lesions may primarily be comedonal, papulopustular, cystic, or a combination of different types. The severity of acne can also be modulated by hormonal changes; hence, the onset during puberty. Other exacerbating factors include use of cosmetics such as hair pomade, occupational exposure to oils or occlusive chemicals, and use of medications like lithium and phenytoin (Dilantin). Clinically, acne vulgaris is most commonly con-

fused with acne rosacea. However, acne rosacea primarily affects middle-aged adults, and comedones are not present.

Treatment: The standard treatment for acne is a combination of retinoids, antibiotics, and benzoyl peroxide. Topical retinoids help unclog the pores and prevent comedo formation; benzoyl peroxide has bacteriostatic and comedolytic activity; and antibiotics kill *Propionibacterium acnes*. Topical therapy with azelaic acid and sulfur preparations is also effective. In severe nodular-cystic and scarring acne, oral therapy with a vitamin A derivative, *cis*-retinoic acid (Accutane), is very effective.

ACNE ROSACEA

Definition and etiology: Rosacea, like acne, is a follicular disease of unknown origin. However, unlike acne, a vascular component is present, and comedones are not seen. The cause of rosacea is unclear. Various potential etiologic factors include familial predisposition, psychogenic factors, sunlight, *Demodex* organisms, vasoactive peptides, and cell-mediated and humoral immunity.

Clinical features: Acne rosacea is an asymptomatic but cosmetically bothersome disease of adults. Four clinical stages have been described in rosacea. In the first stage, intermittent flushing occurs. In the next stage, the erythema becomes persistent, and telangiectasias develop.

In the third stage, papules and pustules develop. In the final stage (which rarely occurs), rhinophyma, which is enlargement of the nasal connective tissue, develops, producing an enlarged, distorted nose.

Clinically, because of the presence of papules, rosacea can be confused with acne. Acne rosacea is also commonly misdiagnosed as systemic lupus erythematosus because of the presence of erythema. The malar erythema in systemic lupus erythematosus is transient, and patients also suffer from systemic symptoms. Raynaud's phenomenon is commonly experienced. In discoid lupus erythematosus, atrophy, pigmentary changes, and follicular plugging occur.

Treatment: Treatment options for rosacea include oral tetracycline, topical metronidazole cream, retinoids, and sulfur preparations. In patients with rhinophyma, use of the CO_2 laser or scalpel paring can be effective.

CONTACT DERMATITIS

Definition and etiology: Contact dermatitis is inflammation of the skin resulting from the interaction between the skin and chemicals. Contact dermatitis can be either an irritant type or an allergic type. Irritant contact dermatitis is a nonimmunologic reaction to a chemical that irritates the skin and causes inflammation. Conversely, allergic contact dermatitis is an individualized immunologic response to the chemical (i.e., the person who is allergic to the chemical will develop a rash when the chemical is absorbed through the skin, whereas another person who is not allergic to the chemical will not develop a rash upon contact). Irritant contact dermatitis is most frequently seen in the hands, whereas allergic contact dermatitis can occur in any part of the body in contact with the allergen.

Clinical features: In acute cases, erythema, scaling, vesicles, and swelling can be found. In patients with persistent disease, the erythema and scaling persist even though vesicles can no longer be found, and the skin becomes lichenified. The differential diagnosis includes acne rosacea (p. 40), seborrheic dermatitis (p. 44), perioral dermatitis (p. 43), lupus erythematosus, pemphigus erythematosus, and tinea faciei. In pemphigus erythematosus, erosions may be found, and a biopsy for immunofluorescence demonstrates characteristic intercellular immunofluorescent staining pattern. Tinea faciei can be excluded by a negative potassium hydroxide (KOH) scraping or fungal culture. Since both irritant and allergic contact dermatitis can morphologically appear identical, patch testing remains the test of choice in confirming the diagnosis of allergic contact dermatitis.

Contact dermatitis of the face can be a result of direct application of a pharmaceutical product, contact with a surface such as a pillow, or contact with airborne vapors, droplets, or dust particles. Rarely, contact dermatitis can also be transmitted from direct contact with other people ("consort" dermatitis). The allergen can also be transferred to the facial area from the hands. Eyelid dermatitis frequently occurs secondary to exposure to cosmetics in nail polish or adhesive resin used to glue on artificial nails.

Treatment: Contact dermatitis can be cured by avoidance of the appropriate allergen or irritant. Topical and oral steroids hasten the resolution of the rash.

IMPETIGO CONTAGIOSA

Definition and etiology: Impetigo contagiosa is a superficial blistering skin infection caused by either *Staphylococcus aureus* or *Streptococcus.*

Clinical features: Impetigo can occur on any cutaneous surface but frequently is seen in a perioral distribution, especially in children. Early on, a flaccid pus-filled blister may be present. Usually, since the blister occurs within the stratum corneum, it easily ruptures, and only erosions remain. The erosions are covered with an orange-colored crust. The major disease in the differential diagnosis is herpes simplex, especially since herpetic lesions can occasionally become secondarily infected. Unlike the lesions of herpes, the erosions and blisters in impetigo are large (centimeter-sized rather then millimeter-sized). The vesicles in herpes are also clustered and have scalloped borders with central umbilication. Patients with herpes infection also frequently have prodromal symptoms before lesions appear. In a primary infection, patients may also have a high fever with associated lymphadenopathy. In addition, herpes simplex may recur in the same site, whereas impetigo generally is not recurrent. In cases in which there is a diagnostic dilemma, a Tzanck preparation and culture should be performed.

Treatment: Impetigo can be treated either with topical mupirocin ointment or with a systemic antibiotic such as penicillin, dicloxacillin, or erythromycin.

HERPES FACIALIS

Definition and etiology: Herpes facialis is a herpes simplex virus type 1 or (rarely) type 2 infection of the oral mucosa most commonly seen in children and young adults.

Clinical features: The eruption starts 2 to 10 days after subclinical exposure to herpes simplex virus. Usually, patients develop prodromal symptoms of burning, discomfort, or itching at the site of the impending eruption. In a primary episode, patients develop fever and malaise. The lesions start out as red macules on the vermilion border that rapidly become vesiculated and develop into widespread erosions. On closer inspection, the erosions are grouped and have scalloped borders characteristic of a herpesvirus infection. The lesions heal spontaneously in a few weeks.

The major diseases in the differential diagnosis are impetigo and contact dermatitis. Systemic and prodromal symptoms are rare in impetigo, the vesicles are not grouped, and scalloped borders are not seen. The golden-orange crust is also characteristic. However, clinicians should remember that herpetic lesions can become secondarily infected. In contact dermatitis, the vesicles are not grouped, bullae may be present, the rash is usually more widespread, and pruritus is very severe. In diagnostically difficult cases, the Tzanck smear should be performed; in herpes lesions, multinucleated giant cells are present. In older lesions, the Tzanck preparation results may be negative, and culture is more sensitive.

Treatment: Oral acyclovir, valacyclovir, or famciclovir, if started during the first 2 days of the infection, can limit the severity and duration of disease. Topical pencyclovir cream is effective for recurrent lesions.

LUPUS ERYTHEMATOSUS

Definition and etiology: Lupus erythematosus is an inflammatory autoimmune disease that affects the skin and extracutaneous tissue. It can be divided into relatively different homogeneous subsets. In one subset, discoid lupus erythematosus (DLE), the skin findings are the only manifestation. In subacute cutaneous lupus erythematosus, patients present with a photosensitive eruption that in approximately 50% of patients is associated with systemic disease. Systemic lupus erythematosus is a multiorgan disease. Patients can be classified into the appropriate subset based on a combination of clinical and laboratory data.

Clinical features: Lupus erythematosus occurs most frequently in young adult females. Classification of disease is independent of the morphology of the cutaneous eruption. For example, the skin lesions of discoid lupus erythematosus can be seen in patients with no systemic disease but can also be found in approximately 10% of patients with systemic disease.

The American Rheumatologic Association has established criteria for the diagnosis of systemic lupus erythematosus. Four of the following 11 criteria should be present:

1. Malar rash
2. Discoid lesions
3. Photosensitivity
4. Oral ulcers
5. Arthritis
6. Proteinuria
7. Seizures or psychosis
8. Pleuritis or pericarditis
9. Low white blood cell count, low platelet count, or hemolytic anemia
10. Antibodies to double-stranded DNA or Sm antigen or false-positive serologic syphilis test
11. Positive antinuclear antibody test

The classic butterfly-shaped malar rash is commonly known to be the cutaneous feature of systemic lupus erythematosus. Confluent erythematous macules overlying the cheeks form the wings of the butterfly, while erythema of the nose forms the body. The rash may be precipitated by sun exposure and lasts several hours to several days.

The word "discoid" is derived from the Greek word *diskoides*, meaning flat and circular. The cutaneous lesions of discoid lupus erythematosus are red, well-demarcated, scaly macules or papules that evolve into coin-shaped (discoid) plaques covered by an adherent scale, which is more prominent around dilated follicular orifices. By removing the scale, one can see keratotic spikes similar to carpet tacks. With time, the lesions expand, leaving atrophic telangiectatic scars in the center. Areas of hyper- and hypopigmentation also develop. The lesions of discoid lupus erythematosus most commonly occur on the face, scalp, ears, V area of neck, and arms. Unlike seborrheic dermatitis, the nasolabial area is usually spared. Scarring occurs in DLE.

In subacute cutaneous lupus erythematosus, patients present with a history of photosensitivity and antibodies against Ro (SS-A) and La (SS-B) antigens. Morphologically, the rash may appear to be either papulosquamous or annular polycyclic on sun-exposed skin. Unlike in discoid lupus erythematosus, the lesions heal without scarring, but postinflammatory hypopigmentation can be seen. The papulosquamous rash may clinically mimic psoriasis, but the lesions are less well-demarcated, have a papular component, and, unlike psoriasis, predominantly occur on sun-exposed skin. The annular polycyclic from of lupus can be confused with granuloma annulare, erythema multiforme, or erythema figuratum. The presence of slight scaling and photodistribution are helpful differentiating features.

Differential diagnosis: Although occasionally the rash may be persistent, most cases of chronic malar erythema in otherwise healthy patients are not due to lupus erythematosus. Persistent erythema of the face with overlying telangiectasias is most commonly seen in acne rosacea. The rash of dermatomyositis may also be confused with lupus erythematosus. In dermatomyositis, the erythema contains a violaceous hue, and periorbital erythema is a prominent feature. Gottron's papules, red papules and plaques overlying the knuckles, are seen in dermatomyositis. In cutaneous lupus, however, if skin lesions are present on the hands, they are more prominent between the joints.

Treatment: The treatment of lupus erythematosus is predicated on the extent of systemic involvement. For cutaneous lupus erythematosus, commonly used therapies include sun protection and avoidance, topical steroids, intralesional steroids, and oral antimalarials.

PERIORAL DERMATITIS

Definition and etiology: Perioral dermatitis is an idiopathic acneiform eczematous eruption characterized by a perioral distribution. The cause of perioral dermatitis is not known, but in one large series of 259 patients with the disease, 250 had been using topical corticosteroids. The topical steroids had been started for a variety of other rashes. The authors postulated that steroids may diminish the patients' tolerance to irritants in cosmetics or other contactants. Another hypothesis is that steroids may change the natural skin flora, thereby producing an acneiform eruption.

Clinical features: Perioral dermatitis is most commonly seen in adult women. A history of pruritus and cosmetic use can commonly be obtained. Papules, vesicles, and pustules on an erythematous base are seen surrounding the mouth. Some scaling resembling dermatitis is also commonly present. Rarely, perioral dermatitis can occur on the eyes, producing "periocular dermatitis." A characteristic clinical finding is a rim of uninvolved normal skin surrounding the vermilion border of the lips. Clinically, perioral dermatitis can be confused with contact dermatitis because of the presence of erythema and scaling or with an acneiform eruption such as acne vulgaris or acne rosacea if a papular or pustular component is prominent.

Treatment: Perioral dermatitis can be effectively treated with oral tetracycline or erythromycin. If patients have been taking potent topical steroids, a low-potency steroid preparation like 1% hydrocortisone may be used to prevent rebound upon stopping the high-potency steroid. Various topical creams or gels such as metronidazole gel, clindamycin, and sulfur preparations can also be used as adjunctive agents.

POLYMORPHOUS LIGHT ERUPTION

Definition and etiology: Polymorphous light eruption is the most common idiopathic photodermatosis in the United States and England.

Clinical features: As the word "polymorphous" implies, the rash can assume a variety of different shapes; however, the appearance of the rash in a specific patient is relatively monomorphous. The disease starts in young adults, but in genetically predisposed individuals such as

American Indians and the Scottish, the disease commonly starts in childhood. Females are more frequently affected than males. The eruption first appears in springtime and has a delayed onset of 24 to 48 hours after sun exposure. With chronic sun exposure, hardening and improvement occur. The morphologic patterns include papulovesicles, eczematous lesions, edematous plaques, excoriated nodules, erythema multiforme-like lesions, and occasionally petechiae and hemorrhage. Pruritus is usually present, and lichenification due to chronic scratching can be seen.

Differential diagnosis: Polymorphous light eruption can be distinguished from systemic lupus erythematosus by the lack of systemic symptoms, and it can be distinguished from discoid lupus erythematosus by the absence of atrophy, telangiectasias, and follicular plugging. In other diseases that can be confused with polymorphous light eruption (such as erythema multiforme, sarcoidosis, and tinea faciei), photosensitivity does not occur.

In diagnostically challenging cases, a skin biopsy may be helpful. Finally, a photocontact or phototoxic eruption should always be excluded by taking a thorough history, including questions about topical or parenteral contact with a photosensitizing agent or by performing patch testing.

Treatment: Treatment consists of sun avoidance and broad-spectrum sunscreens. Topical steroids can be used during acute exacerbations. In severe cases, antimalarial therapy can be effective. Desensitization light therapy can also be used.

PSEUDOFOLLICULITIS BARBAE

Definition and etiology: Pseudofolliculitis barbae is inflammation of the skin in the beard area of adult men caused by penetration of the skin by ingrown curved hair.

Clinical features: Pseudofolliculitis is a common problem in patients with curly hair and is seen most commonly in blacks. Physical examination reveals papules and pustules in the beard area. Closer examination will demonstrate curved and ingrown hairs. Scarring may form. The major diseases in the differential diagnosis are acne vulgaris and folliculitis. In pseudofolliculitis barbae, the eruption is localized to the beard area, and the rest of the face will not be involved (unlike in acne vulgaris). Comedones are not present. Infectious folliculitis most commonly involves the thigh and buttocks area. Culture of a pustule will be positive for *Staphylococcus aureus*.

Treatment: The treatment of pseudofolliculitis is very difficult. Growing a beard will solve the problem, but this is not a desirable solution for everyone. Since shaving in itself can be irritating, shaving at nighttime instead of in the morning can give the skin some time to recover. Topical antibiotic and retinoid preparations offer some benefit. A low-potency hydrocortisone cream applied after shaving may also reduce some of the irritation.

SEBORRHEIC DERMATITIS

Definition and etiology: Seborrheic dermatitis is a common form of dermatitis localized to areas with an increased number of sebaceous glands and increased sebum production such as the scalp, nasolabial folds, eyebrows, cheeks, anterior chest, axilla, and groin. The oil produced by the sebaceous glands facilitates the growth of pityrosporum organisms, thereby producing inflammation and a dermatitis. In neonates, seborrheic dermatitis is called *cradle cap*, but it is most commonly seen in adults, with dandruff being its mildest manifestation. Severe seborrheic dermatitis is sometimes referred to as *tinea amiantacea*, but this term is confusing and is avoided here.

Clinical features: Seborrheic dermatitis is characterized by erythematous plaques covered with yellow, greasy scales. If seborrheic dermatitis involves the cheek, clinically it can be confused with systemic or discoid lupus (p. 42) or contact dermatitis (p. 41). A seborrheic dermatitis-like rash can also occur in patients with riboflavin deficiency. The incidence of seborrheic dermatitis is increased in patients with human immunodeficiency virus infection, Parkinson's disease, dementia, or cardiac failure, as well as in alcoholics. Male patients are also more frequently affected than female patients.

Treatment: Seborrheic dermatitis on the face usually responds well to low-potency topical steroids and imidazole creams such as ketoconazole. The scalp involvement can be treated with antidandruff shampoos containing ketoconazole, zinc oxide, and selenium sulfide. Benzoyl peroxide, zinc pyrithione, and selenium sulfide cleaners are also helpful.

Suggested Readings

ACNE VULGARIS
Kaminer MS, Gilchrest BA. The many faces of acne. J Am Acad Dermatol 1995;32:S6–14.
Thiboutot DM, Lookingbill DP. Acne: acute or chronic disease? J Am Acad Dermatol 1995;32:S2–5.

ACNE ROSACEA
Marks R. Concepts in the pathogenesis of rosacea. Br J Dermatol 1968;80:170–77.

Miller SR, Shalita AR. Topical metronidazole gel (0.75%) for the treatment of perioral dermatitis in children. J Am Acad Dermatol 1994;31:847–48.
Rebora A. Rosacea. J Invest Dermatol 1987;88:56s–60s.
Thiboutot DM. Acne rosacea. Am Fam Physician 1994; 50:1691–97, 1701–2.
Wilkin JK. Rosacea. Pathophysiology and treatment (editorial). Arch Dermatol 1994;130:359–62.

CONTACT DERMATITIS
Dooms-Goossens A. The red face: contact and photocontact dermatitis. Clin Dermatol 1993;11:289–95.

IMPETIGO CONTAGIOSA
Dagan R. Impetigo in childhood: changing epidemiology and new treatments. Pediatr Ann 1993;22:235–40.
Darmstadt GL, Lane AT. Impetigo: an overview. Pediatr Dermatol 1994:11:293–303.
Shriner DL, Schwartz RA, Janniger CK. Impetigo. Cutis 1995;56:30–32.

HERPES FACIALIS
Higgins CR, Schofield JK, Tatnall FM et al. Natural history, management and complications of herpes labialis. J Med Virol 1993;1:22–26.
Spruance SL. The natural history of recurrent oral-facial herpes simplex virus infection. Semin Dermatol 1992; 11:200–6.
Vestey JP, Norval M. Mucocutaneous infections with herpes simplex virus and their management. Clinical Exp Dermatol 1992;17:221–37.

LUPUS ERYTHEMATOSUS
Dubois EL, Tuffanelli DL. Clinical manifestations of systemic lupus erythematosus. Computer analysis of 520 cases. JAMA 1964;190:104–11.

PERIORAL DERMATITIS
Coskey RJ. Perioral dermatitis. Cutis 1984;34:55–56, 58.
Jillson OF. Perioral dermatitis (editorial). Lancet 1980; 12:75.
Jillson OF. Perioral dermatitis. Cutis 1984;34:457–58.
Wilkinson DS, Kirton V, Wilkinson JD. Perioral dermatitis. A 12 year review. Br J Dermatol 1979;101:245–57.

POLYMORPHOUS LIGHT ERUPTION
Morison WL, Stern RS. Polymorphous light eruption: a common reaction uncommonly recognized. Acta Derm Venereol 1982;62:237–40.

PSEUDOFOLLICULITIS BARBAE
Brown LA Jr. Pathogenesis and treatment of pseudofolliculitis barbae. Cutis 1983;32:373–75.
Coquilla BH, Lewis CW. Management of pseudofolliculitis barbae. Mil Med 1995;160:263–69.

Dunn JF Jr. Pseudofolliculitis barbae. Am Fam Physician 1988;38:169–74.

Halder RM. Pseudofolliculitis barbae and related disorders. Dermatol Clin 1988;6:407–12.

SEBORRHEIC DERMATITIS

Barba A, Piubellow W, Vantini I et al. Skin lesions in chronic alcoholic pancreatitis. Dermatologica 1982; 164:322–26.

Janniger CK, Schwartz RA. Seborrheic dermatitis. Am Fam Physician 1995;52:149–55, 159–60.

Marino CT, McDonald E, Romano JF. Seborrheic dermatitis in acquired immunodeficiency syndrome. Cutis 1991;48:217–18.

3 *Oral Mucosa*

ALGORITHM FOR ORAL RASHES

Localized lesions

Ulcer

White patches/plaques

Chronic

Leukoplakia

Other causes
- Cheek biting
- Genodermatosis
  - Darier's disease
  - White sponge nevus
  - Pachonychia congenita, etc.
- Nicotine stomatitis
- Oral hairy leukoplakia

Yes

No

Biopsy

Trauma

Malignant

Benign

Squamous cell carcinoma

Leukokeratosis

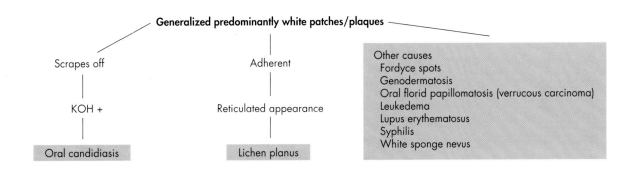

Generalized predominantly white patches/plaques

Scrapes off

Adherent

Other causes
- Fordyce spots
- Genodermatosis
- Oral florid papillomatosis (verrucous carcinoma)
- Leukedema
- Lupus erythematosus
- Syphilis
- White sponge nevus

KOH +

Reticulated appearance

Oral candidiasis

Lichen planus

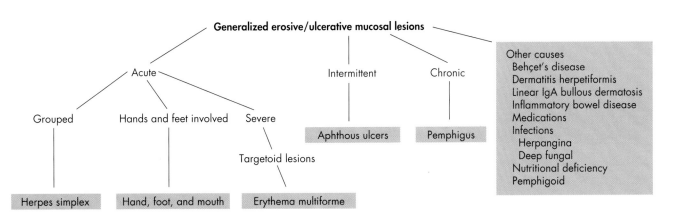

Generalized erosive/ulcerative mucosal lesions

Acute

Intermittent

Chronic

Other causes
- Behçet's disease
- Dermatitis herpetiformis
- Linear IgA bullous dermatosis
- Inflammatory bowel disease
- Medications
- Infections
  - Herpangina
  - Deep fungal
- Nutritional deficiency
- Pemphigoid

Grouped

Hands and feet involved

Severe

Aphthous ulcers

Pemphigus

Targetoid lesions

Herpes simplex

Hand, foot, and mouth

Erythema multiforme

DIFFERENTIAL DIAGNOSIS

DISEASE DISCUSSION

Introduction

Mucosal epithelium is different from the integument in that an outer keratinizing layer (stratum corneum) is not made in the absence of disease, adnexal structures are not present, and there is more rapid epithelialization. There is a limited repertoire of responses that mucosal epithelium can have to diseases. Therefore, oral diseases tend to look identical, and diagnoses made from clinical appearance and history may need to be supported by biopsy and blood test results. For example, white patches can be seen in entirely disparate diseases such as lichen planus, candidiasis, and squamous cell carcinoma. Oral lesions are especially important, since they can interfere with eating. In some diseases such as pemphigus, oral lesions may be the harbinger of a potentially fatal disease.

1. LICHEN PLANUS
VERSUS
ORAL CANDIDIASIS

Features in common: White mucosal lesions.

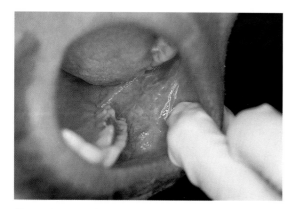

Figure 3.1.1 Lichen planus.

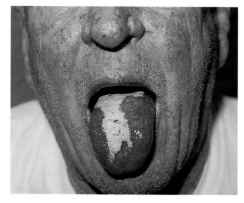

Figure 3.1.2 Oral candidiasis.

Distinguishing features

	LICHEN PLANUS	CANDIDIASIS
Physical examination		
Morphology	White, reticulated plaque	White strands become confluent, forming plaques
	Ulcers commonly present	Ulcers rarely seen
	White plaques do not rub off	White plaques easily rub off
Distribution	Buccal mucosa, tongue, gingiva, palate, lips	Buccal mucosa, tongue, gingiva, palate, pharynx
History		
Symptoms	Asymptomatic or painful if ulcerated	Asymptomatic; occasionally burning mouth
Exacerbating factors	Iatrogenic: antimalarials, quinidine, β-blockers, diuretics, hypoglycemic agents	Iatrogenic: steroids, antibiotics
	Dental amalgams	Immunosuppressant
		Dentures and implants
Associated findings	Violaceous papules and plaques on wrists, ankles, elsewhere in half of patients	Endocrine diseases: diabetes, thyroid, hypoparathyroidism
	Nail dystrophy	Systemic diseases: lymphomas, autoimmune, immunodeficiencies (HIV)
Epidemiology	Adults	Any age
Biopsy	Yes	No
	Lichenoid infiltrate, irregular epidermal hyperplasia with sawtooth-like appearance, hypergranulosis	Spores and pseudohyphae on surface of epithelium (highlighted by periodic acid-Schiff stains)
Laboratory	None; KOH negative	Positive KOH
Treatment	Topical therapy: corticosteroids, cyclosporine swish and swallow, retinoids	Topical therapy: nystatin swish and spit, miconazole troches
	Systemic therapy: retinoids	Systemic therapy: ketoconazole, fluconazole (Diflucan)
Outcome	Chronic course	Good response to therapy

Abbreviations: HIV, human immunodeficiency virus; KOH, potassium hydroxide.

Differential diagnosis of white oral plaques (leukoplakia)

Common causes
 Cheek biting (Morsicatio buccarum)
 Fordyce's spots
 Lichen planus
 Oral candidiasis
 Oral hairy leukoplakia
 Nicotine stomatitis
 Squamous cell carcinoma or dysplasia

Rarer causes
 White sponge nevus
 Oral florid papillomatosis
 Focal epithelial hyperplasia
 Leukoedema
 Mucous patch of syphilis
 White patches of genodermatosis: Darier's disease, pachyonychia congenita, dyskeratosis congenita

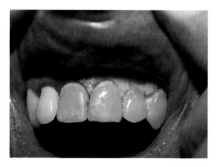

Figure 3.1.3 Lichen planus. *Clue to diagnosis:* Reticulated white plaque on gingiva.

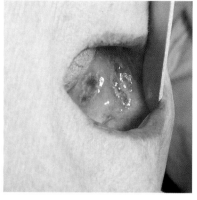

Figure 3.1.4 Lichen planus. *Clue to diagnosis:* Ulcers in buccal mucosa with surrounding white reticulated plaques.

2. APHTHOUS ULCERS
VERSUS
PEMPHIGUS VULGARIS

Features in common: Oral ulcer.

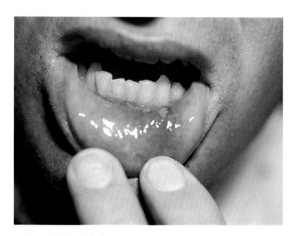

Figure 3.2.1 Aphthous stomatitis.

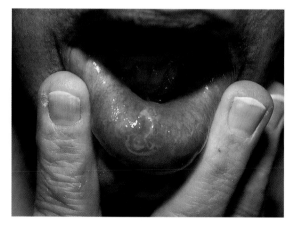

Figure 3.2.2 Pemphigus vulgaris.

Distinguishing features

	APHTHOUS ULCERS	PEMPHIGUS VULGARIS
Physical examination Morphology	Minor aphthae: 4–8 mm round or oval lesions, yellow center and erythematous rim Major aphthae: similar appearance but large 1–3 cm ulcers	Large (often several centimeters in in size) coalescent ulcers and erosions

Distinguishing features (Continued)

	APHTHOUS ULCERS	PEMPHIGUS VULGARIS
Morphology (continued)	Herpetiform: grouped small 1-mm erosions that coalesce into large ulcers	Vesicles not grouped
Distribution	Buccal mucosa and occasionally tongue, soft palate, oropharynx	Buccal mucosa, tongue, palate, gingiva, occasionally oropharynx
History Symptoms	Intermittent oral sores Four stages: premonitory, preulcerative, ulcerative, healing Premonitory stage: asymptomatic or paresthesia and burning sensation Preulcerative and ulcerative stage: pain	Chronic oral sores Severe pain and discomfort
Exacerbating factors	Stress, nutritional deficiencies, food allergy, infections, trauma	Occasionally drug-induced: penicillamine, penicillin, captopril, phenobarbital
Associated findings	Ulcers of genital mucosa occasionally (if uveitis, consider Behçet's disease)	Erosions in glabrous skin Positive Nikolsky's sign
Epidemiology	Common Can occur at any age, but most prevalent in young adults	Rare Primarily affects middle-aged adults
Biopsy	No Nonspecific ulceration	Yes Epidermal acantholysis, eosinophilic infiltrate, tombstoning of the basal epithelial layer
Laboratory	Occasionally vitamin B_{12}, folic acid, iron deficiency	Positive indirect and direct immunofluorescence results
Treatment	Viscous lidocaine, tetracycline, topical corticosteroids, topical tannic acid	Prednisone, immunosuppresive agents: azathioprine, cyclosporine
Outcome	Chronic relapsing course	Mortality of 60%–90% prior to glucocorticoid treatment Chronic disease

Differential diagnosis of oral ulcers

Aphthous stomatitis
Autoimmune blistering
  Cicatricial pemphigoid
  Dermatitis herpetiformis
  Linear IgA bullous dermatosis
  Pemphigus vulgaris
Behçet's syndrome
Cytotoxic drugs (e.g., methotrexate, 6-mercaptopurine)

Epidermolysis bullosa
Infections
  Herpetic gingivostomatitis
  Candidiasis
  Herpangina
  Hand-foot-and-mouth disease
  Deep fungal infections
Lichen planus
Neoplasia carcinoma

Nutritional deficiency
  Noma
Trauma
Ulcerative colitis
Vasculitis
  Wegener's granulomatosis

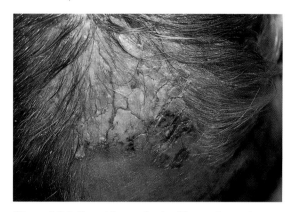

Figure 3.2.3 Pemphigus vulgaris. *Clue to diagnosis:* Erosions on integument.

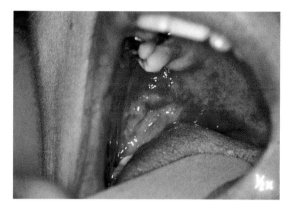

Figure 3.2.4 Pemphigus vulgaris. *Clue to diagnosis:* Chronic unremitting oral ulcers.

3. LICHEN PLANUS
VERSUS
LEUKOPLAKIA

Features in common: White mucosal lesions.

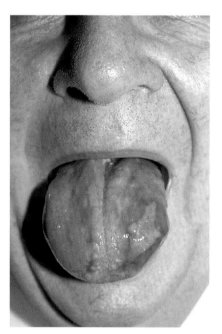

Figure 3.3.1 Lichen planus.

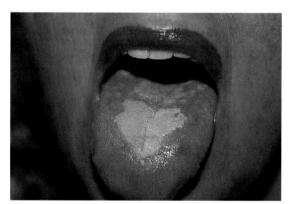

Figure 3.3.2 Leukoplakia.

Distinguishing features

	LICHEN PLANUS	LEUKOPLAKIA
Physical examination		
Morphology	White reticulated plaque	*Localized* white patch/plaque
		Lesions may be small or large
	Erosions/ulcers commonly present	Ulcers only after long-standing duration or trauma
		Lesions become leathery and thick with time
		Erythematous speckled or warty appearance in premalignant lesions
Distribution	Buccal mucosa, tongue, gingiva, palate, lips	Buccal mucosa, retrocommissural mucosa, alveolar ridge, tongue, hard palate, rarely sublingual area and gingiva
History	Not related to tobacco products	Smokers or tobacco chewers
Symptoms	Asymptomatic or painful if ulcerated	Asymptomatic
Exacerbating factors	Iatrogenic: antimalarials, quinidine, β-blockers, diuretics, hypoglycemic agents	None
	Dental amalgams	
Associated findings	Violaceous papules and plaques on wrists, ankles, elsewhere in half of patients	Squamous cell carcinoma
		Occasionally poor dental hygiene
	Nail dystrophy	
Epidemiology	Men and women	Predominantly men
Biopsy	Occasionally	Yes
	Lichenoid infiltrate, sawtoothing of epithelium, hypergranulosis	Epithelial acanthosis with varying amounts of dysplasia
Laboratory	None	Occasionally candida overgrowth found on potassium hydroxide test
Treatment	Topical or systemic steroids	Topical retinoids
	Topical or systemic retinoids	Surgery, laser surgery
	Cyclosporine suspension	
Outcome	Chronic disease	May regress upon stopping tobacco use or may develop into squamous cell carcinoma

Differential diagnosis: See p. 47.

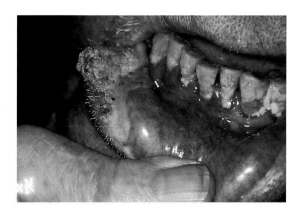

Figure 3.3.3 Squamous cell carcinoma arising within a plaque of leukoplakia. *Clue to Diagnosis:* Crusted nodule and erythema within an area of leukoplakia.

4. HERPES STOMATITIS
VERSUS
ERYTHEMA MULTIFORME

Features in common: Oral erosions and vesicles.

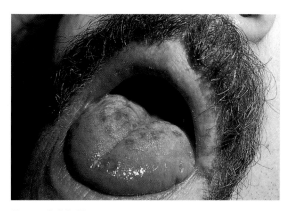

Figure 3.4.1 Herpes stomatitis.

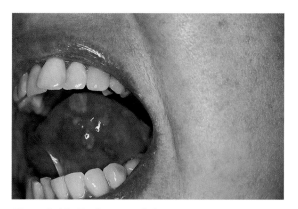

Figure 3.4.2 Erythema multiforme.

Distinguishing features

	HERPETIC GINGIVOSTOMATITIS	ERYTHEMA MULTIFORME
Physical examination		
Morphology	Generalized mucosal grouped vesicles and erosions	Generalized erosions and ulcers with pseudomembrane formation
	Scalloped border may be present	No scalloped border
Distribution	Entire oral mucosa in primary infection	Entire oral mucosa
	Other mucosal surfaces not involved	Involvement of other mucosal surface common (eyes, nose)
	No target lesions	Targetoid lesions on skin
	Localized lymphadenopathy	Generalized lymphadenopathy

Continues

Distinguishing features (*Continued*)

	HERPETIC GINGIVOSTOMATITIS	ERYTHEMA MULTIFORME
History	History of exposure to herpesvirus 2 to 10 days previously (in some cases)	Occasional prodromal upper respiratory tract infection Ingestion of new medication
Symptoms	Fevers, malaise commonly present Cannot eat or drink Pain and discomfort	Fever rarely, presents more commonly with prodrome, malaise Cannot eat or drink Pain and discomfort
Exacerbating factors	Immunosuppression	None
Associated findings	None	Over 50 reported associations including the following: Infections: *Mycoplasma pneumoniae*, herpes simplex Most common medications: nonsteroidal anti-inflammatory agents, antibiotics, barbiturates Rarely associated with neoplasm or connective tissue disease
Epidemiology	Primarily involves children	Primarily involves young adults aged 20–40 years
Biopsy	No Ballooning necrosis of epidermis Multinucleated giant cells within epidermal vesicles	Occasionally Necrotic keratinocytes with areas of epidermal necrosis, interface lymphocytic dermatitis
Laboratory	Positive culture for herpes simplex; Tzanck preparation: multinucleated giant cells	Chest x-ray if pulmonary symptoms Tzanck test and culture negative unless secondary to herpes infection
Treatment	Early on, antiviral therapy (acyclovir, famciclovir, valacyclovir) helpful	Questionably role for oral steroids Discontinuation of drugs
Outcome	Good Resolves over 1–2 weeks No scarring	Usually good Resolves over 4–6 weeks May have residual scarring Eye involvement may lead to blindness Occasionally fatal due to secondary sepsis

Differential diagnosis of erosive oral disease: See p. 49.

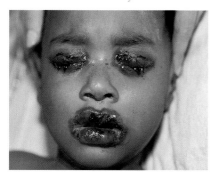

Figure 3.4.3 Erythema multiforme. *Clue to diagnosis:* Involvement of other mucosal skin.

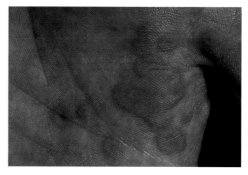

Figure 3.4.4 Erythema multiforme. *Clue to diagnosis:* Targetoid lesions on palms.

Discussion

APHTHOUS STOMATITIS

Definition and etiology: Recurrent aphthous stomatitis, commonly called a canker sore, is an ulcerative disease of the oral mucosa of unknown cause.

Clinical features: Aphthous ulcers are the most common ulcerative disease of the oral mucosa. Twenty percent of the general population may suffer from aphthous ulcerations at some time in their lives.

Patients with aphthous ulcers commonly experience a tingling or burning sensation at the site of the initial lesions. The ulcers are most commonly seen on the buccal mucosa but can also involve the lips, tongue, soft palate, and oropharynx. Morphologically, aphthous ulcers can be classified as minor, major, or herpetiform lesions. Minor aphthae, the most common form, are characterized by small ulcers a few millimeters in size covered with a yellow scab and surrounded by erythema. The lesions usually heal without scarring in 7 to 10 days, but recurrences are common. Major aphthous ulcers (Sutton's disease) have a similar appearance to minor aphthae; however, they are a few centimeters in size and persist up to one month. Scarring can also occur. In patients with the herpetiform variant, small, grouped papular vesicles that coalesce into a larger plaque are present. Herpes culture is negative.

The differential diagnosis includes other ulcerating diseases such as herpes simplex stomatitis and pemphigus vulgaris. Herpes gingival stomatitis usually involves children. Skin involvement is not seen, and the lesions have a characteristic grouped appearance. The herpetiform variant of aphthous ulcers can be distinguished only by means of culture or skin biopsy; however, herpes gingivostomatitis, unlike herpes labialis, is usually not a recurrent disease. Autoimmune blistering diseases such as pemphigus vulgaris and cicatricial pemphigoid usually are chronic, not recurrent. In both pemphigus vulgaris and cicatricial pemphigoid, skin involvement can occur. In cicatricial pem-

phigoid, conjunctival, nasal, or pharyngeal involvement occurs in a majority of patients. Other causes of oral ulcers (such as medications, a nutritional deficiency state, or inflammatory bowel disease) can usually be excluded based upon the history.

Treatment: Since the ulcers in aphthous stomatitis are usually self limited, treatment is usually only palliative. Hot, spicy, and acidic foods should be avoided. A mixture of viscous lidocaine, antacids, and sucralfate (Carafate) can provide temporary relief from the pain.

ORAL CANDIDIASIS

Definition and etiology: Oral candidiasis, also known as oral thrush or acute pseudomembranous candidiasis, is infection of the oropharyngeal cavity with *Candida albicans*, a yeast.

Clinical features: Oral candidiasis can be seen in any age group. Candidiasis starts as small, white, droplike macules and papules on the buccal mucosa, tongue, gingiva, palate, and pharynx. The lesions have been described as resembling milk curds or cottage cheese. With time and in severe cases, large plaques with pseudomembranes, erosions, or ulcers may develop. The base and surrounding mucosa are often erythematous.

Other diseases with white plaques include morsicatio buccarum (cheek biting), lichen planus, leukoplakia, leukoedema, oral florid papillomatosis, white sponge nevus, and squamous cell carcinoma. Unlike in the other diseases, the white plaques in candidiasis usually are easily rubbed off. In morsicatio buccarum, white plaques are produced owing to chronic cheek biting of the buccal mucosa, and white patches are oriented parallel to the gum line. Leukoedema is an idiopathic, asymptomatic swelling of the oral mucosa and lips. The diffuse white discoloration of the mucosa disappears upon stretching the skin. White sponge nevus is an autosomal dominant disease in which white patches are found mainly on the buccal mucosa. In oral florid papillomatosis, a cancerous condition of the oral cavity caused by a papillomavirus infection, localized white papillomatous cauliflower-like vegetations are seen on the buccal mucosa. In lichen planus (discussed in greater detail later in this chapter), the white plaques are arranged in a reticular and lacelike pattern. Finally, in both leukoplakia and squamous cell carcinoma, localized white plaques are found. The plaques may ulcerate or may have a vegetative appearance.

Oral candidiasis is commonly seen in newborns and infants when the mucosa becomes colonized by yeast from the mother's birth canal. In children and adults, oral candidiasis is commonly secondary to underlying systemic disease or is iatrogenically produced. Some common systemic diseases associated with candidiasis include endocrine disorders (diabetes, hypoparathyroidism, hypothyroidism), immune deficiencies (human immunodeficiency virus infection, acquired immunodeficiency syndrome), nutritional deficiencies, and malignancies. Iatrogenic factors include broad-spectrum antibiotics, corticosteroid therapy, immunosuppressive agents, cytotoxic agents, dentures, and other prostheses.

Treatment: The first caveat of treatment is to identify and, when possible, eliminate any predisposing factors. The next step is to eliminate the causative organisms by using either topical or systemic therapy. Topically, a 2- to 3-week course of nystatin suspension or clotrimazole troches is effective. For more severe, recurrent, or chronic cases, oral ketoconazole or fluconazole may be used.

ERYTHEMA MULTIFORME

Definition and etiology: Erythema multiforme is an inflammatory reactive skin disease secondary to a wide variety of triggers. Common causes include medications and infections, such as *Mycoplasma pneumoniae* or herpes simplex. The possible triggers include the following:

Infections: viral, bacterial, mycobacterial,
    fungal (especially coccidioidomycosis and
    histoplasmosis), protozoal
Medications: sulfonamides, penicillins,
    nonsteroidal anti-inflammatory agents,
    barbiturates, phenytoin (Dilantin),
    hydralazine, penicillamine, tetracycline,
    allopurinol
Neoplasms (especially lymphoma)
Connective tissue diseases
Physical agents: radiation therapy
Foods
Contactants: bromofluorine, fire sponge,
    toxixcondendrol

Topical agents
Miscellaneous: pregnancy, sarcoidosis,
    inflammatory bowel disease

Clinical features: Erythema multiforme commonly involves both mucosal and glabrous skin. Generalized erosions with formation of pseudomembrane and crust are seen in the mouth. Sometimes the mucosal involvement can precede the skin findings, which typically include symmetric urticarial macules and papules. Rarely, mucosal involvement is the only manifestation of erythema multiforme. Within the first few days, some of the lesions develop concentric color changes owing to necrosis. This produces the characteristic "target" or "iris" lesion. Blisters may also develop. The lesions appear first on extremities and then extend to the trunk. Patients complain of pain from the mucosal involvement, along with mild malaise or itching. In the severe form, known as *erythema multiforme* major, fevers, arthralgia, severe malaise, and even death due to secondary infection can occur. Erythema multiforme major is defined by mucous membrane involvement (oral, nasal, or eye), as well as severe and widespread skin involvement (Stevens-Johnson syndrome). The relationship between erythema multiforme and toxic epidermal necrolysis (TEN), a disease with widespread tissue desquamation, continues to be debated. In TEN, target lesions are not present. If skin involvement is present, erythema multiforme can be easily diagnosed. If only mucosal involvement is present, the differential diagnosis includes herpetic gingivostomatitis (see later) or other erosive diseases like aphthous ulcers (see p. 54).

Treatment: Erythema multiforme usually resolves spontaneously with supportive care if the precipitating factor is eliminated. Some physicians advocate the use of systemic steroids in the first few days of disease involvement, but the efficacy of steroids has been controversial. Prolonged steroid use is not advised because signs of underlying infection may be missed. Ophthalmologic consultation should be obtained if eye involvement is suspected to prevent synechiae development or scarring. Topical dressings may help lesions to heal. In severe cases, patients should be treated in a burn unit, and electrolyte and fluid balance must be closely monitored.

HERPETIC GINGIVOSTOMATITIS

Definition and etiology: Acute herpetic gingivostomatitis is a primary herpes simplex virus infection of the oral mucosa most commonly seen in children and young adults. It occurs in only a small number of patients with first-time exposure to herpes simplex.

Clinical features: The eruption starts 2 to 10 days after exposure to herpes simplex virus. Many patients are unaware of their source of exposure. Patients develop fever, malaise, and painful erosive stomatitis and pharyngitis. Lesions frequently start in the interdental gingival papillae and spread to involve the entire mucosal surface. The lesions start out as red macules that rapidly become vesiculated and develop into widespread erosions. Intact blisters are rarely found because moisture and maceration in the mouth cause vesicles to rupture. On closer inspection, the erosions are grouped and have scalloped borders characteristic of a herpesvirus infection. The lesions heal spontaneously within a few weeks. The major disease in the differential diagnosis is aphthous stomatitis, which usually is recurrent, unlike herpes gingivostomatitis. Other common blistering diseases in the differential diagnosis are discussed in the section on aphthous stomatitis. A Tzanck preparation or biopsy can help confirm the diagnosis by revealing multinucleated giant cells. A culture or immunofluorescent tests for herpes can also quickly confirm the diagnosis.

Treatment: Oral acyclovir, valacyclovir, or famciclovir, if started during the first 2 days of the infection, can limit the severity and duration of disease. Viscous lidocaine can be used for pain and discomfort.

LEUKOPLAKIA

Definition and etiology: Leukoplakia is a descriptive term, not a disease entity. Leukoplakia is defined as a persistent white patch of the oral mucosa that can be either idiopathic or produced by external irritants. The most common etiologic factor is tobacco smoking or use of chewing tobacco.

Clinical features: The clinical features depend on both the severity of disease and its duration. The lesions start out as small white patches resembling candle wax and with time can become thick, leathery plaques. The lesions usually are sharply demarcated and involve the buccal mucosa. Other sites of involvement include the alveolar ridge, tongue, lips, gingiva, and palate. Squamous cell carcinoma can develop in foci of leukoplakia. Lesions of leukoplakia that are evolving into squamous cell carcinomas frequently have a red color and are called erythroplakia.

The differential diagnosis includes other white patches and plaques of the oral mucosa, such as lichen planus and candidiasis. Areas of leukoplakia can frequently become secondarily infected with candidiasis; however, unlike in candidiasis, the white plaques are adherent and do not scrape off. In lichen planus, the lesions usually have a reticulated appearance, and glabrous skin may be involved. Other rarer entities in the differential diagnosis include the mucous patch of syphilis, white sponge nevus,

leukoedema, cheek biting (morsicatio buccarum), and oral florid papillomatosis. A biopsy should be performed in all cases of suspected leukoplakia to confirm the diagnosis and to rule out underlying squamous cell carcinoma.

Treatment: In many cases, the lesions can resolve spontaneously if the stimulus (such as smoking) is removed. Good dental hygiene can also help. In persistent lesions, topical retinoids and surgery have been used.

LICHEN PLANUS

Definition and etiology: Lichen planus is an idiopathic inflammatory dermatitis that may involve both glabrous skin and mucosa. The cause of lichen planus is not known, but certain drugs such as methyldopa, β-blockers, thiazide diuretics, gold, penicillamine, and nonsteroidal anti-inflammatory agents can produce an oral eruption indistinguishable from classic idiopathic lichen planus. Lichen planus-like eruptions have also been related to use of gold in dental restorations. Associations between oral lichen planus and hepatitis C infection have been reported, and rare reports suggest that lichenoid lesions indistinguishable from lichen planus may be seen as a paraneoplastic phenomenon. These findings need to be confirmed.

Clinical features: Lichen planus most commonly occurs between the ages of 30 and 60 years and affects both sexes equally. The buccal mucosa is the most frequently involved intraoral site, but lichen planus can also involve the tongue, lips, palate, and gingiva. Approximately 15% to 25% of patients with oral lichen planus do not have skin lesions. Conversely, mucous membranes are affected in approximately half of patients with skin lesions.

If the characteristic white reticulated pattern is present, the diagnosis of oral lichen planus can be made clinically. In other cases, a biopsy is necessary to exclude entities such as candidiasis, contact stomatitis, leukoplakia, leukoedema, white sponge nevus, and oral florid papillomatosis. (See discussion of candidiasis.)

Treatment: Treatment of oral lichen planus is usually unsatisfactory. Any suspected causative drug should be eliminated. Drug-induced lichen planus may take a few months to subside after discontinuation of the offending drug. In rare cases, removal of gold or amalgam dental restorations may also be helpful, especially in patients proven by patch testing to be sensitive to mercuric compounds or gold. Irritants like tobacco and alcohol should be avoided. Topical steroid gels or pastes are applied to lesions 3 to 4 times daily. Other therapies include topical cyclosporine, topical or systemic retinoids, and oral griseofulvin.

PEMPHIGUS VULGARIS

Definition and etiology: Pemphigus vulgaris is an intraepidermal autoimmune blistering disease. Blisters can be found both in the oral cavity and on glabrous skin.

Clinical features: Pemphigus vulgaris is rare, occurring in approximately 1 of 100,000 persons. It can occur at any age but most commonly affects middle-aged adults. A genetic predisposition in people of Jewish heritage is present. Pemphigus affects both glabrous and mucosal skin but starts in the oral mucosa in approximately 50% to 70% of patients. The most common intraoral site of involvement is the buccal mucosa, but the palate, pharynx, larynx, and gingiva can also be involved. Physical examination reveals generalized ulcers and erosions that may be several centimeters in diameter and that can be extended with peripheral pressure (Nikolsky's sign). In cases with involvement of glabrous skin, intact blisters are less commonly found, since they easily rupture and leave superficial erosions.

The major disease in the differential diagnosis of oral pemphigus vulgaris is aphthous stomatitis. The ulcers and erosions in aphthous stomatitis are usually intermittent and of short duration (1 to 3 weeks), unlike those of pemphigus vulgaris, which are persistent. The lesions of pemphigus are usually symmetric; if asymmetric ulcers are found, malignancy or trauma should be suspected. Other rarer causes of generalized ulcers, such as medications (e.g., methotrexate, bismuth, chlorpromazine, phenytoin), nutritional deficiency, inflammatory bowel disease, infections (such as herpes), or deep fungi, should also be considered.

The differential diagnosis of pemphigus vulgaris includes other forms of pemphigus such as pemphigus foliaceus, pemphigus erythematosus, pemphigus vegetans, endemic pemphigus (fogo selvagem), and paraneoplastic pemphigus. In pemphigus foliaceus and pemphigus erythematosus, the blister is more superficial on biopsy specimens. The mucosal surface is rarely involved. Malar involvement resembling lupus erythematosus is seen in pemphigus erythematosus. Pemphigus vegetans is a variant of pemphigus vulgaris in which blisters occur predominantly in intertriginous folds. Lesions develop a vegetating appearance. Paraneoplastic pemphigus is a variant of pemphigus associated with internal malignancies, usually lymphomas, in which severe mucosal ulcerations occur along with an erythema multiforme-like skin eruption. Fogo selvagem is a form of pemphigus endemic to parts of Brazil and is thought to be secondary to an infectious agent yet to be identified.

Although the diagnosis of pemphigus vulgaris can be suspected on clinical grounds, it should always be confirmed with biopsy and immunofluorescent studies. Biopsy reveals a blister with intraepidermal acantholysis (disruption of the normal attachments between keratinocytes). Indirect immunofluorescent studies show circulating autoantibodies directed against epidermal adhesion molecules in approximately 90% of patients. Samples for direct immunofluores-cent studies should be taken from perilesional inflamed skin. Intercellular staining for IgG and C3 will occur in approximately 90% of biopsy specimens. Lesional skin or long-standing lesions have many secondary changes that obscure the characteristic immunofluorescent findings.

Treatment: The treatment of choice for pemphigus vulgaris is oral prednisone. Immunosuppressive agents such as azathioprine, cyclophosphamide, and methotrexate are frequently used as either primary agents or steroid-sparing agents. Other therapies include topical steroids, cyclosporine, dapsone, parenteral gold, and plasmapheresis.

Suggested Readings

APHTHOUS STOMATITIS
Balciunas BA, Kelly M, Siegel MA. Clinical management of common oral lesions. Cutis 1991;47:31–36.
Hutton KP, Rogers RS III. Recurrent aphthous stomatitis. Dermatol Clin 1987;5:761–68.

ORAL CANDIDIASIS
Fotos PG, Ray TL. Oral and perioral candidosis. Semin Dermatol 1994;13:118–24.
Janniger CK, Kihiczak TC. Childhood oral candidiasis (oral thrush). Cutis 1994;53:30–32.
Ray TL. Oral candidasis. Dermatol Clin 1987;5:651–73.

ERYTHEMA MULTIFORME
Huff JC, Weston WL, Tonnesen MG. Erythema multiforme: a critical review of characteristics, diagnostic criteria and causes. J Am Acad Dermatol 1983;8: 763–75.

HERPETIC GINGIVOSTOMATITIS
Rowe NH. Diagnosis and treatment of herpes simplex virus disease. Compendium-Suppl. 1988;9:S292–95.

LEUKOPLAKIA
Randle HW. White lesions of the mouth. Dermatol Clin 1987;5:641–50.
Wright JM. Oral precancerous lesions and conditions. Semin Dermatol 1994;13:125–31.

LICHEN PLANUS
Bricker SL. Oral lichen planus: a review. Semin Dermatol 1994;13:87–90.
Conklin RJ, Blasberg B. Oral lichen planus. Dermatol Clin 1987;5:663–73.

PEMPHIGUS VULGARIS
Helm KF, Peters MS. Immunodermatology update: the immunologically mediated vesiculobullous diseases. Mayo Clin Proc 1991;66:187–202.
Siegel MA, Balciunas BA, Kelly M, Serio FG. Diagnosis and management of commonly occurring oral vesiculo-erosive disorders. Cutis 1991;47:39–43.

4 *Hands/Feet*

ALGORITHM FOR INFLAMMATORY DISEASES OF THE HANDS/FEET

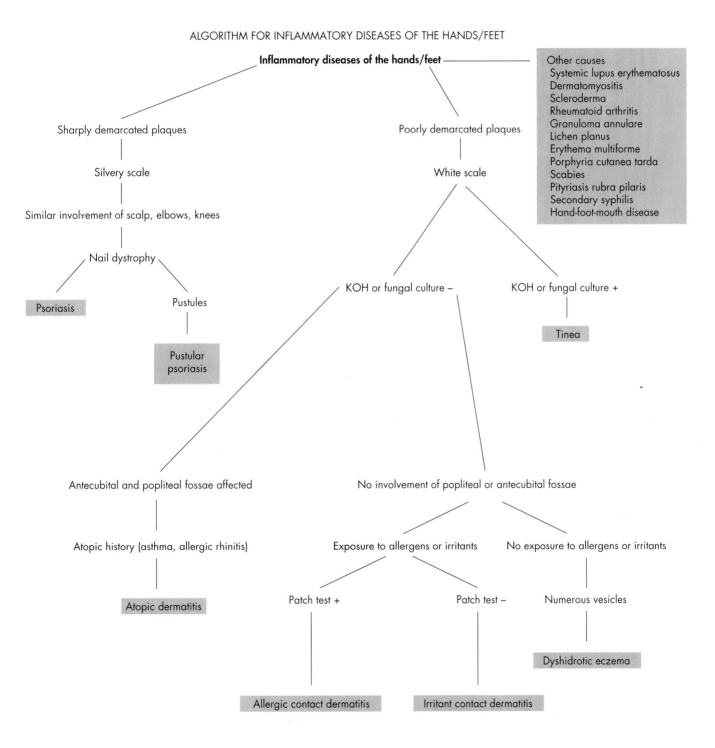

Inflammatory diseases of the hands/feet

Other causes
Systemic lupus erythematosus
Dermatomyositis
Scleroderma
Rheumatoid arthritis
Granuloma annulare
Lichen planus
Erythema multiforme
Porphyria cutanea tarda
Scabies
Pityriasis rubra pilaris
Secondary syphilis
Hand-foot-mouth disease

Sharply demarcated plaques

Poorly demarcated plaques

Silvery scale

White scale

Similar involvement of scalp, elbows, knees

Nail dystrophy

Psoriasis

Pustules

Pustular psoriasis

KOH or fungal culture –

KOH or fungal culture +

Tinea

Antecubital and popliteal fossae affected

No involvement of popliteal or antecubital fossae

Atopic history (asthma, allergic rhinitis)

Exposure to allergens or irritants

No exposure to allergens or irritants

Atopic dermatitis

Patch test +

Patch test –

Numerous vesicles

Dyshidrotic eczema

Allergic contact dermatitis

Irritant contact dermatitis

Introduction

Eruptions of the hands and feet are common and frequently are disabling. Inflamed fissured, blistered, and weeping hands or feet make the activities of daily life and work difficult, if not impossible. It is therefore very important to arrive at an accurate diagnosis on which treatment can be based. With the proper diagnosis and treatment, inflammatory diseases of the hand or foot usually markedly improved or clear completely.

The physical examination is often similar and nondistinguishing when examining the hands or feet alone. The complete skin examination sometimes reveals involvement elsewhere, which will secure the diagnosis. For example, psoriasis of the hands or feet may be associated with typical involvement of the elbows, knees, and scalp. Hand and foot eruptions almost always have associated scaling, and a potassium hydroxide (KOH) preparation or fungal culture should be accomplished to rule out a very treatable disease (e.g., tinea pedis or tinea manuum). For eczematous eruptions of the hands and feet, contact dermatitis, atopic dermatitis, and nonspecific or dyshidrotic eczema need to be considered. For any individual with a hand or foot eruption, one should ultimately ask the question, could this be contact dermatitis? Patch testing with appropriate allergens is the most important diagnostic test to rule out allergic contact dermatitis. For these individuals, removal or avoidance of the allergen or irritant is curative.

1. ALLERGIC CONTACT DERMATITIS
VERSUS
IRRITANT CONTACT DERMATITIS

Features in common: Inflamed patches and plaques.

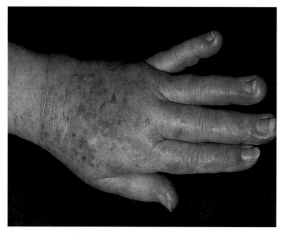

Figure 4.1.1 Allergic contact dermatitis due to a skin care product.

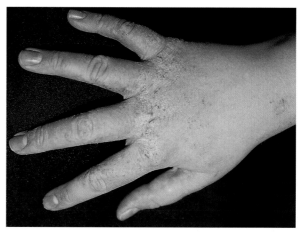

Figure 4.1.2 Irritant contact dermatitis due to detergents.

Distinguishing features

	ALLERGIC CONTACT DERMATITIS	IRRITANT CONTACT DERMATITIS
Physical examination Morphology	Intertriginous areas often uninvolved	Intertriginous areas often involved
History Symptoms	Burning not prominent Pruritus	Burning prominent Pruritus
Exacerbating factors	Exposure to allergen	Exposure to irritant
Associated findings	None	None
Epidemiology	25% of contact dermatitis	75% of contact dermatitis
Biopsy	No	No
Laboratory	Patch test positive	Patch test not done
Treatment	Remove allergen	Remove irritant
Outcome	Curable	Curable

Differential diagnosis of inflamed patches and plaques

Psoriasis

Tinea

Atopic dermatitis

Dyshidrotic eczema

Reiter's disease

Pityriasis rubra pilaris

Lichen planus

Mycosis fungoides

ID reaction

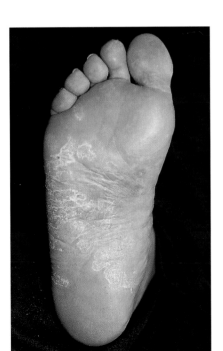

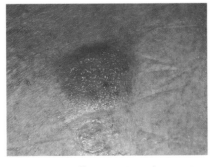

Figure 4.1.4 Allergic contact dermatitis. *Clue to diagnosis:* Positive patch test.

Figure 4.1.3 Allergic contact dermatitis due to insole of shoes. *Clue to diagnosis:* Involvement corresponds to area of contact.

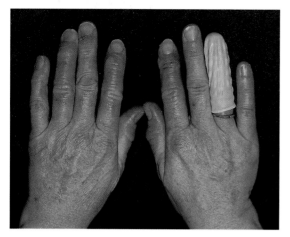

Figure 4.1.5 Allergic contact dermatitis due to finger cot.

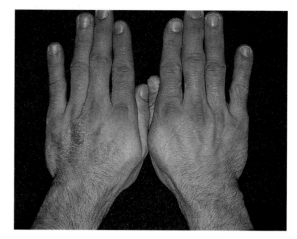

Figure 4.1.6 Irritant contact dermatitis due to glove worn on one hand.

2. DYSHIDROTIC
VERSUS
CONTACT DERMATITIS

Features in common: Inflamed patches and plaques.

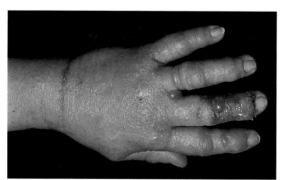

Figure 4.2.1 Dyshidrotic eczema.

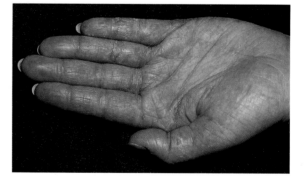

Figure 4.2.2 Allergic contact dermatitis due to permanent hair dye.

Distinguishing features

	DYSHIDROTIC ECZEMA	CONTACT DERMATITIS
Physical examination		
Morphology	Prominent vesicles and bullae Hyperhidrosis frequently present	Less prominent vesicles and bullae No hyperhidrosis
Distribution	Dorsum of hands and feet uninvolved Sides of digits involved	Dorsum of hands and feet involved Sides of digits spared

Continues

Distinguishing features (*Continued*)

	DYSHIDROTIC ECZEMA	CONTACT DERMATITIS
History		
Symptoms	Marked pruritus and burning	Moderate pruritus and burning
Exacerbating factors	Stress	No stress
Associated findings	None	None
Epidemiology	Adults Not occupational	Children and adults 40% is occupational illness
Biopsy	No	No
Laboratory	None	Patch test
Treatment	Steroids	Remove allergen or irritant
Outcome	Chronic with acute flare-ups	Clears

Causes of contact dermatitis of the hands/feet

Allergic

    Medicaments: benzocaine, neomycin, bacitracin

    Preservatives: barrier and moisturizing creams,
      work materials (e.g., metalworking fluids)

    Rubber compounds: gloves, shoes

    Epoxy resins: paints, glues

    Metals: tools, cement

    Fragrances: skin care products

Irritant

    Soaps and detergents

    Solvents

    Acids

    Alkalies

    Wet work

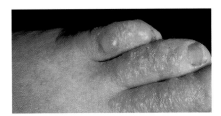

Figure 4.2.3 Dyshidrotic eczema. *Clue to diagnosis:* Numerous vesicles and bullae on digits.

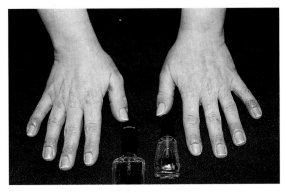

Figure 4.2.4 Allergic contact dermatitis. *Clue to diagnosis:* Involvement where there is contact with nail polish.

3. PSORIASIS
VERSUS
ATOPIC DERMATITIS

Features in common: Scaling patches and plaques.

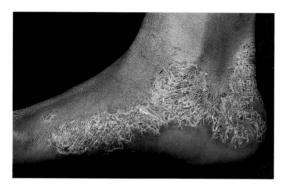

Figure 4.3.1 Psoriasis.

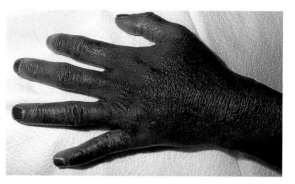

Figure 4.3.2 Atopic dermatitis.

Distinguishing features

		PSORIASIS	ATOPIC DERMATITIS
Physical examination			
	Morphology	Well demarcated	Ill marginated
		Silvery scaling	White scaling
		No lichenification	Lichenification
		Pustules	No pustules
	Distribution	Scalp, elbows, knees, nails	Antecubital and popliteal fossae
History			
	Symptoms	Mild to moderate pruritus	Marked pruritus
		Sunlight improves	Sunlight not helpful
	Exacerbating factors	Skin trauma	Not skin trauma
		Strep throat	Not strep throat
		Not heat or sweating	Sweating, heat
		Not clothes	Clothes, particularly wool
Associated findings		Arthritis	No arthritis
		No allergic respiratory disease	Allergic respiratory disease: asthma and rhinitis
		No secondary infection	Frequent secondary infection with *Staphylococcus aureus*
Epidemiology		Predominantly adults	Predominantly children
Biopsy		No	No
Laboratory		None	None
Treatment		Steroids, tar, and so forth	Steroids, antihistamines
Outcome		Chronic	Chronic
		No remission	Most children "outgrow" their eczema

Differential diagnosis of scaling patches

Contact dermatitis
Tinea
Dyshidrotic eczema
Mycosis fungoides
Lupus erythematosus
Lichen planus

Differential diagnosis of pustular hand dermatoses

Psoriasis
Acrodermatitis
Infected dermatitis
Tinea
Reiter's disease
Drug eruption

Major criteria for diagnosis of atopic dermatitis

1. Pruritus
2. Morphology and distribution:
   Infants: excoriated juicy papules and patches on extensor extremities and face
   Infants, children, adults: excoriated, lichenified patches and plaques on flexor extremities (antecubital and popliteal fossae) and face
3. Chronic relapsing course
4. Atopic disease (asthma, hay fever, eczema) in family or self

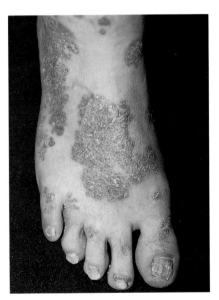

Figure 4.3.3 Psoriasis. *Clue to diagnosis:* Well-demarcated plaques; note nail dystrophy.

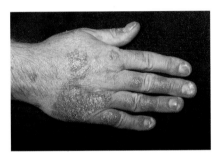

Figure 4.3.4 Psoriasis. *Clue to diagnosis:* Well-demarcated plaques; note nail dystrophy.

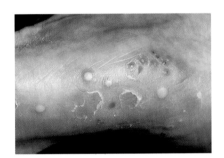

Figure 4.3.5 Pustular psoriasis.

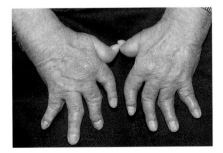

Figure 4.3.6 Psoriatic arthritis.

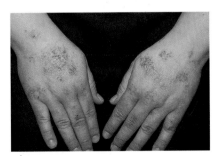

Figure 4.3.7 Atopic dermatitis. *Clue to diagnosis:* Ill-marginated patches and plaques.

4. TINEA
VERSUS
CONTACT DERMATITIS

Features in common: Scaling patches and plaques.

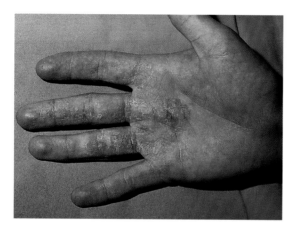

Figure 4.4.1 Tinea.

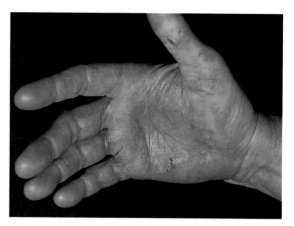

Figure 4.4.2 Contact dermatitis.

Distinguishing features

	TINEA	CONTACT DERMATITIS
Physical examination Morphology	Feet: interdigital maceration, diffuse plantar scaling, vesiculopustular eruptions One hand affected Nails dystrophic, thick	Feet: no maceration, lichenified plaques, no pustules Two hands affected Nails not affected
Distribution	Usually both feet; when hand involvement, one hand and two feet	Dermatitis where contact with allergen or irritant
History Symptoms	Asymptomatic or pruritus	Moderate pruritus and burning
Exacerbating factors	No allergen or irritant	Allergen or irritant
Associated findings	Tinea elsewhere, especially nails No dermatitis	No tinea Dermatitis elsewhere
Epidemiology	Not occupational	40% is occupational illness
Biopsy	No	No
Laboratory	Potassium hydroxide test or culture	Patch test
Treatment	Antifungals	Remove allergen or irritant
Outcome	Clears	Clears

Differential diagnosis of scaling patches of the hands and feet

Psoriasis   Cellulitis
Atopic dermatitis   Xerosis
Dyshidrotic eczema

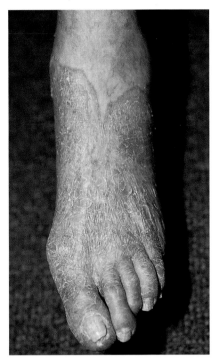

Figure 4.4.3 Tinea pedis. *Clue to diagnosis:* Annular plaque and onychomycosis.

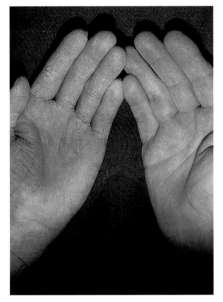

Figure 4.4.4 Tinea manuum. *Clue to diagnosis:* Only one hand infected.

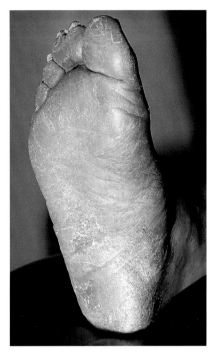

Figure 4.4.5 Tinea pedis. *Clue to diagnosis:* Diffuse plantar scaling in "moccasin" distribution.

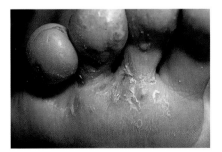

Figure 4.4.6 Tinea pedis with interdigital involvement.

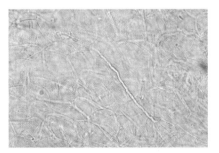

Figure 4.4.7 Tinea pedis and manuum. *Clue to diagnosis:* Positive potassium hydroxide test result.

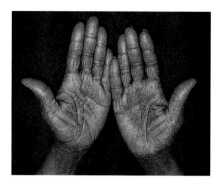

Figure 4.4.8 Contact dermatitis. *Clue to diagnosis:* Involvement where there is contact with hand cream.

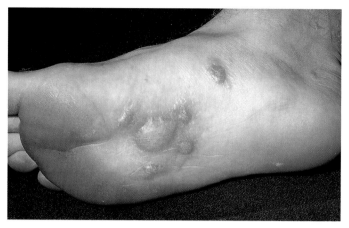

Figure 4.4.9 Contact dermatitis. *Clue to diagnosis:* Involvement with contact with poison ivy.

Discussion

ATOPIC DERMATITIS

Definition and etiology: Atopic dermatitis is a chronic, markedly pruritic, eczematous eruption of unknown cause. It is usually associated with a personal or family history of atopy (e.g., asthma, allergic rhinoconjunctivitis, or atopic dermatitis).

Clinical features: Atopic dermatitis is predominantly a childhood disease, with 5% to 10% of children affected. It usually manifests before 5 years of age. For adults, hand dermatitis may be the most common presentation of atopic dermatitis. It is, however, unusual for adults to develop atopic dermatitis without a history of childhood eczema. Allergic respiratory disease is found in the majority of patients or in their family members. Characteristically, pruritus is the most prominent and distressing symptom in patients with atopic dermatitis. For many, pruritus precedes the eruption and is so severe that it disrupts sleep and other activities of daily life. Atopic dermatitis is a chronic disease punctuated by acute and severe flare-ups.

The examination reveals ill-marginated, lichenified, erythematous scaling patches and plaques that affect the dorsum and the palmar surface of the hands and feet. This may be the only manifestation of atopic dermatitis in adults. Usually, however, there are eczematous patches and plaques scattered elsewhere, particularly affecting the antecubital and popliteal fossae. Generalized dry skin is often found.

The differential diagnosis of atopic hand-and-foot dermatitis includes any eczematous-appearing eruption. This includes contact dermatitis, dyshidrotic eczema, psoriasis, superficial fungal infection, scabies, and rare disorders such as pityriasis rubra pilarias. A skin biopsy is usually not necessary to differentiate among these conditions (with the exception of pityriasis rubra pilaris). If done, the skin biopsy reveals the characteristics of any eczematous eruption. Acute and subacute dermatitis shows epidermal spongiosis and chronic dermatitis hyperkeratosis with acanthosis of the epidermis.

Treatment: Since atopic hand-and-foot dermatitis is a chronic condition, the goal of treatment should be symptomatic relief of itching and control of inflammation. This is accomplished with antihistamines, potent topical steroids, topical psoralens and ultraviolet A light (PUVA), and short bursts of systemic steroids. Compresses or soaks with tar or oatmeal emulsions are soothing and help with oozing, if present. For secondarily infected atopic dermatitis, a 1- to 2-week course of oral antibiotics is indicated. Most important, protection of the hands and avoidance of irritants are necessary to ameliorate the inflammatory process. For those whose occupation requires exposure to irritating chemicals, wearing gloves may be helpful. However, a change in jobs may be necessary. The frequent use of moisturizers for dry and lichenified dermatitis of the hands and feet is also quite helpful.

CONTACT DERMATITIS

Definition and etiology: Contact dermatitis is an inflammatory reaction to an exogenous chemical, irritant, or allergen that comes in contact with the skin. Irritant contact dermatitis is precipitated by a substance that has direct toxic properties, whereas allergic contact dermatitis is triggered by a delayed-type hypersensitivity reaction. Irritating chemicals include acids, alkalies, solvents, and detergents. There are numerous allergens, including plants (poison ivy and oak), metals (nickel), rubber chemicals, cosmetic ingredients (fragrances, preservatives), and topical medicines (neomycin and bacitracin).

Clinical features: Contact dermatitis of the hands is responsible for the great majority of occupational skin diseases. More commonly, the cause is irritant contact dermatitis due to cumulative exposure to wet work, solvents, and detergents, as seen in hairdressers, housewives, nurses, and machinists. These weaker irritants require multiple applications over a period of days before the irritant contact dermatitis appears. For strong irritants, symptoms develop within minutes to hours, and the diagnosis is readily apparent. For allergens, because of the delayed-type hypersensitivity reaction, onset occurs after one day to several days. This makes identification of the allergen more difficult, and it often goes unrecognized. This is particularly true in the case of daily contact with allergens such as rubber chemicals found in gloves or shoes, skin care products, and medicines applied to the hands and feet.

Contact dermatitis varies from acute to chronic, which results in varying appearances. Acute contact dermatitis has marked epidermal edema, or spongiosis, which causes papules, vesicles, bullae, and secondary changes such as oozing and crusting. The hallmark of chronic contact dermatitis is lichenification or thickening of the epidermis associated with scaling and fissuring. The distribution of the dermatitis corresponds with the areas of contact. Streaks, geometric outlines, and sharp margins typically occur, particularly elsewhere on the body (e.g., where there has been application of the contactant or brushing of the leaf or stem of posion ivy or oak). For gloves, both the palmar and the dorsal surface may be involved. Since the stratum corneum is much thinner on the dorsum of the hands and allows penetration of the allergen more easily, however, the dorsum is more commonly affected. For the feet, the distribution depends on what portion of the shoe is causing the contact dermatitis. For example, the insole of the shoe causes diffuse dermatitis on the soles of the feet.

On physical examination, contact dermatitis of the hands and feet can be acute, subacute, or chronic, depending on the strength of the contactant and the nature of exposure. Strong irritants and allergens cause acute contact dermatitis, manifested by a vesicular bullous eruption. Weaker irritants and allergens to which there has been repeated exposure cause chronic lichenified contact dermatitis. Contact dermatitis elsewhere may occur owing to transmission of the irritant or allergen via the hands by touching other areas of the body, such as the face.

Since the morphology of different dermatitic eruptions is identical, dyshidrotic (nonspecific) eczema and atopic dermatitis should be considered. Other eczematous-appearing dermatoses that should be ruled out include superficial fungal infection, psoriasis, and cellulitis. The diagnosis of irritant contact dermatitis is one of exclusion. There is no standard testing for irritation. For allergic contact dermatitis, the allergen can be identified by patch testing.

Treatment: The management of contact dermatitis should emphasize prevention by complete avoidance of the offending irritants or allergens. This may require a change in occupation or lifestyle. Protective clothing such as gloves may be helpful. Substitution of less toxic materials may be accomplished. The principal treatment is topical steroids of medium to potent strength applied twice a day. For those individuals with severe or widespread contact dermatitis, a short course of systemic steroids is indicated. General majors such as astringent soaks or compresses, applied 15 minutes twice a day are used to reduce weeping. Colloidal oatmeal or tar emulsion baths or compresses reduce inflammation and itching. Antihistamines such as diphenhydramine, 25 to 50 mg four times a days or hydroxyzine, 10 to 25 mg four times a day, may be taken as necessary for itching.

DYSHIDROTIC ECZEMA

Definition and etiology: Dyshidrotic eczema, also known as pompholyx, is characteristically a vesicular eruption of the hands and feet of unknown cause.

Clinical features: The characteristic appearance of dyshidrotic eczema is deep-seated vesicles that resemble the pearls in tapioca pudding and involve the palms, soles, and sides of the digits. The vesicles usually occur bilaterally and symmetrically. Vesicles may coalesce, forming bullae or, when slow in resolving, may be replaced by the chronic eczematous changes of erythema, scaling, and lichenification. This disease often has a waxing and waning course with sudden flare-ups of vesicles characterized by marked pruritus and burning. Patients often have associated hyperhidrosis.

The differential diagnosis includes other eczematous eruptions such as contact and atopic dermatitis, psoriasis, tinea, mycosis fungoides, lupus erythematosus, and lichen planus. Although a biopsy is usually not necessary, results reveal spongiosis typical of dermatitis.

Treatment: Treatment of dyshidrotic eczema is similar to that of other eczematous eruptions, with steroids being the mainstay. For symptomatic relief, soaks or compresses with astringents as well as oral antihistamines are helpful.

PSORIASIS

Definition and etiology: Psoriasis is an inflammatory disease characterized by increased epidermal proliferation. The cause of psoriasis is unknown, but abnormal epidermal kinetics as well as the activation of the immune system within the skin must be taken into account.

Clinical features: Approximately one-third of patients have a family history positive for psoriasis. This is a relatively common skin disease affecting about 2% of the population in the United States. The most common age of onset is in the third decade, but it can present at any time. The major precipitating or aggravating factors include streptococcal pharyngitis, trauma to the skin, emotional stress, use of drugs such as β-blocking agents and lithium, and human immunodeficiency virus infection.

The examination of the hands and feet reveals sharply demarcated, erythematous, silvery, scaling plaques. Pustules within these plaques are found in pustular psoriasis. Dystrophic nail changes (pits, onycholysis, brown discoloration, and thickened nail plate) often occur. Typical involvement elsewhere includes the extensor surfaces of the elbows and knees and the scalp.

The differential diagnosis of hand-and-foot psoriasis includes contact dermatitis, tinea, dyshidrotic eczema, atopic dermatitis, mycosis fungoides, lupus erythematosus, and lichen planus. Usually, a skin biopsy is not necessary, but if one is done, findings reveal characteristic hyperkeratosis, parakeratosis, acanthotic epidermis, inflammatory infiltrate in the dermis, and neutrophils migrating into the epidermis, forming microabscesses.

Treatment: Treatment modalities include topical preparations containing steroids, tars, anthralin, and calcipotriol. When the disease is severe, PUVA, methotrexate, etretinate, and cyclosporine are used.

TINEA MANUUM AND PEDIS

Definition and etiology: Tinea manuum and tinea pedis are superficial fungal infections of the hands and feet, respectively, caused by dermatophytes, usually *Trichophyton rubrum*, *Trichophyton mentagrophytes*, or *Epidermophyton floccosum*.

Clinical features: Tinea manuum is relatively uncommon, whereas tinea pedis affects approximately 4% of the general population. Spread of tinea pedis occurs easily in settings such as locker rooms, where high spore counts and bare feet are found. Hot, humid climates; sweating; and occlusive shoes encourage fungal infections.

Tinea manuum typically affects one hand and is associated with bilateral tinea pedis in what is called "one hand, two feet" syndrome. The reason for involvement of only one hand is unknown. The palmar surface is usually affected by mild, diffuse, white scaling. Tinea pedis can appear as interdigital maceration, diffuse plantar scaling, or a vesiculopustular eruption. Often, onychomycosis is associated with tinea manuum and pedis.

The differential diagnosis of tinea manuum and pedis includes atopic and dyshidrotic eczema, psoriasis, xerosis, and occasionally cellulitis. Although usually an infection of adults, tinea should be considered in the differential diagnosis of children with an eczematous eruption of the feet. A KOH preparation or fungal culture confirms the diagnosis.

Treatment: Topical therapy for tinea manuum and pedis is usually effective in controlling or clearing the eruption. When the disease is associated with onychomycosis, oral antifungal agents are required to clear the nails. The most effective agent is probably terbinafine (Lamisil), but also very effective are the azoles, such as ketoconazole (Nizoral). Measures to reduce recurrence of tinea pedis include using topical antiperspirants to reduce sweating, wearing nonocclusive shoes, changing socks frequently, and not going barefoot in public areas such as locker rooms.

Suggested Readings

ATOPIC DERMATITIS
Cooper KD. Atopic dermatitis: recent trends in pathogenesis and therapy. J Invest Dermatol 1994;102:128–37.

Halbert AR, Weston WL, Morelli JG. Atopic dermatitis: is it an allergic disease? J Am Acad Dermatol 1995;33: 1008–18.

Leung DYM. Atopic dermatitis: the skin as a window into the pathogenesis of chronic allergic diseases. J Allergy Clin Immunol 1995;96:302–18.

CONTACT DERMATITIS
Drake LA, Dorner W, Goltz RW et al. Guidelines of care for contact dermatitis. J Am Acad Dermatol 1995;32: 109–13.

Marks JG, DeLeo VA. Contact and Occupational Dermatology. 2nd Ed. Mosby-Year Book, St. Louis, 1997.

Marks JG, Martini MC. Contact dermatitis and contact urticaria. In Sams WM, Lynch PJ (eds): Principles and Practice of Dermatology. 2nd Ed. pp. 419–30. Churchill Livingstone, New York, 1996.

DYSHIDROTIC ECZEMA
Kutzner H, Wurzel RM, Wolff HH. Are acrosyringia involved in the pathogenesis of "dyshidrosis"? Am J Dermatopathol 1986;8:109–16.

Yokozeki H, Katayama I, Nishioka K et al. The role of metal allergy and local hyperhidrosis in the pathogenesis of pompholyx. J Dermatol 1992;19:964–67.

PSORIASIS
Cram DL. Psoriasis: current advances in etiology and treatment. J Am Acad Dermatol 1981;4:1–14.

Drake LA, Ceilley RI, Cornelison RL et al. Guidelines of care for psoriasis. J Am Acad Dermatol 1993;28:632–37.

Griffiths CEM. Cutaneous leukocyte trafficking and psoriasis. Arch Dermatol 1994;130:494–99.

TINEA MANUUM AND PEDIS
Drake LA, Dinehart SM, Farmer ER et al. Guidelines of care for superficial mycotic infections of the skin: tinea corporis, tinea cruris, tinea faciei, tinea manuum, and tinea pedis. J Am Acad Dermatol 1996;34: 282–86.

Elewski BE, Weil ML. Dermatophytes and superficial fungi. In Sams MW, Lynch PJ (eds): Principles and Practice of Dermatology. 2nd Ed. pp. 149–58. Churchill Livingstone, New York, 1996.

5 *Nail Diseases*

ALGORITHM FOR NAIL DYSTROPHY

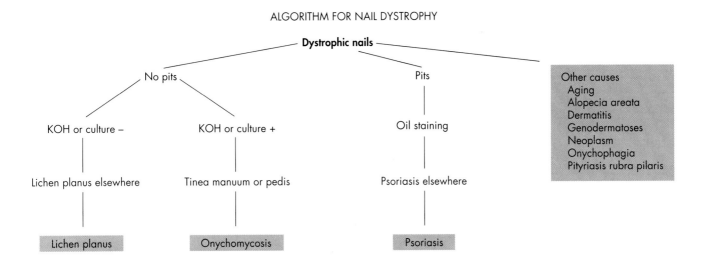

Dystrophic nails

No pits

KOH or culture −

Lichen planus elsewhere

Lichen planus

KOH or culture +

Tinea manuum or pedis

Onychomycosis

Pits

Oil staining

Psoriasis elsewhere

Psoriasis

Other causes
  Aging
  Alopecia areata
  Dermatitis
  Genodermatoses
  Neoplasm
  Onychophagia
  Pityriasis rubra pilaris

dystrophy. The dystrophic physical appearance of the nail cannot be used reliably to make a diagnosis. For the three diseases discussed in this chapter—onychomycosis, psoriasis, and lichen planus—other entities in the differential diagnosis include aging, trauma, and secondary changes due to dermatitis. A history, skin examination, and appropriate laboratory tests are required to arrive at a definite diagnosis. This is particularly important with respect to onychomycosis, since it is treatable with systemic antifungals.

Introduction

In addition to having significant cosmetic value, the nail protects the distal end of the fingers and toes from trauma and is used for fine grasping and scratching. The nail unit is not a static horny appendage but a dynamic growing structure consisting of matrix, bed, folds, hyponychium, and plate. These components of the nail unit are affected by a number of diseases, which ultimately can alter the appearance of the nail plate and cause nail

1. ONYCHOMYCOSIS
VERSUS
PSORIASIS

Features in common: Dystrophic nails.

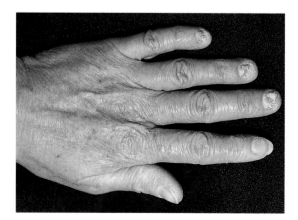

Figure 5.1.1 Onychomycosis.

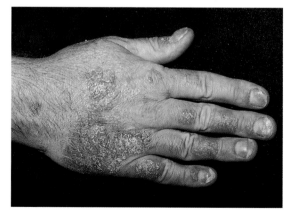

Figure 5.1.2 Psoriasis.

Distinguishing features

	ONYCHOMYCOSIS	PSORIASIS
Physical examination		
Morphology	No pits No oil spots	Pits Oil spots
Distribution	No elbow, knee involvement	Elbow, knee involved
History		
Symptoms	Asymptomatic or some discomfort	Asymptomatic or some discomfort
Exacerbating factors	Not stress Sweating	Stress Not sweating
Associated findings	Tinea manuum and pedis No arthritis	No tinea manuum or pedis Arthritis
Epidemiology	Common	Common
Biopsy	No	No
Laboratory	KOH or culture positive	KOH or culture negative
Treatment	Oral antifungals	None
Outcome	Cure	Chronic

Abbreviation: KOH, potassium hydroxide.

Differential diagnosis of dystrophic nails

Aging
Trauma
Dermatitis
Lichen planus

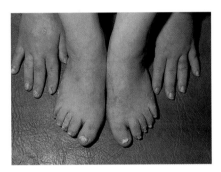

Figure 5.1.3 Onychomycosis. *Clue to diagnosis:* One hand, two foot involvement.

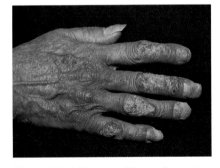

Figure 5.1.4 Psoriasis. *Clue to diagnosis:* Associated psoriasis of fingers.

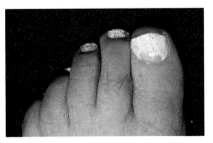

Figure 5.1.5 Onychomycosis with superficial white infection.

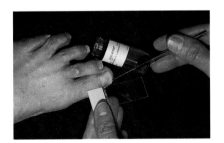

Figure 5.1.6 Onychomycosis. Confirm diagnosis with potassium hydroxide test and culture.

2. PSORIASIS
VERSUS
LICHEN PLANUS

Features in common: Dystrophic nails.

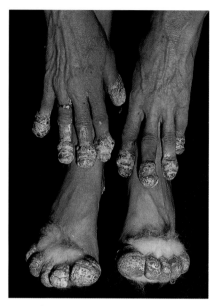

Figure 5.2.1 Psoriasis.

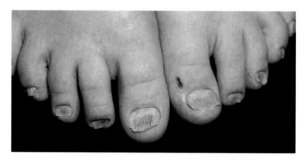

Figure 5.2.2 Lichen planus.

Distinguishing features

	PSORIASIS	LICHEN PLANUS
Physical examination		
Morphology	Pits	No pits
	No pterygium	Pterygium
Distribution	Elbows, knees involved	No elbow, knee involvement
	Mouth uninvolved	Mouth involved
History		
Symptoms	Asymptomatic or some discomfort	Asymptomatic or some discomfort
Exacerbating factors	Physical or emotional stress or illness	None
Associated findings	Arthritis	No arthritis
Epidemiology	Common	Uncommon
Biopsy	No	No
Laboratory	No	No
Treatment	None	None
Outcome	Chronic	Chronic

Differential diagnosis of dystrophic nails

Aging
Trauma
Dermatitis
Lichen planus

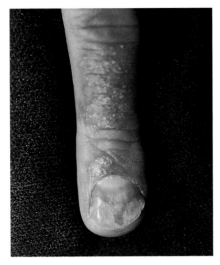

Figure 5.2.3 Psoriasis. *Clue to diagnosis:* Oil stain and nail fold involvement characteristic of psoriasis.

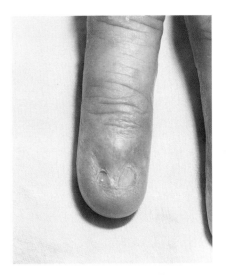

Figure 5.2.4 Lichen planus. *Clue to diagnosis:* Pterygium formation.

Discussion

LICHEN PLANUS

Definition and Etiology: Lichen planus is an idiopathic inflammatory process affecting the nails, hair, skin, and and mucous membranes.

Clinical features: Lichen planus is a relatively uncommon disorder, usually of adults. The skin is most commonly affected by pruritic papules, and the mucous membranes develop asymptomatic white patches or painful erosions. A minority of cases (approximately 10%) have nail involvement. Rarely, lichen planus involves only the nails without associated skin or mucous membrane findings.

The nail affected by lichen planus has a variety of appearances. Most commonly, the nail plate is thickened or thinned and is separated from the nail bed (onycholysis). Occasionally, scarring occurs with formation of a characteristic pterygium.

The differential diagnosis of lichen planus of the nails includes psoriasis, onychomycosis, aging, trauma, and dermatitis. Some entities in the differential diagnosis include genodermatoses, alopecia areata, onychophagia, and 20-nail dystrophy, which is a nail disorder primarily seen in children that is thought to be a variant of lichen planus only affecting the nails. Associated lichen planus found elsewhere, particularly on the wrists, ankles, and mucous membranes of the mouth, confirms the diagnosis. A negative potassium hydroxide (KOH) test result or fungal culture will rule out onychomycosis.

Treatment: There is no good treatment for lichen planus affecting the nails. Topical steroids are usually ineffective but may be tried.

ONYCHOMYCOSIS

Definition and etiology: Onychomycosis, also termed tinea unguium, is a superficial fungal infection of the nail caused by the dermatophytes *Trichophyton rubrum* and *Trichophyton mentagrophytes.*

Clinical features: Onychomycosis is almost always associated with tinea pedis or manuum. Infection of the toenails is more common than infection of the fingernails. It is uncommon for all 10 toenails to be involved at the same time or to the same degree. There are three patterns of nail involvement: proximal, distal, and white superficial.

The examination of an onychomycotic nail reveals white, yellow, or brown discoloration. In the distal type, which is the most common, the plate is usually thickened with distal subungual debris, and it may be crumbling. Occasionally, the dermatophyte infects only the top surface of the nail plate, causing a white, crumbling superficial onychomycosis. Rarely, the thickening and debris occur in the proximal nail plate. Usually, both feet are affected. On occasion, a typical presentation will be the so-called "one hand, two feet" syndrome, in which the nails of one hand and both feet are infected in association with tinea manuum and pedis.

The differential diagnosis of onychomycosis includes psoriasis, lichen planus, and other causes of dystrophic nails such as aging, trauma, and dermatitis. Onychomycosis cannot be diagnosed reliably by physical examination alone; a KOH test or a fungal culture *must* be done to confirm the diagnosis.

Treatment: Treatment must be with an oral antifungal. Itraconazole (Sporanox), fluconazole (Diflucan), or terbinafine (Lamisil) given continuously or pulsed for 6 weeks for fingernails and 12 weeks for toenails is usually effective. Preventative measures to reduce recurrence include applying topical agents to reduce sweating, wearing nonocclusive shoes, changing damp socks frequently, and not going barefoot in public areas such as locker rooms.

PSORIASIS

Definition and etiology: Psoriasis is an inflammatory disease characterized by increased epidermal proliferation. The cause of psoriasis is unknown, but abnormal epidermal kinetics as well as the activation of the immune system within the skin must be taken into account.

Clinical features: Approximately one-third of patients have a family history positive for psoriasis. This is a relatively common skin disease affecting about 2% of the population in the United States. The most common age of onset is in the third decade, but it can present at any time. The major precipitating or aggravating factors include streptococcal pharyngitis, trauma to the skin, emotional stress, and use of drugs such as β-blocking agents and lithium.

The examination of the psoriatic nail typically reveals pitting, yellow oil staining, thickening, and separation of the nail plate from the nail bed (onycholysis). All or just a few nails may be involved. It is uncommon for psoriasis to affect only the nails without associated cutaneous disease.

The differential diagnosis of psoriatic nails includes other causes of dystrophic nails such as onychomycosis, lichen planus, aging, and dystrophy secondary to eczema or another inflammatory process of the nail fold. Typical psoriatic involvement elsewhere, such as the extensor surface of the elbows and knees and the scalp, confirms the diagnosis. Biopsy of the nail is rarely done.

Treatment: Psoriasis of the nail is chronic, with a waxing and waning course. Treatment is difficult and rarely effective. Systemic medications used to control psoriasis elsewhere often help the nail involvement. However, nail involvement alone does not warrant use of these potentially toxic drugs.

Suggested Readings

André J, Achten G. Onychomycosis. Int J Dermatol 1987; 26:481–90.

Daniel CR. The diagnosis of nail fungal infection. Arch Dermatol 1991;127:1566–67.

Drake LA, Dinehart SM, Farmer ER et al. Guidelines of care for nail disorders. J Am Acad Dermatol 1996; 34:529–33.

Scher RK, Daniel CR. Nails: Therapy, Diagnosis, Surgery. WB Saunders, Philadelphia, 1990.

Zaias N. The Nail in Health and Disease. Norwalk, CT, Appleton & Lange, 1980.

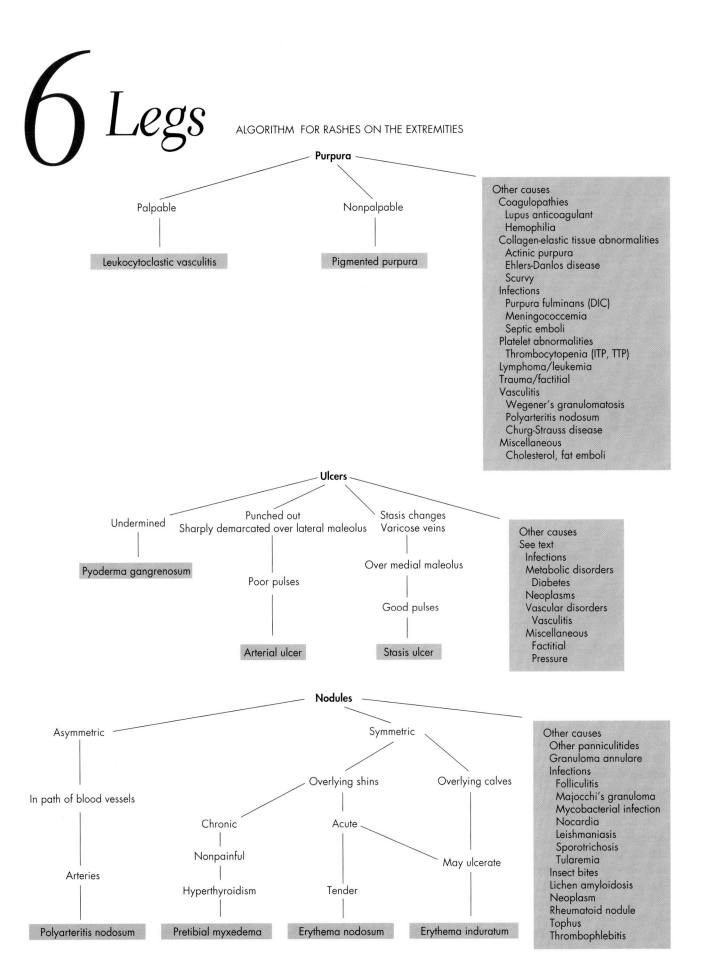

6 Legs

ALGORITHM FOR RASHES ON THE EXTREMITIES

Purpura

Palpable

Leukocytoclastic vasculitis

Nonpalpable

Pigmented purpura

Other causes
 Coagulopathies
  Lupus anticoagulant
  Hemophilia
 Collagen-elastic tissue abnormalities
  Actinic purpura
  Ehlers-Danlos disease
  Scurvy
 Infections
  Purpura fulminans (DIC)
  Meningococcemia
  Septic emboli
 Platelet abnormalities
  Thrombocytopenia (ITP, TTP)
 Lymphoma/leukemia
 Trauma/factitial
 Vasculitis
  Wegener's granulomatosis
  Polyarteritis nodosum
  Churg-Strauss disease
 Miscellaneous
  Cholesterol, fat emboli

Ulcers

Undermined

Pyoderma gangrenosum

Punched out
Sharply demarcated over lateral maleolus

Poor pulses

Arterial ulcer

Stasis changes
Varicose veins

Over medial maleolus

Good pulses

Stasis ulcer

Other causes
See text
 Infections
 Metabolic disorders
  Diabetes
 Neoplasms
 Vascular disorders
  Vasculitis
 Miscellaneous
  Factitial
  Pressure

Nodules

Asymmetric

In path of blood vessels

Arteries

Polyarteritis nodosum

Symmetric

Overlying shins

Chronic

Nonpainful

Hyperthyroidism

Pretibial myxedema

Acute

Tender

Erythema nodosum

Overlying calves

May ulcerate

Erythema induratum

Other causes
 Other panniculitides
 Granuloma annulare
 Infections
  Folliculitis
  Majocchi's granuloma
  Mycobacterial infection
  Nocardia
  Leishmaniasis
  Sporotrichosis
  Tularemia
 Insect bites
 Lichen amyloidosis
 Neoplasm
 Rheumatoid nodule
 Tophus
 Thrombophlebitis

Introduction

Circulatory diseases most often present on the legs. Gravity, distance from the heart, increased venous pressure, and the lower temperature of the limbs compared with core body temperature all compromise the function of blood vessels in the legs and predispose them to the development of lesions. Gravity and increased venous pressure affect the venous circulation and lead to venous insufficiency. Over time, valves become incompetent, and varicosities develop. Eventually, venous incompetence results in extravasation of blood into the skin, producing stasis dermatitis, fibrosis, and ulceration. Emboli may lodge in arteries because they end in capillary beds without adequate collateral circulation. Venous insufficiency and resultant stasis dermatitis need to be differentiated from arterial disease or pyoderma gangrenosum because the treatments for these disorders are different. In patients with vasculitis, circulating immune complexes lodge in small vessels in dependent sites, producing palpable purpura. Nonpalpable purpura due to capillaritis (i.e., pigmented purpura) is also most commonly found on the legs. Panniculitis frequently presents on the shins and calves. Other rashes with a predilection for the shins include necrobiosis lipoidica diabeticorum and pretibial myxedema. Each of these disorders shares an affinity for the legs and is associated with certain clues that allow for accurate differentiation among them. This chapter outlines helpful clues in their differential diagnosis.

1. ERYTHEMA NODOSUM
VERSUS
ERYTHEMA INDURATUM

Features in common: Red nodules and plaques on lower extremities.

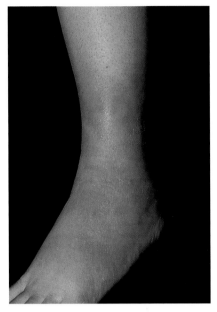

Figure 6.1.1 Erythema nodosum.

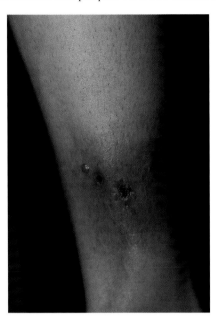

Figure 6.1.2 Erythema induratum.

Distinguishing features

	ERYTHEMA NODOSUM	ERYTHEMA INDURATUM
Physical examination		
Morphology	*Lesions do not ulcerate*	*Lesions frequently ulcerate*
		Ulcers have ragged violaceous margin
	Resolving lesions: purpuric bruiselike nodules	No purpuric lesions
Distribution	Pretibial area, rarely elsewhere	Predilection for calves
		Occasionally shins and thighs
History		
Symptoms	Pain	Pain
Exacerbating factors	Prolonged standing, limb dependencies	None
Associated findings	Medications: oral contraceptives	No medications
	Infections: streptococcal infections, deep fungal infections, *Yersinia*, *Campylobacter*	Infections: tuberculosis
	Immunologic diseases: sarcoidosis, Behçet's disease	No immunologic disease
	Inflammatory bowel disease	No bowel disease

Continues

Distinguishing features (Continued)

	ERYTHEMA NODOSUM	ERYTHEMA INDURATUM
Epidemiology	More common in females Common	More common in females Rare

Biopsy	Occasionally
	Septal panniculitis with mixed
	    inflammatory infiltrate
		Yes
		Lobular panniculitis with histiocytes
		    and caseation necrosis, vasculitis
		    of medium-sized venules and
		    occasionally arteries

Laboratory	Anti-streptolysin O titer, chest x-ray	Purified protein derivative, chest x-ray

Treatment	Rest, nonsteroidal anti-inflammatory
	    drugs, dapsone, oral corticosteroids
	Treat underlying disease
		Occasionally resolves with
		    antituberculous therapy
		Oral corticosteroids

Outcome	Self-limited, resolves over several weeks	Chronic

Differential diagnosis of leg nodules

Common causes
    Erythema nodosum
    Furunculosis
    Thrombophlebitis
    Insect bites
    Infections: Majocchi's granuloma

Rarer causes
    Granuloma annulare
    Gouty tophus
    Infections: leishmaniasis, myco-
        bacterial infection, *Nocardia*,
        parasitic infection, sporotrichosis,
        tularemia
    Rheumatoid nodule
    Erythema induratum

Rarer causes (*continued*)
    Polyarteritis nodosa
    Malignant neoplasms: lymphoma,
        metastases
    Benign neoplasms: lipoma,
        adnexal tumors
    Lichen amyloidosis
    Lupus profundus

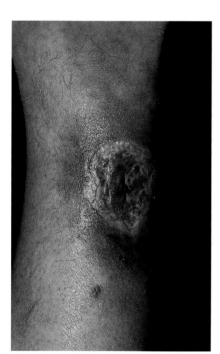

Figure 6.1.3 Erythema induratum. *Clue to diagnosis*: Location over the calves and ulceration.

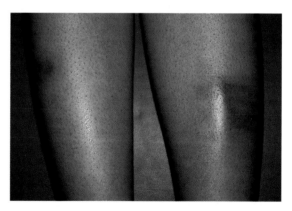

Figure 6.1.4 Erythema nodosum. *Clue to diagnosis*: A lesion with a bruiselike appearance (erythema contusiformis).

2. LEUKOCYTOCLASTIC VASCULITIS
VERSUS
PIGMENTED PURPURA

Features in common: Purpura on lower legs.

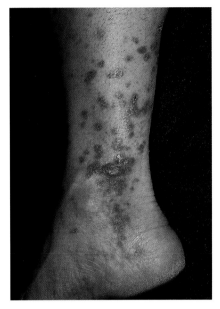

Figure 6.2.1 Leukocytoclastic vasculitis.

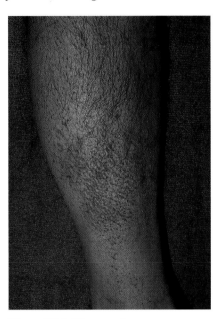

Figure 6.2.2 Pigmented purpura.

Distinguishing features

	LEUKOCYTOCLASTIC VASCULITIS	PIGMENTED PURPURA
Physical examination		
Morphology	Urticarial lesions	No urticarial lesions
	Lesions palpable	Lesions not palpable
	No cayenne-pepper-like macules	Orange-brown cayenne-pepper-like macules
Distribution	Occasionally ulcers and vesicles	No ulcers or vesicles
	Lower legs and dependent areas	Lower legs
History		
Symptoms	Fever, malaise, pain, burning, itching	Asymptomatic or mild itching
Exacerbating or causative factors	Drugs	Occasionally drugs
	Infections	
	Collagen vascular diseases	
	Malignancies	
	Miscellaneous: paraproteinemia, cryoglobulinemia	
Associated findings	Occasionally extracutaneous vasculitis: kidney, central nervous system, gastrointestinal tract, lung, joints, heart	No systemic vasculitis

Continues

Distinguishing features (Continued)

	LEUKOCYTOCLASTIC VASCULITIS	PIGMENTED PURPURA
Epidemiology	Uncommon No sex predominance	Uncommon Slight male predominance
Biopsy	Yes Fibrinoid necrosis of blood vessels, neutrophilic infiltrate, leukocytoclasis, endothelial swelling, extravasated erythrocytes	No Superficial lymphochytic infiltrate, extravasated erythrocytes, hemosiderin
Laboratory	Anti-streptolysin O titer, erythrocyte sedimentation rate, complete blood count with differential, cryoglobulins, serum protein electrophoresis, antinuclear antibody, hepatitis screen in suggestive clinical history, chest x-ray	None
Treatment	Treating underlying disease Oral steroids, dapsone, colchicine, and nonsteroidal anti-inflammatory agents, potassium iodine	Topical steroids
Outcome	Acute or chronic depending on associated disease or cause	Chronic

Differential diagnosis of purpura

Connective tissue abnormality
  Actinic purpura
  Scurvy
  Ehlers-Danlos syndrome
Vascular abnormality
Vasculitis—usually palpable
  Henoch-Schönlein purpura
  Leukocytoclastic (allergic) disease
  Finkelstein's disease
  Wegener's granulomatosis
  Polyarteritis nodosa
  Thrombophlebitis
Pigmented purpura

Hematologic abnormality
  Thrombocytopenia
  Idiopathic thrombocytopenic purpura
  Thrombotic thrombocytopenia
  Coagulopathies (hemophilia)
  Purpura fulminans (disseminated intravascular coagulation)
  Leukemia
Infections
  Meningococcemia
  Rocky Mountain spotted fever
  Endocarditis
  Acute hemorrhagic fever

Miscellaneous
  Amyloidosis
  Cholesterol/fat emboli
  Drug-induced (corticosteroid) disorder
  Dysproteinemia
  Trauma/bites
  Panniculitis
  Wiskott-Aldrich syndrome
  Langerhans cell granulomatosis
  Increased intravascular pressure: coughing, Valsalva's maneuver

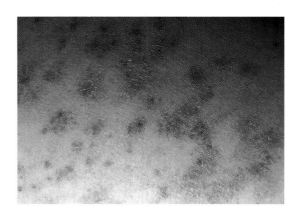

Figure 6.2.3 Pigmented purpura. *Clue to diagnosis:* Cayenne-pepper-like appearance.

3. ERYTHEMA NODOSUM
VERSUS
POLYARTERITIS NODOSA

Features in common: Red nodules on lower extremities.

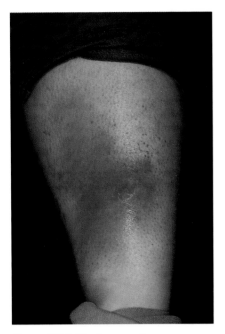

Figure 6.3.1 Erythema nodosum.

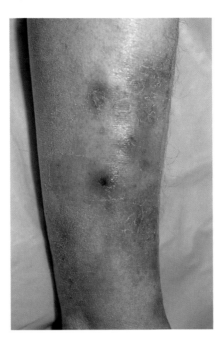

Figure 6.3.2 Polyarteritis nodosa.

Distinguishing features

	ERYTHEMA NODOSUM	POLYARTERITIS NODOSA
Physical examination		
Morphology	No ulcers	Ulcers (occasionally)
	Lesions do not follow arteries	Lesions follow course of arteries
	No livedo pattern	Livedo pattern occasionally present
Distribution	Pretibial area, rarely elsewhere	Variable, most common on lower legs
History	Pain	Pain
Symptoms	No suppuration	Suppuration
	No fever or malaise	Fever, malaise
	No central nervous system symptoms	Central nervous system symptoms
Exacerbating factors	Prolonged standing, limb dependencies	Prolonged standing, limb dependency
Associated findings/causes	Medications: oral contraceptives	No medications
	Infections: streptococcal infection, deep fungal infections, *Yersinia*, *Campylobacter*	Infections: hepatitis B infection
	Malignancies	No malignancies

Continues

Distinguishing features (Continued)

	ERYTHEMA NODOSUM	POLYARTERITIS NODOSA
Associated findings/causes	Immunologic diseases: sarcoidosis, Behçet's disease	No immunologic disease
Epidemiology	Uncommon Young female predominance	Rare
Biopsy	No Septal panniculitis with mixed inflammatory infiltrate	Yes Vasculitis of medium-sized arteries
Laboratory	Anti-streptolysin O titer, chest x-ray	Hepatitis B screen Childhood variant: ASO positive Angiography Erythrocyte sedimentation rate
Treatment	Treat underlying cause; rest, leg elevation, oral steroids, dapsone, potassium iodide (SSKI), nonsteroidal anti-inflammatory drugs	Oral steroids Immunosuppressive agents
Outcome	Self-limited, resolves over several weeks	Variable with significant morbidity and mortality; patients with only cutaneous manifestations have a good prognosis

Some causes of erythema nodosum

Medications
   Oral contraceptives
   Bromides
   Sulfonamides
Inflammatory bowel disease
   Ulcerative colitis, Crohn's disease
Infections
   Bacterial: *Streptococcus, Yersinia*, enterocolitis,
      Mycoplasma pneumoniae, leptospirosis,
      tularemia, cat-scratch disease
   Fungal: coccidioidomycosis, blastomycosis,
      histoplasmosis, dermatophytosis
   Viruses: hepatitis
Malignancies
   Lymphoma
   Rarely solid tumors
Autoimmune diseases
   Sarcoidosis
   Behçet's disease
Miscellaneous
   Postradiation therapy
Idiopathic factors

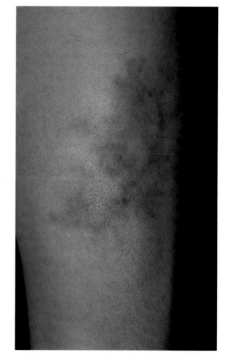

Figure 6.3.3 Polyarteritis nodosa. *Clue to diagnosis:* Poikilodermatous skin with underlying nodules.

4. PYODERMA GANGRENOSUM
VERSUS
STASIS ULCER

Features in common: Ulcers on lower extremities.

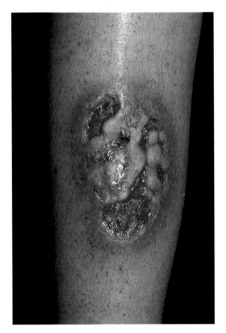

Figure 6.4.1 Pyoderma gangrenosum.

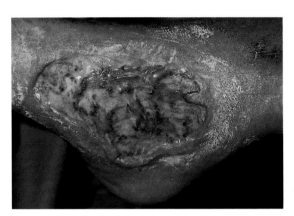

Figure 6.4.2 Stasis ulcer.

Distinguishing features

	PYODERMA GANGRENOSUM	STASIS ULCER
Physical examination		
Morphology	No dermatitis	Surrounding dermatitis
	Ulcer with undermined purple edge	No undermined edge
	No venous insufficiency	Venous insufficiency: varix
	No papillomatosis	Chronic lesions: papillomatosis, elephantiasis
Distribution	71% multiple lesions: Lower legs > thighs > buttocks > chest	Lower legs: most commonly overlying medial malleolus
History		
Symptoms	Severe pain not helped by leg elevation	Dull pain that improves with leg elevation
Exacerbating factors	Active bowel disease	Standing

Continues

Distinguishing features (Continued)

	PYODERMA GANGRENOSUM	STASIS ULCER
Associated findings	Ulcerative colitis Crohn's disease Rheumatoid arthritis Idiopathic Leukemia	Deep vein phlebitis
Epidemiology	Variable age, equally male and female	Elderly; multiparous females

Biopsy	Yes
	Dermal abscess that early on is follicular
	  centered, lymphocytic vasculitis in periphery
		No
		Dermal edema, fibrosis, hemosiderin
		  deposition and spongiosis

Laboratory	Rheumatoid factor, erythrocyte
	  sedimentation rate, serum
	  protein electrophoresis
		Ultrasound

Treatment	Systemic steroids, steroid injections,
	  dapsone, cyclosporine
		Leg elevation, pressure stockings,
		  topical steroids, acetylsalicylic acid,
		  dipyridamole

Outcome	Chronic course, lesions heal with
	  cribriform scarring
		Chronic; stasis papillomatosis
		  (elephantiasis verrucosum nostras)

Differential diagnosis of ulcers

Infections
  Abscess
  Anthrax
  Amebiasis
  Ecthyma gangrenosum
  Deep fungal: histoplasmosis,
    chromoblastomycosis,
    cryptococcosis, mycetoma
  Fournier's gangrene
  Mycobacterial infection
  Sexually transmitted disease:
    syphilis, chancroid
Metabolic disorders
  Diabetes
  Necrobiosis lipoidica diabeticorum
  Prolidase deficiency
Miscellaneous
  Bites (human, pet, and insect,
    especially brown recluse spider)

Miscellaneous (continued)
  Pyoderma gangrenosum
  Neuropathic disorders
  Pressure/decubitus ulcers
  Factitial disorders
  Erythema induratum or
    other panniculitis
  Sickle cell anemia
Neoplasms
  Lymphoma
  Squamous cell carcinoma
  Basal cell carcinoma
  Other
Vascular disorders
  Stasis ulcer (atrophie blanche)
  Arterial ulcer
  Vasculitis
  Calciphylaxis

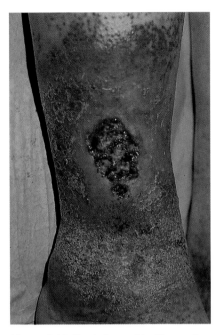

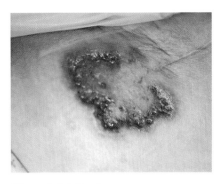

Figure 6.4.4 Pyoderma gangrenosum.
Clue to diagnosis: Ulcer that heals with
cribriform scar.

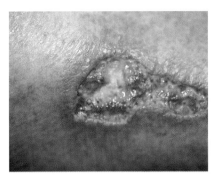

Figure 6.4.5 Pyoderma gangrenosum.
Clue to diagnosis: Violaceous rim of skin
surrounding ulcer.

Figure 6.4.3 Stasis dermatitis. *Clue to diagnosis:* Eczematous skin surrounding ulcer.

5. STASIS ULCER
VERSUS
ARTERIAL ULCER

Features in common: Ulcers in lower extremities.

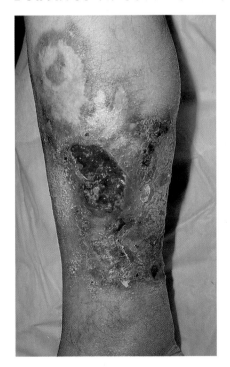

Figure 6.5.1 Stasis ulcer.

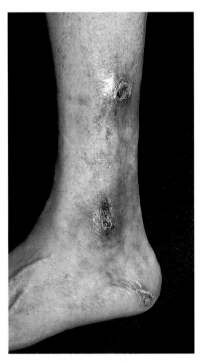

Figure 6.5.2 Arterial ulcer.

Distinguishing features

	STASIS ULCER	ARTERIAL ULCER
Physical examination Morphology	Skin erythematous Good capillary refill Prominent varix Pitting edema No hair loss Surrounding dermatitis Elephantiasis may develop	Skin pale, cyanotic Poor capillary refill No prominent varix No pitting edema Hair loss occasionally present No surrounding dermatitis No elephantiasis
Distribution	Lower legs: most commonly overlying medial malleolus	Most common over lateral malleolus
History Symptoms	Dull pain that improves with leg elevation No claudication	Severe pain, worsens with leg elevation Claudication
Exacerbating factors	Deep vein phlebitis	Hypertension, renal disease, arteriosclerosis, smoking
Associated findings	Venous insufficiency Good pulses No murmur Extremities cold Lipodermatosclerosis	Arterial insufficiency Poor pulses Vascular murmur Extremities warm No lipodermatosclerosis
Epidemiology	Elderly; multiparous females	Elderly men
Biopsy	No Dermal edema, fibrosis, lobular proliferation of blood vessels, hemosiderin deposition, epidermal acanthosis and spongiosis	No Thickened blood vessels
Laboratory	Photoplethysmography Venous hypertension on ultrasound occasionally	Arteriogram, Doppler ultrasound
Treatment	Support/pressure stockings, dressings and wound care, topical steroids for dermatitis	Vascular surgery, low-dose, acetylsalicylic acid, dipyridamole
Outcome	Chronic Elephantiasis	Chronic Untreated: gangrene

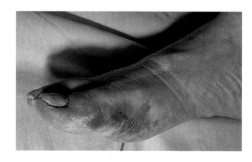

Figure 6.5.3 Arterial ulcer. *Clue to diagnosis:* Cyanotic skin due to peripheral vascular disease.

6. PRETIBIAL MYXEDEMA
VERSUS
STASIS DERMATITIS

Features in common: Red plaques on lower extremities.

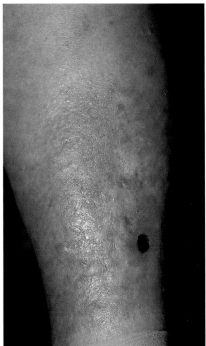

Figure 6.6.1 Pretibial myxedema.

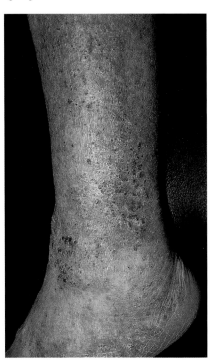

Figure 6.6.2 Stasis dermatitis.

Distinguishing features

	PRETIBIAL MYXEDEMA	STASIS DERMATITIS
Physical examination	Primarily dermal changes No scales	Primarily epidermal changes Scales present
Morphology	Nonpitting edema Does not ulcerate Chronic lesions: waxy thickened skin with woody feel and peau d'orange	Pitting edema May ulcerate Chronic lesions: papillomatosis, elephantiasis
Distribution	Shins	Lower legs
History Symptoms	Asymptomatic	Dull pain that improves with leg elevation
Exacerbating factors	Hyperthyroidism	Deep vein phlebitis
Associated findings	Exophthalmos, thyroid disease	Thrombophlebitis

Continues

Distinguishing features (Continued)

	PRETIBIAL MYXEDEMA	STASIS DERMATITIS
Epidemiology	Adult females	Elderly; multiparous females
Biopsy	Yes Epidermal acanthosis and papillomatosis in old lesions, dermal mucin, frequently grenz zone of uninvolved collagen in superficial papillary dermis	No Dermal edema, fibrosis, lobular proliferation of blood vessels, hemosiderin and mucin deposition, epidermal acanthosis and spongiosis
Laboratory	Thyroid receptor antibodies, thyroid-stimulating hormone, long-acting thyroid-stimulating hormone	Venous hypertension, ultrasound
Treatment	Inadequate: topical steroids	Compression/pressure stockings and topical steroids
Outcome	Chronic and persistent, poor response to therapy	Chronic, stasis papillomatosis

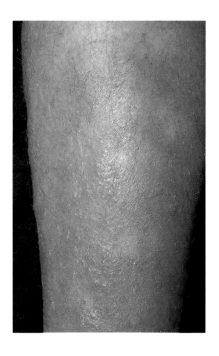

Figure 6.6.3 Pretibial myxedema. *Clue to diagnosis:* Erythematous papular-nodular skin overlying shins.

Discussion

ARTERIAL ULCER

Definition and etiology: Arterial ulcers occur secondary to necrosis of skin and soft tissue owing to insufficient arterial circulation.

Clinical features: The ulcers occur commonly in adult men who smoke. Coexisting atherosclerotic coronary artery disease is frequently present. Examination reveals poor pulses; pale, cold extremities; and poor capillary refill. Occasionally, vascular murmurs can be heard in the inguinal area over the femoral artery. The ulcers commonly are very painful at rest and frequently made worse with leg elevation. The ulcers are sharply punched out and commonly occur overlying the lateral malleolus. Loss of hair on the toes and the dorsum of the foot may occur. The toenails may become thick and dystrophic. The end result of chronic untreated arterial insufficiency is dry gangrene with loss of toes or part of the extremity.

The major disease in the differential diagnosis is stasis ulcer. Stasis ulcers most commonly occur in the medial malleolus and do not have a punched-out appearance. The surrounding skin is erythematous, not pale, and dermatitis is frequently present. The skin may also be indurated owing to inflammation in the fat (i.e., lipodermatosclerosis, hypodermatitis sclerodermiformis). Varicose veins and a history of thrombophlebitis are common features. Stasis ulcers are painful; however, unlike with arterial ulcers, the pain can be relieved by leg elevation. In severe cases, pitting edema and chronic thickening of the skin producing elephantiasis verrucosum nostras occur. Other diseases in the differential diagnosis include pyoderma gangrenosum, factitial, infectious, vasculitic, diabetic, pressure, and malignant ulcers. The ulcers of pyoderma gangrenosum have an undermined violaceous border and heal with a characteristic cribriform scar. Diabetic ulcers most commonly occur on the plantar surface of the foot as a result of neuropathy and trauma due to walking in poorly fitting shoes. The lesions of necrobiosis lipoidica diabeticorum can also ulcerate, but the surrounding atrophic yellow-colored plaques should not be confused with other entities. Ulcers due to vasculitis, such as arterial ulcers, are sharply punched out, and palpable purpura is usually present. Pressure ulcers occur at sites of pressure on the skin (such as over the heel) owing to chronic immobility. Pressure ulcers occur in comatose patients as well as in those with neuropathy or central nervous system disease, since these patients cannot feel the pain caused by the chronic pressure. Malignant ulcers have a rough irregular base and, frequently, heaped-up borders; however, since squamous cell carcinoma can also develop in chronic stasis ulcer, malignancy should be considered in any nonhealing ulcer and must be excluded by biopsy. Infectious ulcers usually occur secondary to trauma and have purulent drainage.

Treatment: The crux of the treatment is to improve the arterial circulation. Patients should stop smoking. Aspirin and dipyridamole (Persantine) may be helpful. Severe cases require vascular surgery.

ERYTHEMA NODOSUM

Definition and etiology: Erythema nodosum is panniculitis characterized by tender, red nodules and plaques on the pretibial surface. Erythema nodosum can be caused by a variety of different entities. The most common causes include oral contraceptives, streptococcal infections, sarcoidosis, inflammatory bowel disease, and gastrointestinal infections due to *Salmonella*, *Campylobacter*, or *Yersinia*.

Clinical features: Females are more commonly affected than males. Most cases occur in young adults.

Patients present with sudden onset of tender, red nodules overlying the extensor surface of the legs. The lesions may last 3 to 6 weeks; lesions older then 2 weeks become purpuric, resembling an old bruise. Rarely, the upper extremities or other cutaneous surfaces can be involved. Arthralgia may be present.

The major clinical diseases in the differential diagnosis are erythema induratum, other panniculitides, polyarteritis nodosa, insect bites, cellulitis, Majocchi's granuloma, and thrombophlebitis. Unlike erythema nodosum, erythema induratum involves the calves and frequently ulcerates. The lesions of erythema nodosum never ulcerate. The lesions of thrombophlebitis predominantly affect the sides of the legs, are hard and firm, and are attached to a vein. Venous insufficiency is usually apparent. Early on, the acute lesions of erythema nodosum can resemble cellulitis, but cellulitis is usually unilateral. In addition, nodules are not present in cellulitis, and patients are febrile. Majocchi's granuloma is a fungal infection involving hair follicles and is usually asymmetric and slightly scaly. These patients have been exposed to a source of tinea. Insect bites may also present with dermal nodules, on closer inspection, however, a central punctum can be found, and the lesions are not symmetric. Other panniculitides such as lupus pernio can also be confused with erythema nodosum. Helpful distinguishing features in the case of lupus pernio are the association with exposure to cold and the location of the lesions predominantly over distal extremities. Patients with polyarteritis usually have systemic manifestations of disease such as fever or renal insufficiency. The lesions most commonly follow the course of blood vessels and are frequently found in the popliteal fossa. Sometimes, however, an excisional biopsy is needed to exclude these other diseases.

Treatment: Patients with erythema nodosum should be evaluated for an underlying cause. The routine work-up is a throat culture, measurement of anti-streptolysin O antibody or streptozyme levels to exclude a streptococcal infection, and chest x-ray to exclude sarcoidosis or other pulmonary infection. A gastroenterology work-up should also be performed if there are gastrointestinal symptoms. Once the underlying cause is eliminated, the lesions will spontaneously improve. To hasten the resolution, systemic steroids, topical steroids, nonsteroidal anti-inflammatory agents, dapsone, and potassium iodide (SSKI) can be helpful. Patients should also elevate their legs and avoid prolonged standing or physical activity.

ERYTHEMA INDURATUM

Definition and etiology: Erythema induratum is a form of chronic recurrent panniculitis. In Europe, it is frequently secondary to tuberculosis. In the United States, the association between erythema induratum and tuberculosis is rare. More commonly, erythema induratum is believed to be an indiopathic vasculitis and is often termed *nodular vasculitis*.

Clinical features: Females are affected more commonly. Erythema induratum presents with erythematous, tender, subcutaneous nodules with a predilection for the calf area. Ulceration is common, and the lesions heal with scarring. In cases associated with tuberculosis, there is a strongly positive result with purified protein derivative testing. The major disease in the differential diagnosis is erythema nodosum. Erythema nodosum predominantly affects the shins, not the calves, and the lesions do not ulcerate or heal with scarring, as in erythema induratum. As in erythema nodosum, the differential diagnosis would also include other panniculitides, infections, polyarteritis nodosa, and thrombophlebitis. Although the disease may be clinically suspected, the diagnosis of erythema induratum requires pathologic examination. Histologic analysis demonstrates lobular panniculitis with caseation necrosis and with vasculitis of a medium-sized blood vessel.

Treatment: Cases associated with tuberculosis can be successfully treated with triple antituberculid therapy. The idiopathic form can be treated with topical, intralesional, or systemic steroids, dapsone, and SSKI.

LEUKOCYTOCLASTIC VASCULITIS

Definition and etiology: Leukocytoclastic vasculitis (necrotizing vasculitis, hypersensitivity vasculitis) represents an inflammatory destructive process of postcapillary venules due to deposition of immune complexes. The stimuli for immune complex formation are protean, including collagen vascular diseases, infections, medications, cryoglobulins, paraprotein, and malignancies.

Clinical features: During the first few hours, urticarial papules develop in dependent sites, such as the lower legs and buttocks. The lesions rapidly develop into the classic palpable purpuric macules and papules. In severe cases, necrosis, ulcers, livedo reticularis, and even vesicles occur. Commonly associated symptoms include fever and arthralgias. Rarely, glomerulonephritis and gastrointestinal symptoms such as nausea, vomiting, diarrhea, and pain can occur.

   The pigmented purpuras can be distinguished from leukocytoclastic vasculitis by their lack of palpable lesions and lack of systemic symptoms. In questionable cases, biopsy can be helpful. The differential diagnosis could also include other types of vasculitis. The lesions of Henoch-Schönlein purpura (HSP) are identical to those of leukocytoclastic vasculitis. HSP is most commonly

seen in children, and abdominal pain and renal involvement occur more frequently than in leukocytoclastic vasculitis. The definitive diagnosis of HSP can be made only if direct immunofluorescent studies demonstrate IgA immunoreactants in blood vessels. In Wegener's granulomatosis, palpable purpura can also be found along with ulcers, papules, and plaques. If respiratory tract symptoms occur along with renal involvement, Wegener's granulomatosis should be suspected. In polyarteritis nodosa, nodules are found along the course of arteries. Erythema elevatum diutinum is a chronic variant of leukocytoclastic vasculitis in which nodules are found overlying hand, elbow, and knee joints.

Treatment: In all cases of leukocytoclastic vasculitis, an underlying cause should be sought, eliminated, and treated. Treatments include nonsteroidal anti-inflammatory agents, dapsone, and brief courses of systemic steroids.

PIGMENTED PURPURA

Definition and etiology: Pigmented purpura is a benign, usually idiopathic, capillaritis that can appear in several different overlapping clinical patterns. Rarely, a pigmented purpuric eruption can be attributed to a medication.

Clinical features: The pigmented purpuras are characterized by nonpalpable purpura, most commonly on the lower extremities. The purpura is associated with yellow-to-red petechiae and eczematous plaques. If petechiae predominate, this is called *Schamberg's disease*. Sometimes the lesions have an annular distribution, then the eponym *Majocchi's disease* (purpura annularis telangiectodes) applies. Other variants includes Gougerot-Blum syndrome (pigmented purpuric lichenoid dermatitis), in which small red papules can be found, and lichen aureus, in which the lesions have a golden rust-colored hue. Histologically, all the different subtypes have similar findings a superficial perivascular lymphocytic infiltrate, extravasated erythrocytes, and hemosiderin deposition. An overlying dermatitis can be found in Majocchi's disease, and the inflammation is denser and more lichenoid in Gougerot-Blum syndrome and lichen aureus variant.

   The major diseases in the differential diagnosis are stasis dermatitis, leukocytoclastic vasculitis, and petechiae secondary to thrombocytopenia. The lesions of pigmented purpura are nonpalpable, unlike the lesions of leukocytoclastic vasculitis. Systemic involvement and an early urticarial phase are also not present. Although in stasis dermatitis, petechiae and yellow plaques can also be found, signs of venous insufficiency such as edema and varicose veins are prominent features. Petechiae secondary to thrombocytopenia are usually widespread and involve the mucous membranes, and epistaxis and internal bleeding can be present.

Treatment: Since the pigmented purpuras are only of cosmetic concern, no treatment is necessary; however, topical steroids can be beneficial in severe cases.

PYODERMA GANGRENOSUM

Definition and etiology: Pyoderma gangrenosum is a clinically distinct, painful skin ulcer related to a variety of systemic diseases. The most commonly associated systemic diseases are inflammatory bowel disease and rheumatoid arthritis. Other rarer associations include leukemia, myeloma, and paraproteinemia.

Clinical features: The first lesions usually develop in a site of trauma, most commonly in the lower legs, but can be found in any cutaneous surface. Pyoderma gangrenosum starts out as a follicular-based papulovesicle or pustule that over a few days becomes necrotic, enlarged, and ulcerated. Upon presentation, large ulcers with a violaceous undermined border are present. The ulcers characteristically are very painful and heal with a cribriform scar. The characteristic clinical course and appearance allow easy differentiation from other causes of ulcers discussed previously. A biopsy is occasionally helpful to rule out other causes of ulcers, such as infections or malignancies. The histologic findings in pyoderma gangrenosum are not diagnostic. Early lesions may show a follicular-centered abscess. The base of the ulcer in pyoderma gangrenosum shows an abscess, but a biopsy specimen taken from the edge of the ulcer will show lymphocytic vasculitis.

Treatment: Underlying systemic diseases should be sought and appropriately treated. The most commonly used treatment is high-dose oral prednisone. Cyclosporine is also highly effective in refractory cases. Other therapies include intralesional steroid injection, cyclophosphamide, chlorambucil, thalidomide, dapsone, minocycline, occlusive dressings, topical cromolyn, and hyperbaric oxygen.

POLYARTERITIS NODOSA

Definition and etiology: Polyarteritis nodosa is vasculitis of medium-sized arteries. The commonly affected organs include skin, kidneys, central nervous system, peripheral nervous system, lungs, heart, and gastrointestinal tract. A rare variant primarily affecting the skin, joints, and peripheral nervous system can also occur. The cause is unclear, but some cases have been associated with hepatitis B infection.

Clinical features: Patients are usually sick and suffer from multiple systemic complaints. The most common findings are fever, weight loss, arthritis, mononeuritis multiplex, cutaneous disorders, renal involvement, gas-

trointestinal symptoms, asthma, hypertension, and cardiac failure. Cutaneous findings include erythematous nodules that follow the course of the superficial arteries. The nodules are most prominent in the popliteal fossa, anterior lower leg, and dorsum of the foot. Severe involvement can lead to ulcer formation, necrosis, and gangrene. Purpuric lesions due to extravasated erythrocytes can also frequently be found along with livedo reticularis. The major diseases in the differential diagnosis are thrombophlebitis and panniculitides such as erythema nodosum. The lesions of thrombophlebitis follow the course of veins, not arteries, and varicose veins are usually present. Systemic symptoms are also lacking. The lesions of erythema nodosum are unrelated to vasculature pattern and predominantly occur overlying the shins. Livedo reticularis, ulcers, and necrosis do not occur in erythema nodosum. Purpura only occurs in old resolving lesions.

Treatment: The therapy for polyarteritis nodosa is high-dose systemic steroids. Immunosuppressive agents such as cyclophosphamide and cyclosporine can also be used.

PRETIBIAL MYXEDEMA

Definition and etiology: Pretibial myxedema is the deposition of mucin in the pretibial area in patients with Graves' disease.

Clinical features: Early on, patients develop symmetric bilateral erythema overlying the shins. With time, the lesions become indurated, firm, nonpitting plaques. The follicular orifices become prominent, and localized hypertrichosis may be present. The associated clinical findings due to Graves' disease includes exophthalmos, thyroid acropachy, and a diffuse goiter. Laboratory examination reveals circulating antibody against thyroid-stimulating hormone receptor in the majority of patients.

Pretibial myxedema needs to be differentiated from stasis dermatitis. In stasis dermatitis, pitting edema, pigmentary changes due to dermal melanin and hemosiderin deposition, and eczematous scaly plaques are present. Although upon biopsy of the lesions, mucin can be found in both stasis dermatitis and pretibial myxedema, in pretibial myxedema a grenz zone of normal-appearing collagen is present in the superficial papillary dermis.

Treatment: There is no adequate treatment for pretibial myxedema. Topical and intralesional steroids have been of limited benefit.

STASIS ULCER

Definition and etiology: A stasis ulcer is an ulcer found on the lower extremities secondary to chronic venous insufficiency.

Clinical features: Stasis ulcers most commonly occur overlying the medial aspect of the shin and medial malleolus. The ulcers start as small, millimeter-sized defects, frequently secondary to trauma, but can grow to several centimeters in size. Signs of venous insufficiency are present around the ulcer such as edema, fibrosis, and varicose veins. The surrounding skin frequently exhibits stasis dermatitis (e.g., red and scaly irregular-colored plaques and patches due to melanin and hemosiderin deposition).

The differential diagnosis includes other forms of ulcer such as diabetic ulcer, arterial ulcer, pyoderma gangrenosum, infectious ulcer, neoplastic ulcer, and vasculitic ulcer. Arterial ulcers are very painful, sharply demarcated, and most prominent over the lateral malleolus. Signs of arterial insufficiency are also present such as pallor, poor pulses, loss of hair, and atrophic skin. Other types of ulcers were discussed previously in the section on arterial ulcers.

Treatment: A variety of treatments exist. Circulation can be improved with use of pressure stockings and leg elevation. Low-dose aspirin or dipyridamole has been effective in some patients. Use of occlusive dressings can also speed up the healing process. In large refractory ulcers, skin grafts may be helpful.

Suggested Readings

ARTERIAL ULCERS
Baker SR, Stacey MC, Singh G et al. Aetiology of chronic leg ulcers. Eur J Vasc Surg 1992;6:245–51.

Ennis WJ, Meneses P. Leg ulcers: a practical approach to the leg ulcer patient. Ostomy Wound Man 1995;41 (suppl 7A):52S–62S.

Henderson CA, Highet AS, Lane SA et al. Arterial hypertension causing leg ulcers. Clin Exp Dermatol 1995; 20:107–14.

ERYTHEMA NODOSUM
Fox MD, Schwartz RA. Erythema nodosum [see comments] [review]. Am Fam Physician 1992; 46:818–22.

Hannuksela M. Erythema nodosum [review]. Clin Dermatol 1986;4:88–95.

ERYTHEMA INDURATUM
Ollert MW, Thomas P, Korting HC et al. Erythema induratum of Bazin. Evidence of T-lymphocyte hyperresponsiveness to purified protein derivative of tuberculin: report of two cases and treatment. Arch Dermatol 1993;129:469–73.

Schneider JW, Geiger DH, Rossouw DJ et al. *Mycobacterium tuberculosis* DNA in erythema induratum of Bazin [letter]. Lancet 1993;342:747–48.

LEUKOCYTOCLASTIC VASCULITIS
Gibson LE, Su WP. Cutaneous vasculitis [review]. Rheum Dis Clin North Am 1990;16:309–24.

Smith JG Jr. Vasculitis [review]. J Dermatol 1995;22: 812–22.

PIGMENTED PURPURA
Nishioka K, Katayana I, Masuzawa M et al. Drug-induced chronic pigmented purpura. J Dermatol 1989;16: 220–22.

Ratnam KV, Su WP, Peters MS. Purpura simplex (inflammatory purpura without vasculitis): a clinicopathologic study of 174 cases. J Am Acad Dermatol 1991;25: 642–47.

POLYARTERITIS NODOSA
Bacon PA. Systemic vasculitic syndromes [review]. Curr Opin Rheumatol 1993;5:5–10.

Chen KR. Cutaneous polyarteritis nodosa: a clinical and histopathological study of 20 cases. J Dermatol 1989;16: 429–42.

Minkowitz G, Smoller BR, McNutt NS. Benign cutaneous polyarteritis nodosa. Relationship to systemic polyarteritis nodosa and to hepatitis B infection. Arch Dermatol 1991;127:1520–23.

Siberry GK, Cohen BA, Johnson B. Cutaneous polyarteritis nodosa. Reports of two cases in children and review of the literature [review]. Arch Dermatol 1994;13: 884–89.

PRETIBIAL MYXEDEMA
Fatourechi V, Pajouhi M, Fransway AF. Dermopathy of Graves disease (pretibial myxedema). Review of 150 cases. Medicine 1994;73:1–7.

Somach SC, Helm TN, Lawlor KB et al. Pretibial mucin. Histologic patterns and clinical correlation. Arch Dermatol 1993;129:1152–56.

PYODERMA GANGRENOSUM
Chow RK, Ho VC. Treatment of pyoderma gangrenosum. J Am Acad Dermatol 1996;34:1047–60.

Duguid CM, Powell FC. Pyoderma gangrenosum. Clin Dermatol 1993;11:129–33.

Graham JA, Hansen KK, Rabinowitz LG et al. Pyoderma gangrenosum in infants and children. Pediatr Dermatol 1994;11:10–17.

Powell FC, Su WP, Perry HO. Pyoderma gangrenosum: classification and management. J Am Acad Dermatol 1996;34:395–409; quiz 410–12.

STASIS ULCERS
Black SB. Venous stasis ulcers: a review [review]. Ostomy Wound Man 1995;41:20–22.

Gourdin FW, Smith JG Jr. Etiology of venous ulceration [review]. South Med J 1993;86:1142–146.

Miller WL. Chronic venous insufficiency [review]. Curr Opin Cardiol 1995;10:543–48.

7 Genitalia

ALGORITHM FOR GENITAL RASHES

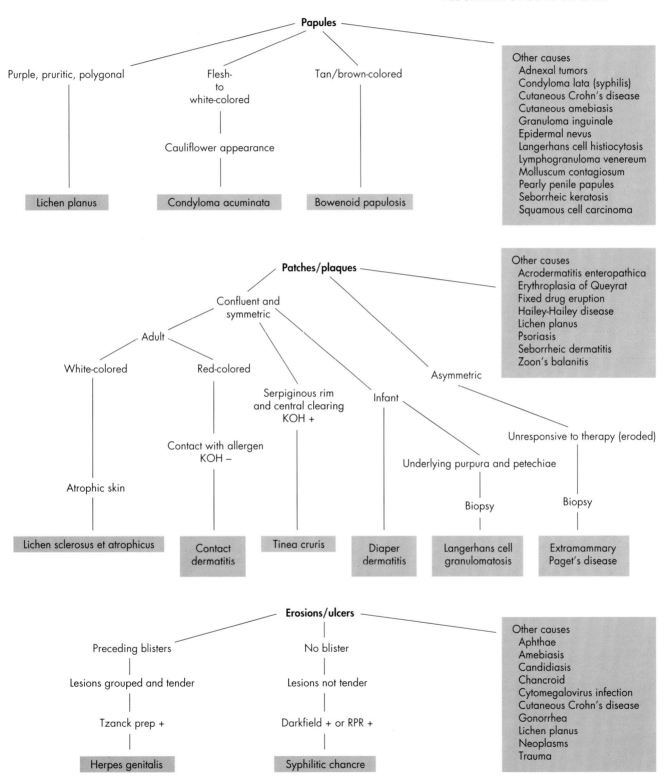

Papules

Purple, pruritic, polygonal

Flesh-to white-colored

Tan/brown-colored

Cauliflower appearance

Lichen planus

Condyloma acuminata

Bowenoid papulosis

Other causes
 Adnexal tumors
 Condyloma lata (syphilis)
 Cutaneous Crohn's disease
 Cutaneous amebiasis
 Granuloma inguinale
 Epidermal nevus
 Langerhans cell histiocytosis
 Lymphogranuloma venereum
 Molluscum contagiosum
 Pearly penile papules
 Seborrheic keratosis
 Squamous cell carcinoma

Patches/plaques

Confluent and symmetric

Adult

White-colored

Red-colored

Serpiginous rim and central clearing KOH +

Infant

Asymmetric

Contact with allergen KOH −

Unresponsive to therapy (eroded)

Atrophic skin

Underlying purpura and petechiae

Biopsy

Biopsy

Lichen sclerosus et atrophicus

Contact dermatitis

Tinea cruris

Diaper dermatitis

Langerhans cell granulomatosis

Extramammary Paget's disease

Other causes
 Acrodermatitis enteropathica
 Erythroplasia of Queyrat
 Fixed drug eruption
 Hailey-Hailey disease
 Lichen planus
 Psoriasis
 Seborrheic dermatitis
 Zoon's balanitis

Erosions/ulcers

Preceding blisters

No blister

Lesions grouped and tender

Lesions not tender

Tzanck prep +

Darkfield + or RPR +

Herpes genitalis

Syphilitic chancre

Other causes
 Aphthae
 Amebiasis
 Candidiasis
 Chancroid
 Cytomegalovirus infection
 Cutaneous Crohn's disease
 Gonorrhea
 Lichen planus
 Neoplasms
 Trauma

Introduction

The genital region is subject to a variety of different rashes. In adults, the genital region, not surprisingly, is the location where cutaneous manifestations of a variety of sexually transmitted diseases can be found. Other common problems found in the genital region because of its moist environment are tinea cruris and candidiasis. In babies and toddlers, the combination of diapers, wetness, friction, and incontinence of urine and stool can produce diaper dermatitis. Diaper dermatitis also needs to be distinguished from Langerhans cell granulomatosis. Although all dermatoses (e.g., seborrheic dermatitis, atopic dermatitis) can occur in the genital region, some (like lichen planus) seem to have a predilection for this site. In adults and, rarely, in children, the genital area is where where the rash of lichen sclerosus et atrophicus can be most commonly found. Finally, the manifestations of extramammary Paget's disease, a malignant tumor, can mimic and be misdiagnosed as tinea cruris or dermatitis.

1. BOWENOID PAPULOSIS
VERSUS
CONDYLOMA ACUMINATUM

Features in common: Warty-appearing papules in genitalia.

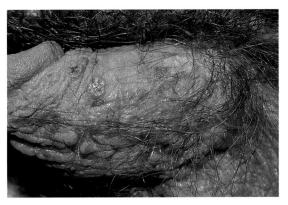

Figure 7.1.1 Bowenoid papulosis.

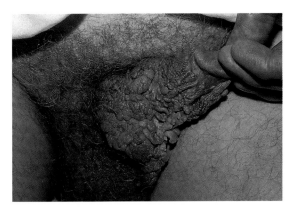

Figure 7.1.2 Condyloma acuminatum.

Distinguishing features

	BOWENOID PAPULOSIS	CONDYLOMA ACUMINATUM
Physical examination		
Morphology	Brown Papules No cauliflower-like appearance	Flesh colored Papillomatous papules and plaques Frequent cauliflower-like appearance
Distribution	Genital area	Genital area
History		
Symptoms	Asymptomatic	Asymptomatic
Exacerbating factors	None	Spread in areas of injury (Koebner's phenomenon)
Associated findings	Other sexually transmitted diseases Cervical dysplasia	Other sexually transmitted diseases Cervical dysplasia
Epidemiology	Sexually active adults	Sexually active adults
Biopsy	Yes Epidermal acanthosis and papillomatosis; however, epidermal atypia resembling squamous cell carcinoma in situ present	No Epidermal acanthosis, papillomatosis, koilocytosis, tortuous blood vessels in dermal papilla No atypia
Laboratory	Experimental: HPV typing, HPV types 16, 18, 30, 33	Experimental: HPV typing, HPV types 6, 11, 16, 18

Continues

Distinguishing features (Continued)

	BOWENOID PAPULOSIS	CONDYLOMA ACUMINATUM
Treatment	Liquid nitrogen, laser surgery, 5-fluorouracil, electrosurgical removal	Liquid nitrogen, topical acids, podophyllin, podophyllin toxin, laser surgery, intralesional or subcutaneous interferon
Outcome	Good response to therapy Duration weeks to years Spontaneous regression may occur	Good response to therapy Duration weeks to years Spontaneous regression may occur

Abbreviation: HPV, human papillomavirus.

Differential diagnosis of genital papules

Common causes
   Bowenoid papulosis
   Condyloma acuminatum
   Lichen planus
   Molluscum contagiosum
   Pearly penile papules
   Seborrheic keratosis

Rarer causes
   Cutaneous amebiasis
   Cutaneous Crohn's disease
   Condyloma latum (syphilis)
   Eruptive syringoma
   Granuloma inguinale
   Langerhans cell histiocytosis
   Lymphogranuloma venereum
   Squamous cell carcinoma
     (giant condyloma of
     Buschke-Löwenstein)

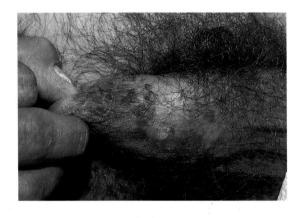

Figure 7.1.3 Bowenoid papulosis. *Clue to diagnosis:* Small size of papules with brown color.

2. LICHEN SCLEROSUS ET ATROPHICUS VERSUS DERMATITIS

Features in common: Both may present with tender white- to red-colored plaques on genitalia.

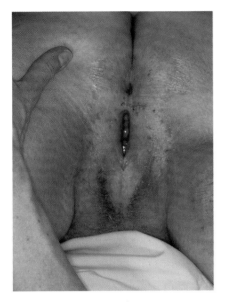

Figure 7.2.1 Lichen sclerosus et atrophicus.

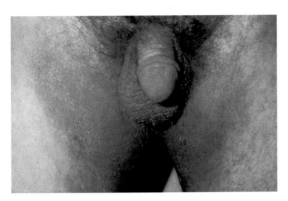

Figure 7.2.2 Allergic contact dermatitis.

Distinguishing features

	LICHEN SCLEROSUS	DERMATITIS
Physical examination		
Morphology	Ivory colored	Red colored
	Atrophy	No atrophy (thickening of skin in chronic cases)
	Little or no scaling	Scaling prominent
	Blisters rare	Blisters common
	Hemorrhage common	Hemorrhage rare
Distribution	Hourglass appearance with involvement of vulva, perineum, perianal skin	In sites of contact or irritation
	20% of time involvement elsewhere	Spares inguinal creases
History		
Symptoms	Soreness, dyspareunia	Pruritus
Exacerbating factors	Intercourse	Scratching, secondary infection

Continues

Distinguishing features (Continued)

	LICHEN SCLEROSUS	DERMATITIS
Associated findings	Vitiligo, pernicious anemia, alopecia areata, systemic lupus erythematosus	None
Epidemiology	Females > males approximately 10:1 ratio; average age 45–60 years	No sex predilection, can occur at any age
Biopsy	Yes Epidermal atrophy, occasionally epidermal acanthosis, follicular plugging, homogenized collagen in upper dermis with dermal edema, bandlike lymphocytic infiltrate underneath altered collagen	No Spongiosis, parakeratosis, superficial perivascular inflammatory infiltrate
Laboratory	Usually none Experimentally: antibodies against thyroid, smooth muscle, gastric, and parietal cells	Patch testing if allergic contact dermatitis suspected
Treatment	High-potency topical steroids, topical testosterone, topical retinoids	Avoid allergen or irritant, topical steroids
Outcome	Chronic Rarely squamous cell carcinomas develop within lesions	Good, resolves after elimination of allergens and irritants Not associated with malignancies

Differential diagnosis of genital rashes

Common causes
  Candidiasis
  Contact dermatitis
  Diaper dermatitis
  Intertrigo
  Lichen sclerosus et atrophicus
  Psoriasis
  Seborrheic dermatitis
  Tinea cruris

Rarer causes
  Acrodermatitis enteropathica
  Granulomatous slack skin
  Hailey-Hailey disease
  Langerhans cell granulomatosis
    (histiocytosis X)

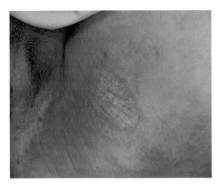

Figure 7.2.3 Lichen sclerosus et atrophicus. *Clue to diagnosis:* Atrophic white patch.

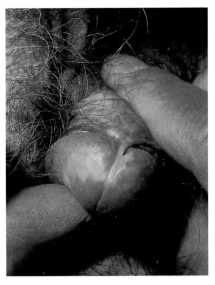

Figure 7.2.4 Balanitis xerotica obliterans (lichen sclerosus et atrophicus of the penis). *Clue to diagnosis:* Porcelain white color.

3. HERPES GENITALIS
VERSUS
PRIMARY SYPHILITIC CHANCRE

Features in common: Papules/erosions/ulcers in genital area.

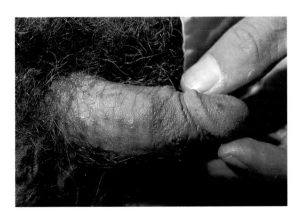

Figure 7.3.1 Herpes genitalis.

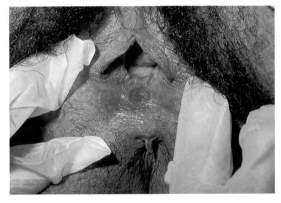

Figure 7.3.2 Syphilitic chancre.

Distinguishing features

	HERPES GENITALIS	SYPHILITIC CHANCRE
Physical examination		
Morphology	Grouped blisters Erosions and ulcer with scalloped border Border not indurated	No grouped blisters Border smooth Border firm, indurated
Distribution	Genital area	Genital area
History		
Symptoms	Prodrome of burning or itching Pain	No prodrome No pain
Exacerbating factors	Immunosuppresion	Immunosuppresion

Associated findings	Lymphadenopathy	Lymphadenopathy
		Occasionally papulosquamous
		  eruption of secondary syphilis
		  may become evident

Epidemiology	Sexually active adults	Sexually active adults

Biopsy	No
	Multinucleated giant cells
		No
		Ulcer with underlying plasma cell
		  infiltrate, Warthin Starry stain
		  positive for spirochetal organisms

Laboratory	Tzanck preparation positive Culture or direct immunofluorescent studies	Tzanck preparation negative Darkfield or rapid plasma reagin test positive
Treatment	Antiviral therapy if started in first 1–2 days: acyclovir, valacyclovir, and famciclovir	Penicillin, tetracycline, erythromycin

Outcome	Chronic relapsing course	Curable with therapy; may progress
		  to secondary or tertiary syphilis
		  if untreated

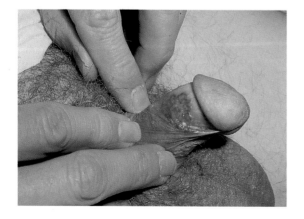

Figure 7.3.3 Herpes genitalis. *Clue to diagnosis:* Scalloped borders.

4. TINEA CRURIS
VERSUS
EXTRAMAMMARY PAGET'S DISEASE

Features in common: Red, scaly patches/plaques in genital region.

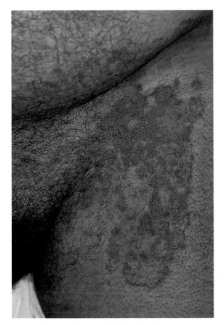

Figure 7.4.1 Tinea cruris.

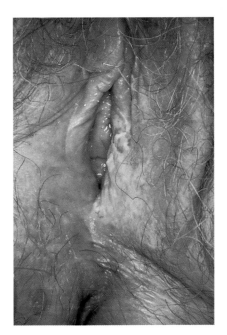

Figure 7.4.2 Extramammary Paget's disease.

Distinguishing features

	TINEA CRURIS	EXTRAMAMMARY PAGET'S DISEASE
Physical examination		
Morphology	Symmetric	Asymmetric
	Serpiginous border common	Serpiginous borders at times
	Central clearing	No central clearing
	Lesions flat	Occasional elevated or nodular areas
Distribution	Genital area	Genital area
	Spares scrotum	May involve scrotum
History		
Symptoms	Pruritus	Asymptomatic
Exacerbating factors	Topical steroid use	None
Associated findings	Tinea pedis	Internal malignancy of genitourinary or gastrointestinal tract in many cases
Epidemiology	Any age, more common in men	Elderly adults

Continues

Distinguishing features (Continued)

	TINEA CRURIS	**EXTRAMAMMARY PAGET'S DISEASE**
Biopsy	No Spores and hyphae within the stratum corneum	Yes Large pale cells spreading in a pagetoid or buckshot pattern within the epidermis
Laboratory	Fungus culture KOH+	Stool guaiac, urinalysis, prostate exam for underlying malignancy Consider cystoscopy, sigmoidoscopy KOH−
Treatment	Topical or systemic antifungal agent	Surgery, laser surgery
Outcome	Resolves with therapy	Frequently recurs, poor prognosis if associated with internal malignancy

Abbreviation: KOH, potassium hydroxide.

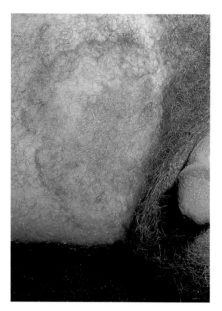

Figure 7.4.3 Tinea cruris. *Clue to diagnosis:* Central clearing with peripheral scaling.

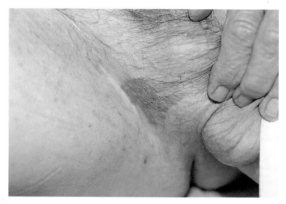

Figure 7.4.4 Extramammary Paget's disease. *Clue to diagnosis:* Asymmetry and irregularly shaped borders.

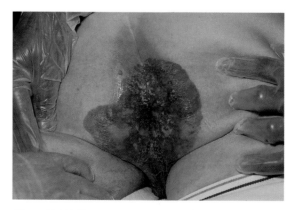

Figure 7.4.5 Extramammary Paget's disease. *Clue to diagnosis:* Erosions in indurated plaque.

5. DIAPER DERMATITIS
VERSUS
LANGERHANS CELL GRANULOMATOSIS

Features in common: Patches/plaques in diaper area in babies and toddlers.

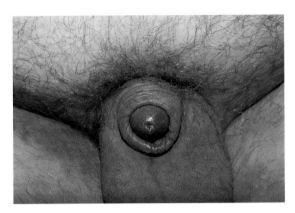

Figure 7.5.1 Candidal diaper dermatitis.

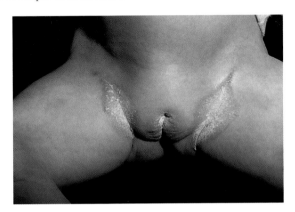

Figure 7.5.2 Langerhans cell granulomatosis.

Distinguishing features

	DIAPER DERMATITIS	LANGERHANS CELL GRANULOMATOSIS
Physical examination		
Morphology	Erythema and scaling	Erythema and scaling
	No papules	Brownish tan papules present
	Lichenification	No lichenification
	If *Candida* present: bright red erythema, satellite papules and pustules	Dusky erythema
		No satellite papules or pustules
	No purpura	Areas of petechiae and purpura
	No crusts/erosions	Crusts/erosions frequently present
	Occasional sparing of skin folds	No sparing of skin folds
	Nodules and ulcers only seen in severe cases (Jacquet's granuloma)	Occasional nodules and ulcers
Distribution	Genital area	Scalp, trunk, genital area
History		
Symptoms	Irritability	Irritability
	No malaise	Generalized malaise may be present
Exacerbating factors	Infrequent diaper changes	None
Associated findings	None	Lymphadenopathy, pancytopenia, hepatosplenomegaly, pulmonary infiltrates, diabetes insipidus, exophthalmos, otitis media
Epidemiology	Infants and toddlers	Infants and toddlers, rarely adults

Continues

Distinguishing features (Continued)

	DIAPER DERMATITIS	LANGERHANS CELL GRANULOMATOSIS
Biopsy	No Dermatitis with epidermal spongiosis and superficial perivascular lymphocytic infiltrate	Yes Bandlike infiltrate with "histiocytic"-appearing cells with cleaved kidney-bean shaped nucleus in dermis and extending into epidermis; foam cells, lymphocytes, and eosinophils also frequently present
Laboratory	KOH+	KOH− Complete blood count with differential, x-rays and systemic work as indicated
Treatment	Mild topical steroids, antifungal creams, barrier creams such as zinc oxide, more frequent diaper changes, superabsorbent diapers	Topical nitrogen mustard Chemotherapy for systemic disease
Outcome	Good	Variable; may resolve or occasionally may be fatal

Abbreviation: KOH, potassium hydroxide.

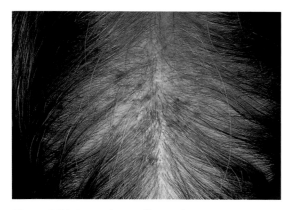

Figure 7.5.3 Langerhans cell granulomatosis. *Clue to diagnosis:* Purpuric crusted papules.

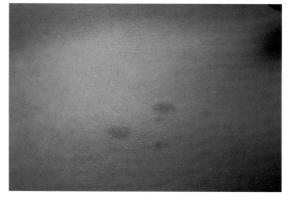

Figure 7.5.4 Langerhans cell granulomatosis. *Clue to diagnosis:* Brown xanthomatous-appearing plaques.

6. LICHEN PLANUS
VERSUS
CONDYLOMA ACUMINATUM

Features in common: Papules in genital area.

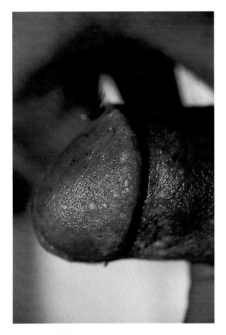

Figure 7.6.1 Lichen planus.

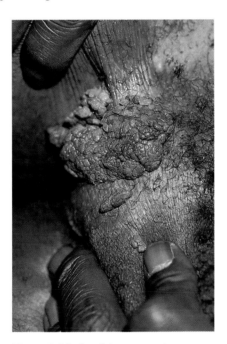

Figure 7.6.2 Condyloma acuminatum.

Distinguishing features

	LICHEN PLANUS	CONDYLOMA ACUMINATUM
Physical examination		
Morphology	Purple polygonal papules	Skin-colored papules and plaques
	Flat topped	Cauliflower-like appearance
	Occasionally erosions and blisters	No erosions or blisters
	White fine scale (Wickham's striae)	No Wickham's striae
Distribution	Shaft of penis, occasionally groin flexures	Anywhere in genital area but predilection for shaft of penis and perivaginal area
History		
Symptoms	Pruritus	Asymptomatic
Exacerbating factors	Trauma, isomorphic response (e.g., Koebner's reaction: lesions develop in traumatized skin)	Trauma, isomorphic response (e.g., Koebner's reaction: lesions develop in traumatized skin)

Continues

Distinguishing features (Continued)

	LICHEN PLANUS	CONDYLOMA ACUMINATUM
Associated findings	Lesions on skin and in mucosa and nail dystrophy Hepatitis, rarely neoplasia Occasionally drug-induced	Other sexually transmitted diseases: syphilis, HIV infection Not drug-induced
Epidemiology	Middle-aged adults	Sexually active adults
Biopsy	Yes Bandlike (lichenoid) inflammatory infiltrate, epidermal acanthosis with sawtooth appearance, wedge-shaped hypergranulosis, colloid bodies	No Epidermal acanthosis, papillomatosis, koilocytosis, tortuous blood vessels in dermal papilla
Laboratory	Hepatitis C virus, occasionally familial	Rapid plasma reagin test HIV test, hepatitis B & C tests
Treatment	Topical steroids	Liquid nitrogen, topical acids, laser electrosurgery, podophyllin, podophyllin toxin, interferons
Outcome	Chronic but usually self-limited, variable response to therapy; isolated reports of associated squamous cell carcinoma	Curable Good response to therapy

Abbreviation: HIV, human immunodeficiency virus.

Discussion

BOWENOID PAPULOSIS

Definition and etiology: Bowenoid papulosis is a human papillomavirus infection of the genitals in which there are warty-appearing papules that demonstrate epithelial atypia reminiscent of squamous cell carcinoma on biopsy.

Clinical features: Multiple small (2- to 20-mm) red- to brown-colored papules and plaques that are warty, chronic, and treatment resistant are found in the genitalia most commonly in sexually active adults. Men are more frequently involved than women. Biopsy results show the changes of Bowen's disease (squamous cell carcinoma in situ). Unlike in Bowen's disease, however, the lesions of bowenoid papulosis are small and slightly brown colored, do not grow in size, and do not progress to become invasive squamous cell carcinoma.

The major clinical disease in the differential diagnosis of bowenoid papulosis is condyloma acuminatum, which is caused by another human papillomavirus infection. The lesions of condyloma acuminatum are usually larger than the papules of bowenoid papulosis and are more skin-colored than the more deeply pigmented lesions of bowenoid papulosis. Atypia are also not present on biopsy of condyloma acuminatum. Lichen planus, like bowenoid papulosis, can present with colored papules in the genitalia; however, the lesions of lichen planus are very pruritic and purple colored. Lichen planus lesions are also frequently present in the oral mucosa and other skin surfaces but may occasionally be limited to genital skin. Other diseases to be considered in the differential diagnosis include psoriasis, granuloma inguinale, lymphogranuloma venereum, molluscum contagiosum, pearly penile papules (penile angiofibromas), and scabies.

Treatment: A variety of different destructive treatments can be used, such as liquid nitrogen, laser surgery, electosurgical removal, excisional surgery, and topical 5-fluorouracil. Radical surgery is not necessary, since bowenoid papulosis biologically behaves in a benign manner.

CONDYLOMA ACUMINATUM

Definition and etiology: Condyloma acuminatum is a sexually trasmitted human papillomavirus infection.

Clinical features: Sessile warty skin-colored papules and plaques in the genital area may progress to become large cauliflower-like masses. Lesions may koebnerize, or develop in sites of trauma. The major disease in the differential diagnosis is bowenoid papulosis. Although the lesions of condyloma acuminatum are usually quite distinctive, they occasionally can be confused with skin tags, seborrheic keratoses, condyloma latum (syphilis), cutaneous Crohn's disease, cutaneous amebiasis, molluscum contagiosum, and squamous cell carcinoma. Skin tags are usually pedunculated, flesh-colored papules with a smooth surface. Seborrheic keratoses have a characteristic tan to brown color and "stuck-on" appearance. Recent studies indicate that some clinically and histologically typical seborrheic keratoses may harbor human papillomavirus and may be "old condylomata." The lesions of condyloma latum (secondary syphilis) are moist, oozing, white-colored papules and always need to be considered in the differential diagnosis. In fact, since condyloma acuminatum is a sexually transmitted disease, most patients should be screened for other sexually transmitted disease such as syphilis, human immunodeficiency virus (HIV) infection, and hepatitis.

Patients with Crohn's disease may develop a combination of skin tags, fissures, fistulas, and ulcers in perianal skin. Cutaneous amebiasis occurs most frequently in patients with HIV infection and presents with perirectal ulcers, abscesses, and, occasionally, condyloma-like papules or plaques. Squamous cell carcinoma secondary to specific human papillomavirus subtypes produces large condyloma-like lesions (given the eponym *giant condyloma of Buschke-Löwenstein*). Unlike condyloma acuminatum, giant condyloma of Buschke-Löwenstein are very firm and develop fistulas and sinus tracts because of invasion into the dermis.

Treatment: A variety of destructive treatments for condyloma acuminatum exist. Liquid nitrogen is usually the first-line treatment. Other therapies include podophyllin, podophyllin toxin, acids, laser surgery, and intralesional or systemic interferon.

CONTACT DERMATITIS

Definition and etiology: Contact dermatitis is inflammation of the skin resulting from interaction between the skin and the environment. Contact dermatitis can be either an irritant type or an allergic type. Irritant contact dermatitis is a nonimmunologic reaction to a chemical that irritates the skin and causes inflammation. Conversely, allergic contact dermatitis is an individualized immunologic response to the chemical (i.e., the person who is allergic to the chemical will develop a rash when the chemical is absorbed through the skin, whereas another person who is not allergic to the chemical will not develop a rash upon contact). Irritant contact dermatitis is most frequently seen in the hands, whereas allergic contact dermatitis can occur in any part of the body in contact with the allergen.

Clinical features: In acute cases, erythema, scaling, vesicles, and swelling can be found. In patients with persistent disease, the erythema and scaling persist, but vesicles disappear and the skin becomes lichenified. It can be difficult to differentiate between irritant and allergic contact dermatitis. Since both irritant and allergic contact dermatitis can appear identical morphologically, patch testing remains the test of choice in confirming the diagnosis of allergic contact dermatitis. The differential diagnosis includes tinea cruris, diaper dermatitis, extramammary Paget's disease, Hailey-Hailey disease, and, in children, Langerhans cell granulomatosis. Tinea cruris can be excluded by a potassium hydroxide (KOH) examination of a skin scraping. The lesions of tinea cruris also have annular serpiginous borders, and some central clearing may be present. In children, allergic contact dermatitis should be considered when diaper dermatitis fails to respond to therapy. The chafing type of diaper dermatitis can be considered a type of irritant contact dermatitis. In Hailey-Hailey disease (benign familial pemphigus), the primary process is a genetically inherited blistering disease that usually presents in adolescence as maceration, erythema, and erosions in body folds. Linear erosions in a background of red patches in the axilla and groin are the characteristic findings. The rash of extramammary Paget's disease can be confused with dermatitis. The eruption is usually asymmetric, may be irregularly shaped, and may have an eroded or nodular component.

Treatment: Contact dermatitis can be cured by avoidance of the triggering allergen or irritant. Topical and oral steroids hasten the resolution of the rash.

DIAPER DERMATITIS

Definition and etiology: Diaper dermatitis is an eczematous eruption in the diaper area caused by a combination of factors, including occlusion, prolonged contact with urine and stool, bacteria, and *Candida*.

Clinical features: The clinical appearance depends on which etiologic factor is most prominent. In the irritant type of "chafing diaper dermatitis," examination reveals erythematous lichenified plaques and patches in area of friction such as the buttocks, genitalia, and lower abdomen. The inguinal creases are commonly spared. Candidal diaper dermatitis presents with bright red plaques with overlying white scaling and satellite papules and pustules. Unlike in the chafing type of diaper dermatitis, inguinal folds are involved in candidiasis.

The differential diagnosis of diaper dermatitis includes seborrheic dermatitis, psoriasis, atopic dermatitis, tinea cruris, bullous impetigo, chronic bullous disease of childhood, acrodermatitis enteropathica, and Langerhans cell granulomatosis. In infantile and, rarely, adult seborrheic dermatitis, the diaper area develops dusky erythematous scaly plaques. Unlike the irritant or candidal type of diaper dermatitis, infants do not appear to be symptomatic. Associated findings include cradle cap and involvement of the armpits. In atopic dermatitis, the diaper area is usually spared because of the moisture produced by the occlusive diaper. Infants usually have a rash elsewhere, such as the cheeks, and they are often irritable. A family history of atopy can be elicited. Psoriasis usually spares the flexural areas and has a characteristic silver-white-colored scale. Tinea cruris primarily occurs in adults with tinea pedis. The rash is serpiginous with central clearing. KOH test results are positive for fungal elements. Acrodermatitis enteropathica may be acquired or may be inherited as an autosomal recessive disease. A sharply demarcated rash is present around the mouth, in the diaper area, and also on the distal extremities. In Langerhans cell granulomatosis, purpuric foci along with brown-colored papules may be present. A biopsy will reveal proliferation of Langerhans cells rather than the characteristic spongiosis of diaper dermatitis.

Treatment: Infants with diaper dermatitis should have their diapers changed frequently to minimize prolonged contact with urine and feces. After a diaper change, a barrier ointment should be applied. If severe inflammation is present, topical cortisone preparations are necessary. If candidiasis is present, a topical antifungal cream is also needed.

EXTRAMAMMARY PAGET'S DISEASE

Definition: Extramammary Paget's disease (EMPD) is a rare cutaneous adenocarcinoma. The adenocarcinoma is localized to the skin in approximately one-third of cases and is secondary to an underlying adnexal adenocarcinoma in one-third of cases. It can also be secondary to an underlying internal malignancy, typically of genitourinary or gastrointestinal tract origin.

Clinical features: Physical examination reveals a sharply demarcated erythematous scaly plaque. The border may be slightly elevated, and the surface may be covered with a slight crust. EMPD frequently can be mistaken for dermatitis, tinea infection, or Bowen's disease. Dermatitis usually is symmetric, and, unless excoriated, blood or crust should not be present. Patients with tinea cruris usually also have tinea pedis. The rash is symmetric with central clearing, and the KOH test result is positive. Bowen's disease usually occurs in sun-exposed sites and does not have a raised border. When extramammary Paget's disease is suspected, a biopsy should be performed. Biopsy results reveal

large clear cells scattered in a buckshot fashion throughout the epidermis.

Treatment: Small localized lesions can be treated with surgical excision. For larger lesions, treatment with CO_2 lasers has been successful. For surgically unresectable tumors or tumors with underlying adenocarcinoma, a variety of different modalities have been used such as chemotherapy, radiation therapy, and surgical approaches.

HERPES GENITALIS

Definition and etiology: Herpes genitalis is a sexually transmitted herpes simplex virus type II or, rarely, type I infection of the genitalia.

Clinical features: The eruption starts 2 to 10 days after exposure to herpes simplex virus. Usually, patients develop prodromal symptoms of burning, discomfort, or itching at the site of the impending eruption. In a primary episode, patients develop fever and malaise. The lesions start out as red macules that rapidly become vesiculated and develop into widespread erosions. On closer inspection, the erosions are grouped and have scalloped borders characteristic of a herpesvirus infection. The lesions heal spontaneously in a few weeks.

The major diseases in the differential diagnosis are other sexually transmitted diseases such as syphilitic chancre, chancroid, lymphogranuloma venereum, and granuloma inguinale. Prodromal symptoms and grouped blisters do not occur in these other entities, and herpes lesions can be recurrent in some patients. Syphilitic chancres characteristically are painless ulcers with firm nonscalloped borders. Chancroid presents with exquisitely tender ulcers with undermined borders. In granuloma inguinale, red friable papules that ulcerate are seen. In questionable cases, the diagnosis of herpes genitalis can be confirmed by finding multinucleated giant cells in a Tzanck preparation, preparing a culture, or obtaining positive results of direct immunofluorescence in a skin swab specimen.

Treatment: Oral acyclovir, valacyclovir, or famciclovir, if started during the first two days of the infection, can limit the severity and duration of disease.

LANGERHANS CELL GRANULOMATOSIS

Definition and etiology: Langerhans cell granulomatosis (histiocytosis X) is an idiopathic group of diseases caused by proliferation of Langerhans cells. Debate exists as to whether the proliferation of Langerhans cells is reactive or neoplastic. Because of morphologic similarity between proliferating Langerhans cells and histiocytes,

Langerhans cell granulomatosis was previously called histiocytosis X. Langerhans cell granulomatosis can present as a localized, multifocal, or generalized process. The localized form of Langerhans cell granulomatosis has been called eosinophilic granuloma. Multifocal disease with bone lesions, exophthalmos, and diabetes insipidus has been called *Hand-Schüller-Christian disease*, and the generalized form with hepatosplenomegaly, lymphadenopathy, and generalized purpura has been called *Letterer-Siwe disease*.

Clinical features: Langerhans cell granulomatosis is primarily a disease of young children but may present in adults in rare cases. Three forms are widely recognized: eosinophilic granuloma, Hand-Schüller-Christian disease, and Letterer-Siwe disease. Skin findings are most commonly seen in the Hand-Schüller-Christian and Letterer-Siwe variants and consist of small red-brown slightly scaly papules several millimeters in size. Purpura and, occasionally, larger ulcerative nodules and plaques can be present. The scalp and diaper area are most commonly involved. However, in severe cases, lesions can be found over the entire tegmentum. The cutaneous lesions of Langerhans cell granulomatosis are frequently misdiagnosed as seborrheic dermatitis or diaper dermatitis in children. Purpura should not be found in either seborrheic dermatitis or diaper dermatitis. In adults, because of their predilection for the groin and the presence of ulcers, the lesions may also be confused with hidradenitis suppurativa. The red-brown-colored papules can be confused with Darier's disease. Ultimately, a biopsy is necessary for definitive diagnosis and will reveal proliferation of Langerhans cells in the dermis. The cells have kidney-bean-shaped nuclei, stain with antibody against S100 protein, and contain Birbeck granules when studied with the electron microscope.

Treatment: For purely cutaneous involvement, topical steroids, nitrogen mustard, radiation therapy, and oral prednisone can be used. If systemic involvement is present, a variety of chemotherapeutic agents, such as methotrexate, vinblastine, doxorubicin, vincristine, etoposide, and cyclophosphamide, have been used. Prognosis is grave if the lung, bone marrow, or liver is involved.

LICHEN PLANUS

Definition and etiology: Lichen planus is an idiopathic inflammatory dermatitis that can involve both glabrous and mucosal skin. The cause of lichen planus is not known. Certain drugs, such as methyldopa, β-blockers, thiazide diuretics, gold, penicillamine, and nonsteroidal anti-inflammatory agents, can occasionally cause lichen planus.

Clinical features: Lichen planus most commonly occurs between the ages of 30 and 60 years and affects both sexes equally. Lichen planus predominantly affects the flexural surfaces of the arms and the extensor surfaces of the legs. The characteristic lesions are purple-colored, flat-topped polygonal papules and are very pruritic. Wickham's striae are delicate networks of fine white-colored scales that can be seen overlying lesions. The lesions resolve with postinflammatory hyperpigmentation. A variety of morphologic variants can be seen, such as bullous, atrophic, hypertrophic, erosive, ulcerative, erythematous, exfoliative, and follicular lichen planus. The lesions may also have annular or linear arrangements. The Koebner's phenomenon is seen, which consists of lesions occurring at sites of injury. Mucous membranes are affected in approximately half of patients with skin lesions. Thickened dystrophic nails may also be found (see Ch. 5). Patients may rarely present with scarring alopecia as the primary sign of lichen planus (see Ch. 1).

Treatment: Treatment of lichen planus is usually difficult. Any suspected causative drug should be eliminated. Drug-induced lichen planus may take a few months to subside after discontinuation of the offending drug. The most common treatment is topical steroids. Other therapies include topical or systemic retinoids and oral griseofulvin.

LICHEN SCLEROSUS ET ATROPHICUS

Definition and etiology: Lichen sclerosus et atrophicus is an idiopathic disease in which white atrophic patches of skin develop.

Clinical features: Lichen sclerosus et atrophicus occurs most commonly in the genital skin of postmenopausal women. However, lichen sclerosus et atrophicus can also develop in children at times and in skin outside the genital area. Extragenital involvement is somewhat more common in children. In men, lichen sclerosus develops most commonly on the penis in uncircumcised individuals; genital involvement in men is called *balanitis xerotica obliterans*. Patients complain of pruritus, soreness, discomfort, oozing, and pain with intercourse. Examination reveals porcelain-white skin that is atrophic. Follicular plugging may be present. In women, the perivaginal and perirectal distribution of the patches imparts an hourglass appearance. The atrophic skin frequently becomes irritated and red, and vesicles and hemorrhage can result from trauma.

The major diseases in the differential diagnosis are contact dermatitis and vitiligo. The lesions of contact dermatitis are red, pruritic rather than painful, not atrophic, and scaly in appearance. Vitiligo is asymptomatic, and atrophy is also not present. Small, residual, pigmented macules may be seen around hair follicles in patches of vitiligo. In newly developing lesions of lichen sclerosus, a biopsy may be necessary to confirm the diagnosis, since there is less atrophy and more erythema. Biopsy results show edema and sclerosis of the collagen bundles in the upper dermis, follicular plugging, and a bandlike lymphocytic infiltrate.

Treatment: The treatment of choice for lichen sclerosus et atrophicus is high-potency topical corticosteroids. Topical treatment with retinoids and testosterone preparations can also be effective.

PRIMARY SYPHILIS

Definition and etiology: Syphilis (except congenital syphilis) is a sexually transmitted disease caused by the spirochete *Treponema pallidum.* Syphilis is one of the great mimickers and can present with a variety of cutaneous and systemic manifestations.

Clinical features: The clinical features of syphilis can be subdivided into four different stages: primary, secondary, latent, and tertiary. The primary stage occurs 9 to 90 days after inoculation, when a painless, firm ulcer (the chancre) usually develops in the genital region. The chancre has an indurated, round border with a fine erythematous rim. Secondary syphilis, which occurs 8 weeks to approximately 2 years after inoculation, has protean manifestations including a truncal papular rash, moth-eaten alopecia (see Ch. 1), and white wartlike lesions in the genitalia, condyloma latum. Without treatment, the lesions of secondary syphilis resolve, and the disease evolves into a latent stage, only to erupt many years later in some patients as tertiary syphilis. The cutaneous manifestations of tertiary syphilis include nodular, psoriasiform, serpiginous plaques and gummas, which are painless, necrotic, ulcerating nodules.

The differential diagnosis of syphilitic chancre includes other sexually transmitted diseases such as herpes genitalis, chancroid, and lymphogranuloma venereum. The lesions of herpes are vesicular, scalloped, and usually multiple, in contrast to the typical syphilis chancres, which are usually single. The lesions of chancroid are very tender and have an undermined border. Granuloma inguinale presents with friable, vascular-appearing papules that ulcerate. The diagnosis in suspected cases should be confirmed with darkfield microscopy or serologic testing (Venereal Disease Research Laboratories, rapid plasma reagin, and fluorescent treponemal antibody absorption tests).

Treatment: In primary or secondary infections, 2.4 million units of intramuscular penicillin can be used. Oral tetracycline or erythromycin tablets are alternative therapies for penicillin-allergic patients.

TINEA CRURIS

Definition and etiology: Tinea cruris is a dermatophyte infection of the groin folds.

Clinical features: Patients with tinea cruris exhibit erythematous, serpiginous plaques with central clearing in the groin and extending down the thigh. Occasionally, if the fungus extends down into a hair follicle, a nodular component can be present. Extension onto the buttock area occurs frequently. In men, the penis and scrotum are usually spared. Tinea cruris is most commonly seen in men because of the higher incidence of tinea pedis in men, a high level of perspiration, and occlusion from clothing and from the scrotum. Tinea cruris is more common in warmer climates.

The differential diagnosis includes contact dermatitis, intertrigo, Langerhans cell granulomatosis, diaper dermatitis, seborrheic dermatitis, Hailey-Hailey disease, and extramammary Paget's disease. In contact dermatitis, vesicles may be present, and central clearing is absent. Intertrigo and diaper dermatitis are due to a combination of factors such as rubbing, moisture, bacteria, and yeast. The lesions are symmetric, and serpiginous borders are not present. In Langerhans cell granulomatosis, purpuric lesions are usually present, and a biopsy will confirm the diagnosis. Hailey-Hailey disease is an autosomal dominant blistering disease in which the primary lesion is an erosion. It most commonly will also affect the axillary area. Extramammary Paget's disease should be suspected if lesions are asymmetric and do not heal. A biopsy is required for accurate diagnosis.

Treatment: A variety of different topical or oral antifungal agents can be used. Commonly used treatments include imidazole or allylamine creams. Oral therapy with griseofulvin, terbinifine, fluconazole, itraconazole, or ketoconazole can be used in particularly severe or refractory cases in which the diagnosis has been firmly established.

Suggested Readings

BOWENOID PAPULOSIS
Carpenter-Kling JT, Jacyk WK. Anogenital flat papules. Bowenoid papulosis of the genitalia. Arch Dermatol 1994;130:1314.

CONDYLOMA ACUMINATUM
Kling AR. Genital warts—therapy [review]. Semin Dermatol 1992;11:247–55.
Ling MR. Therapy of genital human papillomavirus infections. Part I: Indications for and justification of therapy [review]. Int J Dermatol 1992;31:682–86.
Ling MR. Therapy of genital human papillomavirus infections. Part II: Methods of treatment [see comments] [review]. Int J Dermatol 1992;31:769–76.

Sykes NL Jr. Condyloma acuminatum [review]. Int J Dermatol 1995;34:297–302.

DIAPER DERMATITIS
Longhi F, Carlucci G, Belluci R et al. Diaper dermatitis: a study of contributing factors. Contact Dermatitis 1992;26:248–52.
Singalavanija S, Frieden IJ. Diaper dermatitis [review]. Pediatr Rev 1995;16:142–47.

EXTRAMAMMARY PAGET'S DISEASE
Balducci L, Athar M, Smith GF et al. Extramammary Paget's disease: an annotated review [review]. Cancer Invest 1988;6:293–303.
Saida T, Iwata M. "Ectopic" extramammary Paget's disease affecting the lower anterior aspect of the chest [review]. J Am Acad Dermatol 1987;17:910–13.

LANGERHANS CELL GRANULOMATOSIS
Egeler RM, D'Angio GJ. Langerhans cell histiocytosis [review]. J Pediatrics, 1995;127:1–11.
Egeler RM, Nesbit ME. Langerhans cell histiocytosis and other disorders of monocyte-histiocyte lineage [review]. Crit Rev Oncol Hematol 1995;18:9–35.

LICHEN PLANUS
Shai A, Halevy S. Lichen planus and lichen planus-like eruptions: pathogenesis and associated disease [review]. Int J Dermatol 1992;31:379–84.

LICHEN SCLEROSUS ET ATROPHICUS
Helm KF, Gibson LE, Muller SA. Lichen sclerosus et atrophicus in children and young adults [see comments]. Pediatr Dermatol 1991;8:97–101.
Ridley CM. Lichen sclerosus et atrophicus [review]. Semin Dermatol 1989;8:54–63.
Tremaine RD, Miller RA. Lichen sclerosus et atrophicus [review]. Int J Dermatol 1989;28:10–16.

SYPHILIS
Johnson PC, Farnie MA. Testing for syphilis [review]. Dermatol Clin 1994;12:9–17.
Sanchez MR. Infectious syphilis [review]. Semin Dermatol 1994;13:234–42.

TINEA CRURIS
Aly R. Ecology and epidemiology of dermatophyte infections [review]. J Am Acad Dermatol 1994;31:S21–25.
Cohn MS. Superficial fungal infections. Topical and oral treatment of common types [review]. Postgrad Med 1992;91:239–44.
Odom R. Pathophysiology of dermatophyte infections [review]. J Am Acad Dermatol 1993;28:S2–S7.
Rezabek GH, Friedman AD. Superficial fungal infections of the skin. Diagnosis and current treatment recommendations [review]. Drugs 1992;43:674–82.
Smith EB. Topical antifungal drugs in the treatment of tinea pedis, tinea cruris, and tinea corporis. J Am Acad Dermatol 1993;28:S24–S28.

II

Generalized Rashes

8

Papulosquamous Diseases

ALGORITHM FOR PAPULOSQUAMOUS DISEASES

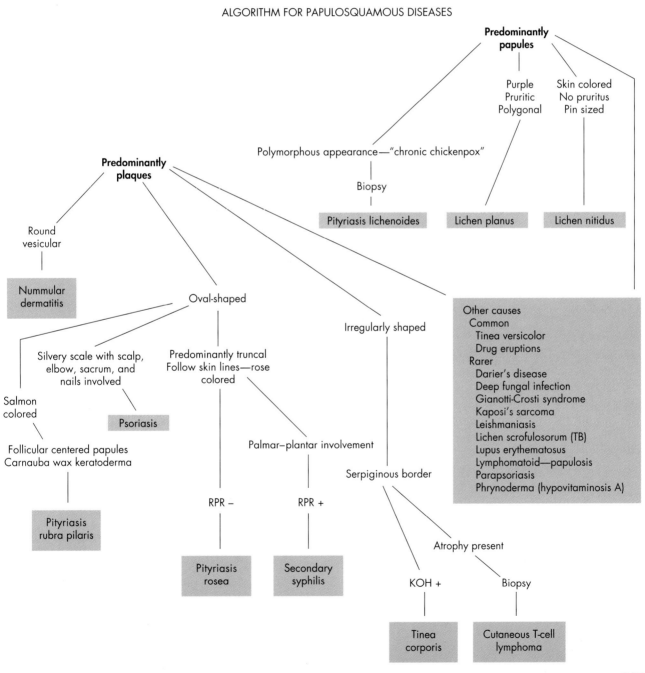

DIFFERENTIAL DIAGNOSIS

DISEASE DISCUSSION

Introduction

A variety of diseases have been classified as papulosquamous disorders. These diseases have the common features of generalized scaling patches, papules, and plaques. The classic papulosquamous diseases include psoriasis, lichen planus, pityriasis rosea, pityriasis rubra pilaris, secondary syphilis, tinea corporis, and nummular dermatitis. The majority of the papulosquamous diseases can be easily diagnosed because of their morphology, distribution, and history. For example, psoriasis predominates on extensor surfaces, has a white silvery scale, and occurs symmetrically. There is often a family history of the disease. Pityriasis rosea is an acute eruption of small pink papules and plaques that follow skin lines on the trunk. The lesions of lichen planus have a purple color and a polygonal appearance and are very pruritic. Tinea corporis can be excluded if skin scrapings treated with potassium hydroxide solution are negative for hyphae. Although the rash of secondary syphilis may mimic pityriasis rosea, an accurate diagnosis can be made by the finding of palmar and plantar papules. These are not found in pityriasis rosea but are characteristic of syphilis. The sexual history, the finding of genital lesions and white mucous patches, and a reactive rapid plasma reagin test all help confirm the diagnosis. Nummular dermatitis usually presents in adults and is characterized by coin-sized eczematous papules and plaques. In this chapter, some uncommon papulosquamous diseases such as lichen nitidus, mycosis fungoides (cutaneous T-cell lymphoma), pityriasis rubra pilaris, and pityriasis lichenoides are also discussed and compared with the diseases they most closely mimic: lichen planus, nummular dermatitis, psoriasis, and scabies infection.

1. PSORIASIS
VERSUS
PITYRIASIS RUBRA PILARIS

Features in common: Red scaly papules and plaques.

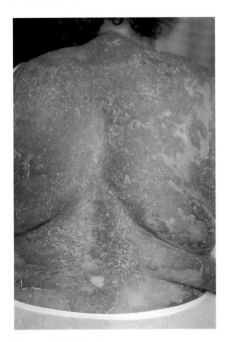

Figure 8.1.1 Psoriasis.

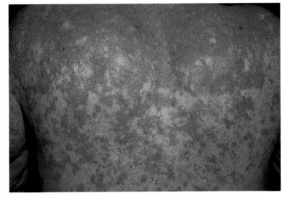

Figure 8.1.2 Pityriasis rubra pilaris.

Distinguishing features

	PSORIASIS	**PITYRIASIS RUBRA PILARIS**
Physical examination	Lesions red-colored	Lesions red-orange in color
	No follicular accentuation	Follicular accentuation
Morphology	When erythrodermic, no islands of normal skin are found	Islands of normal skin when erythrodermic
	Keratoderma uncommon	Keratoderma has a yellow-orange carnauba wax appearance
Distribution	Scalp and extensor surface predilection	Scalp, palmar-plantar surface, and glabrous skin; may be worse in photodistributed areas
Associated findings	Arthritis	No arthritis
	Onychodystrophy	Onychodystrophy
History	Family history in 10% to 20% of patients	Rarely autosomal dominant disorder
	Improves with sun exposure	No improvement with sun exposure
Symptoms	Asymptomatic to moderate pruritus	Asymptomatic to mild pruritus
	Arthritis in some patients	No associated arthritis

Continues

Distinguishing features (Continued)

	PSORIASIS	PITYRIASIS RUBRA PILARIS
History (continued) Exacerbating factors	Infections: streptococcal, HIV, and upper respiratory tract infections Medications: antimalarials, Angiotensin-converting enzyme inhibitors, fluoxetine, β-adrenergic blocking agents, lithium, quinidine, corticosteroid withdrawal; nonsteroidal anti-inflammatory agents	None
Epidemiology	Any age; no sex predilection	Any age; no sex predilection
Biopsy	Usually not necessary Psoriasiform epidermal hyperplasia with neutrophil microabscesses in epidermis and stratum corneum	Yes Chronic dermatitis, parakeratotic mounds around follicular orifices, and alternating areas of parakeratosis in vertical and horizontal pattern within stratum corneum
Laboratory	None	None
Treatment	Topical: steroids, tars, calcipotriene, anthralin Ultraviolet light B, PUVA Systemic treatments: methotrexate, etretinate, cyclosporine	Topical steroids are not effective Ultraviolet light: not effective Systemic treatments: methotrexate, etretinate, accutane
Outcome	Chronic Variable response to therapy	Chronic Poor response to therapy, but eventually remits after months to years

Abbreviations: HIV, human immunodeficiency virus; PUVA, psoralen plus ultraviolet A light.

Differential diagnosis of papulosquamous lesions

Common causes
  Drug eruption
  Lichen planus
  Nummular dermatitis
  Pityriasis rosea
  Psoriasis
  Seborrheic dermatitis
  Tinea corporis/versicolor
  Tinea versicolor
Rarer causes
  Cutaneous T-cell lymphoma
    (mycosis fungoides)

Rarer causes (continued)
  Darier's disease
  Deep fungal infection
    (coccidioidomycosis)
  Erythema annulare centrifugum
  Gianotti-Crosti syndrome
  Kaposi's sarcoma in patients with
    acquired immunodeficiency
    syndrome
  Leprosy
  Leishmaniasis
  Lichen nitidus
  Lichen spinulosus

Rarer causes (continued)
  Lichen scrofulosorum
  Lymphomatoid papulosis
  Lupus erythematosus
  Mycosis fungoides
  Pityriasis lichenoides
  Pityriasis rubra pilaris
  Parapsoriasis
  Phrynoderma (vitamin A
    deficiency)
  Secondary syphilis

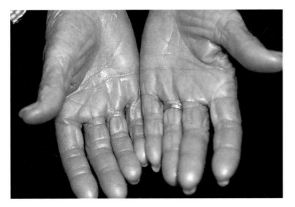

Figure *8.1.3* Pityriasis rubra pilaris. *Clue to diagnosis:* Carnauba-wax-like keratoderma.

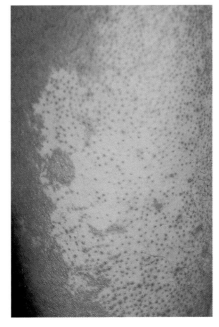

Figure *8.1.4* Pityriasis rubra pilaris. *Clue to diagnosis:* Follicular-based papules.

2. PSORIASIS
VERSUS
NUMMULAR DERMATITIS

Features in common: Scaly plaques.

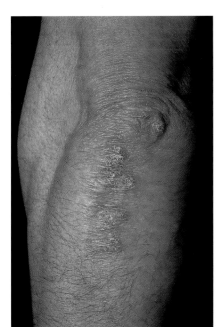

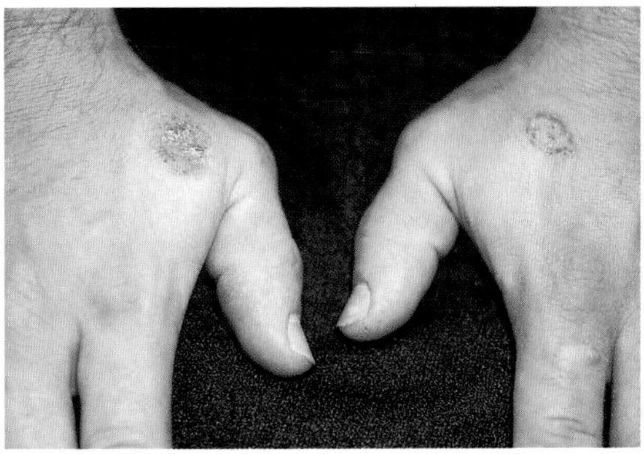

Figure *8.2.2* Nummular dermatitis.

Figure *8.2.1* Psoriasis.

Distinguishing features

	PSORIASIS	NUMMULAR DERMATITIS
Physical examination	No vesicles	Small vesicles and papules within plaques
Morphology	No crust Silvery scale Koebner's phenomenon Lesions range in size from few millimeters to several centimeters	Crust Flesh-colored to white scale No Koebner's phenomenon Lesions the size of a quarter
Distribution	Scalp and predilection for extensor surfaces of body (elbows, knees)	Trunk and extremities
Associated findings	Arthritis Onychodystrophy (often with subungual oil spot and pits) No dry skin	No arthritis No nail dystrophy Dry skin
History	Family history in 10% to 20% of patients	No family history
Symptoms	Improves with sun exposure Asymptomatic to moderate pruritus	No improvement with sun exposure More common in wintertime Asymptomatic to marked pruritus
Exacerbating factors	Infections: streptococcal, HIV, and upper respiratory tract infections Medications: antimalarials, angiotensin-converting enzyme inhibitors, β-adrenergic blocking agents, lithium, quinidine, corticosteroid withdrawal, nonsteroidal anti-inflammatory drugs	Dry skin Not associated with infection No medications
Epidemiology	Any age; no sex predilection	Adult men predominate
Biopsy	Usually not necessary Epidermal hyperplasia with neutrophil microabscesses in epidermis and stratum corneum	No Hyperplasia of the epidermis with prominent spongiosis, scale crust, and a superficial perivascular infiltrate
Laboratory	None	None
Treatment	Topical: steroids, tars, calcipotriol ointment Ultraviolet light Systemic: methotrexate, retinoids, cyclosporine, PUVA	Topical: corticosteroid creams, emollients Systemic: occasionally antibiotics
Outcome	Chronic disease	Self-limited disease with periodic exacerbation

Abbreviations: HIV, human immunodeficiency virus; PUVA, psoralen plus ultraviolet A light.

Drugs producing psoriasiform dermatitis or exacerbating psoriasis

Antimalarials
Angiotensin-converting enzyme inhibitors
β-adrenergic receptor blocking agents
Corticosteroid withdrawal

Lithium
Nonsteroidal anti-inflammatory drugs
  (not well established—isolated reports)
Quinidine

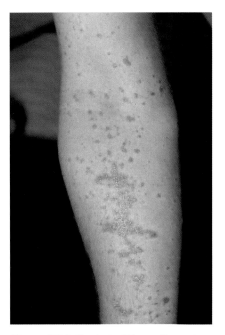

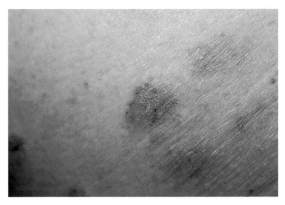

Figure 8.2.4 Nummular dermatitis. *Clue to diagnosis:* Coin-sized eczematous plaques.

Figure 8.2.3 Psoriasis. *Clue to diagnosis:* Koebner's reaction (lesions, in this case linear lesions, develop in sites of scratching).

3. PITYRIASIS ROSEA
VERSUS
SECONDARY SYPHILIS

Features in common: Oval scaly patches and plaques on trunk.

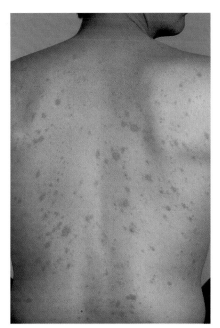

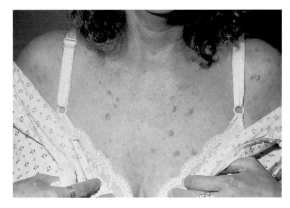

Figure 8.3.2 Secondary syphilis.

Figure 8.3.1 Pityriasis rosea.

Distinguishing features

	PITYRIASIS ROSEA	SECONDARY SYPHILIS
Physical examination	Fine white scale No palmar or plantar lesions	Minimal scale Macules and papules frequently found on palms and soles
Morphology	Disease starts as a single large patch (herald patch) No mucous patch	No herald patch White patches may be found on lips or mouth (mucous patch)
Distribution	Primarily truncal and proximal extremities	Involves entire body
History	Not associated with sexual contact	Sexual contact
Symptoms	Prodrome of fever and malaise in 5% of patients	Generalized malaise common
Exacerbating factors	None (possibly associated with upper respiratory tract infections)	Other sexually transmitted disease Immunosuppression (human immunodeficiency virus)
Associated findings	Lymphadenopathy rare	Lymphadenopathy common Hepatitis, arthritis
Epidemiology	75% of patients between age 10 and 35; most common in fall, winter, and spring	Sexually active
Biopsy	Usually not necessary Epidermal acanthosis, spongiosis, parakeratotic mounds, and superficial perivascular lymphocytic infiltrate	Usually not done Psoriasiform hyperplasia of epidermis with superficial and deep perivascular and bandlike lymphoplasmacytic infiltrate Warthin-Starry stain positive for spirochetes in many cases
Laboratory	RPR negative	RPR positive
Treatment	Antipruritics Ultraviolet light	Antibiotics (penicillin derivatives)
Outcome	Resolves spontaneously	Lesions resolve without treatment, but disease persists in a latent stage and eventually may present as tertiary syphilis

Abbreviation: RPR, rapid plasma reagin.

Drugs producing pityriasis-rosea-like eruption

Barbiturates Gold Metronidazole
Captopril Isotretinoin Penicillamine
Clonidine

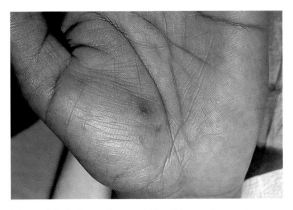

Figure 8.3.3 Secondary syphilis. *Clue to diagnosis:* Palmar lesions.

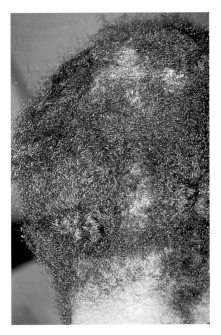

Figure 8.3.4 Secondary syphilis. *Clue to diagnosis:* Moth-eaten alopecia.

4. PITYRIASIS ROSEA
VERSUS
GUTTATE PSORIASIS

Features in common: Small, round, red scaly plaques and patches.

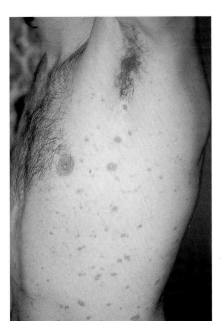

Figure 8.4.1 Pityriasis rosea.

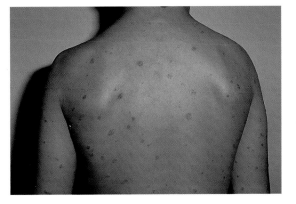

Figure 8.4.2 Guttate psoriasis.

Distinguishing features

	PITYRIASIS ROSEA	GUTTATE PSORIASIS
Physical examination	Pink oval plaques Fine white scale	Red scaly papules and plaques Adherent silvery scale
Morphology	Disease starts as a single large patch (herald patch) Long axis of lesions follows skin lines No Koebner's reaction	No herald patch Lesions do not follow skin lines Koebner's reaction
Distribution	Primarily truncal and proximal extremities Scalp and distal extremities not involved	Trunk and extremities favored (elbows, knees) Scalp commonly involved
History	No family history Prodrome of fever and malaise in 5% of patients	Family history in 10% to 20% of patients Prodrome of streptococcal pharyngitis in majority of children
Symptoms	Asymptomatic or mild pruritus	Asymptomatic to mild pruritus
Exacerbating factors	May improve with sun exposure	Improves with sun exposure
Associated findings	No arthritis No onychodystrophy	Arthritis Onychodystrophy
Epidemiology	75% of patients between age 10 and 35; most common in fall, winter, and spring	Most common in children
Biopsy	Usually not necessary Slight epidermal acanthosis, spongiosis, parakeratotic mounds, and superficial perivascular lymphocytic infiltrate	Usually not necessary Epidermal hyperplasia with neutrophil microabscesses in epidermis and stratum corneum
Laboratory	Rapid plasma reagin negative	Positive anti-streptolysin-O antibody or streptozyme titer
Treatment	Antihistamines Topical corticosteroids Ultraviolet B light	Oral antibiotics (e.g., penicillin, erythromycin) Topicals: steroids, tars, anthralin, calcipotriene Ultraviolet B light, psoralen plus ultraviolet A light
Outcome	Resolves spontaneously	Acute or chronic disease 50% of children with guttate psoriasis may clear with antibiotic therapy only

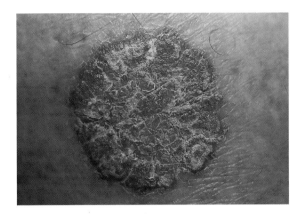

Figure 8.4.3 Psoriasis. *Clue to diagnosis:* White-silvery-colored scale.

5. PITYRIASIS ROSEA
VERSUS
TINEA CORPORIS

Features in common: Scaly papules and plaques.

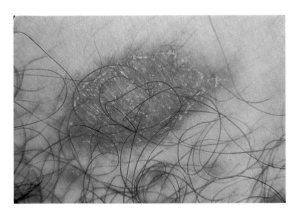

Figure 8.5.1 Herald plaque of pityriasis rosea.

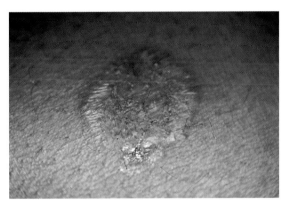

Figure 8.5.2 Tinea corporis.

Distinguishing features

	PITYRIASIS ROSEA	TINEA CORPORIS
Physical examination	Pink oval plaques Fine white scale	Red serpiginous plaques Coarse scale
Morphology	Disease starts as a single large patch (herald patch) Long axis of lesions follows skin lines No central clearing	No herald patch Unrelated to skin lines Central clearing
Distribution	Primarily truncal and proximal extremities	Any glabrous skin

Continues

Distinguishing features (*Continued*)

	PITYRIASIS ROSEA	**TINEA CORPORIS**
History	Prodrome of fever and malaise in 5% of patients	No fever or malaise
Symptoms	Asymptomatic or mild pruritus	Mild to moderate pruritus
Exacerbating factors	None	Immunosuppression Corticosteroids
Associated findings	Arthritis Onychodystrophy No tinea pedis	No arthritis Onychomycosis Tinea pedis
Epidemiology	75% of patients between age 10 and 35; most common in fall, winter, and spring	Any age; more common in wrestlers, people with athlete's foot or with pets
Biopsy	No Slight epidermal acanthosis, spongiosis, parakeratotic mounds, and superficial perivascular lymphocytic infiltrate	No Neutrophilic scale crust, spongiosis, and organisms within stratum corneum
Laboratory	Rapid plasma reagin test negative	Potassium hydroxide test positive and positive culture on DTM (dermatophyte test medium)
Treatment	Antihistamines Topical corticosteroids Ultraviolet light	Topical allylamine or imidazole antifungal agents or in widespread or refractory cases, oral griseofulvin or imidazole agents
Outcome	Resolves spontaneously	Curable with therapy

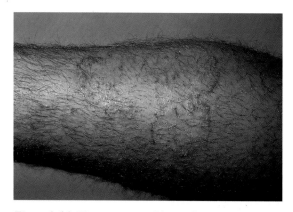

Figure 8.5.3 Tinea corporis. *Clue to diagnosis:* Serpiginous borders with central clearing.

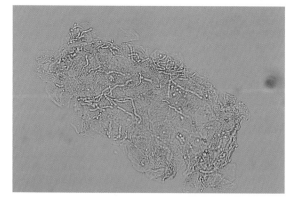

Figure 8.5.4 Tinea corporis. *Clue to diagnosis:* Skin scraping treated with potassium hydroxide (KOH) solution, which accentuates numerous hyphae among keratinocytes.

6. PSORIASIS

VERSUS

LICHEN PLANUS

Features in common: Scaly papules and plaques.

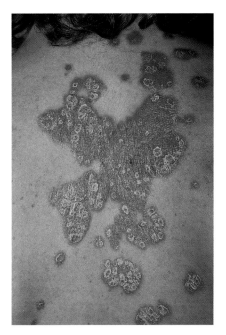

Figure 8.6.1 Psoriasis.

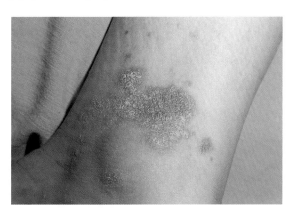

Figure 8.6.2 Lichen planus.

Distinguishing features

	PSORIASIS	LICHEN PLANUS
Physical examination		
Morphology	Red-colored	Purple color
	Coarse white scale	Fine white scale forming a collarette in periphery of lesions (Wickham's striae)
Distribution	Extensor surface of arms and legs (elbows, knees)	Flexural surface of forearms Extensor surface of legs
	Scalp involvement common	Scalp involvement rare
History	Family history in 10% to 20% of patients	No family history
	Improves with sun exposure	Gradual onset
Symptoms	Asymptomatic to moderate pruritus	Moderate to severe pruritus
	Arthritis in some patients	No arthritis

Continues

Distinguishing features (Continued)

	PSORIASIS	LICHEN PLANUS
History (continued) Exacerbating factors	Infections: streptococcal, human immunodeficiency virus, and upper respiratory tract infections Medications: antimalarials, angiotensin-converting enzyme inhibitors, β-adrenergic blocking agents, lithium, quinidine, fluoxetine, corticosteroid withdrawal, nonsteroidal anti-inflammatory drugs	Infections: hepatitis C Medications: angiotensin-converting enzyme inhibitors, nonsteroidal anti-inflammatory drugs, sulfonyl-ureas, gold, penicillamine, thiazides, carbamazepin, methyldopa, lithium, quinidine, quinine, β-blockers
Associated findings	Arthritis Onychodystrophy No oral lesions No associated autoimmune disease or internal malignancy	No arthritis Onychodystrophy White reticulated oral patches Rarely associated with other autoimmune diseases or internal malignancy
Epidemiology	Any age	Mostly middle-aged adults
Biopsy	No Psoriasiform epidermal hyperplasia with neutrophil microabscesses in epidermis and stratum corneum	Yes Irregular epidermal hyperplasia in a "sawtoothed" pattern, colloid bodies, wedge-shaped hypergranulosis, and a dense lymphocytic infiltrate obscuring the dermal epidermal junction
Laboratory	None	None
Treatment	Topicals: steroids, tars, anthralin, calcipotriene Ultraviolet light Systemic: methotrexate, retinoids, cyclosporine	Topical steroids Systemic: rarely oral steroids or retinoids
Outcome	Chronic disease	Resolves over months to years

Common treatments for psoriasis

Topical
  Corticosteroids
  Tars
  Anthralin
  Calcipotriene
  Retinoids
  Zinc pyrithione

Light
  Psoralen plus ultraviolet A or
    ultraviolet B phototherapy
Systemic
  Retinoids
  Methotrexate
  Cyclosporine
  Tacrolimus

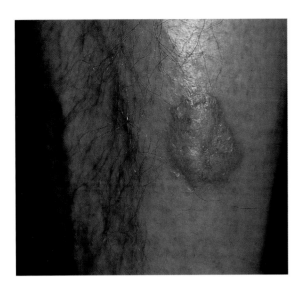

Figure 8.6.3 Lichen planus. *Clue to diagnosis:* Purple color.

7. CUTANEOUS T-CELL LYMPHOMA
VERSUS
NUMMULAR DERMATITIS

Features in common: Erythematous scaly plaques.

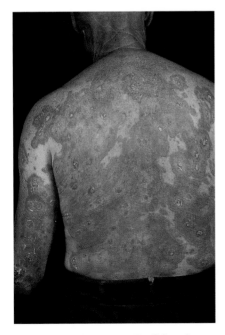

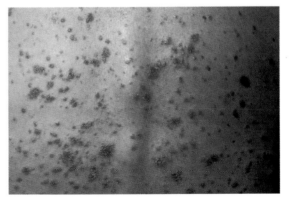

Figure 8.7.2 Nummular dermatitis.

Figure 8.7.1 Cutaneous T-cell lymphoma.

Distinguishing features

	CUTANEOUS T-CELL LYMPHOMA	NUMMULAR DERMATITIS
Physical examination	Red patches, plaques, and nodules No vesicles	Red plaques Small vesicles and papules frequently present within plaques
Morphology	No crust Scale but not prominent Lesions variable in size Lesions frequently have serpiginous borders Telangiectasias and fine wrinkling are present in patches	Crust Prominent scale Lesions the size of a quarter Lesions round No telangiectasias or wrinkling
Distribution	Trunk, extremities	Trunk, extremities
History	Chronic rash refractory to therapy	Rash worsens in winter months
Symptoms	Asymptomatic to severe pruritus	Mild to moderate pruritus
Exacerbating factors	None	Dry skin Emotional stress
Associated findings	Lymphadenopathy Hepatosplenomegaly	No lymphadenopathy No hepatosplenomegaly
Epidemiology	Adult men	Adult men

Biopsy	Yes; often nonspecific early on
	Bandlike infiltrate with atypical
	  cerebriform lymphocytes extending
	  into epidermis
		No
		Dermatitis: psoriasiform
		  hyperplasia of the epidermis with
		  spongiosis, scale crust, and
		  superficial perivascular infiltrate

Laboratory	Sézary prep for circulating atypical lymphocytes	None

Treatment	Topical: steroids, nitrogen mustard
	Light: ultraviolet B, psoralen plus
	  ultraviolet A
	Systemic: methotrexate, chemotherapy
	Radiation therapy (e.g., electron
	  beam therapy)
		Topical steroids
		Emollients
		Short course of systemic
		  corticosteroids

Outcome	Chronic slowly progressive lymphoma;
	  approximately 50% of patients will
	  die of unrelated causes; occasional
	  transformation to anaplastic lymphoma
		Self-limited disease

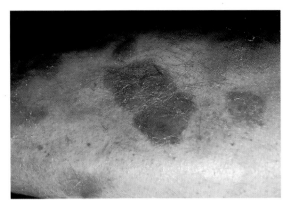

Figure 8.7.3 Cutaneous T-cell lymphoma. *Clue to diagnosis:* Indurated plaques and nodules.

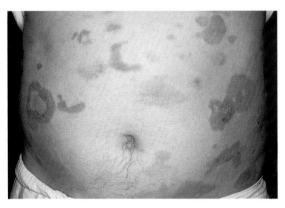

Figure 8.7.4 Cutaneous T-cell lymphoma. *Clue to diagnosis:* Serpiginous annular plaques.

8. LICHEN PLANUS
VERSUS
LICHEN NITIDUS

Features in common: Small scaly papules.

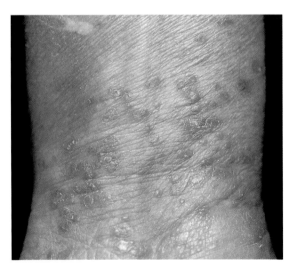

Figure 8.8.1 Lichen planus.

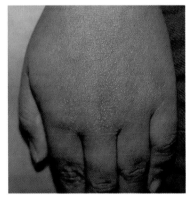

Figure 8.8.2 Lichen nitidus.

Distinguishing features

	LICHEN NITIDUS	LICHEN PLANUS
Physical examination		
Morphology	Pin-sized discrete papules	Papules and plaques
	Skin color	Purple color
	Minimal scale	Fine white scale forming a collarette in periphery of lesions (Wickham's striae)
Distribution	Forearms, extensor surface	Forearms, flexoral surface
	Abdomen, chest, buttocks, and genitals commonly involved	Abdomen, chest, buttocks less frequently involved
	Legs less commonly involved	Extensor surface of legs
History		
Symptoms	Lesions asymptomatic	Moderate to severe pruritus
Exacerbating factors	None	Infections: hepatitis C
		Medications: angiotensin-converting enzyme inhibitors, nonsteroidal anti-inflammatory drugs, β-blockers, sulfonylureas, gold, penicillamine, carbamazepine, methyldopa, lithium, quinidine, quinine
Associated findings	No onychodystrophy	Onychodystrophy
	Mucous membrane lesions rare	White reticulated oral patches
	Occasionally associated with lichen planus	Rarely associated with other autoimmune diseases
	Reported to be seen in Crohn's disease	No association with Crohn's disease
Epidemiology	Children and young adults	Mostly middle-aged adults
	Blacks more commonly involved	
Biopsy	Yes	Yes
	Focal lymphohistiocytic infiltrate surrounded by epidermis forming "ball in claw" appearance	Irregular epidermal hyperplasia in a "sawtooth" pattern, colloid bodies, wedge-shaped hypergranulosis, and a dense lymphocytic infiltrate obscuring the dermal-epidermal junction
Laboratory	None	None
Treatment	Topical steroids	Topical steroids
		Rarely oral steroids or retinoids
Outcome	May resolve within weeks or last years	Resolves over months to years

Possible etiologic factors in lichen-planus-like eruptions

Medications

Angiotensin-converting
enzyme inhibitors

Nonsteroidal anti-inflammatory drugs

β-Blockers

Sulfonylureas

Thiazide diuretics

Medications (continued)

Miscellaneous: gold, penicillamine, carbamazepine,
methyldopa, lithium, quinidine, quinine

Infections

Hepatitis C

Neoplasms

Graft-vs.-host disease

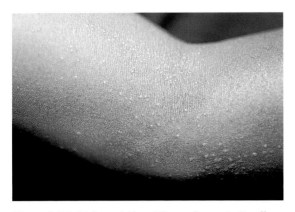

Figure 8.8.3 Lichen nitidus. *Clue to diagnosis:* Small size of papules.

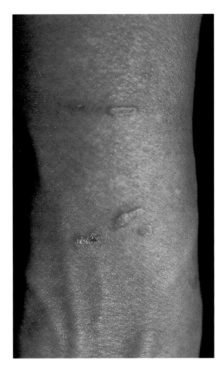

Figure 8.8.4 Lichen planus. *Clue to diagnosis:* Purple color with Koebner's phenomenon.

9. PSORIASIS
VERSUS
PITYRIASIS LICHENOIDES

Features in common: Red scaly papules and plaques.

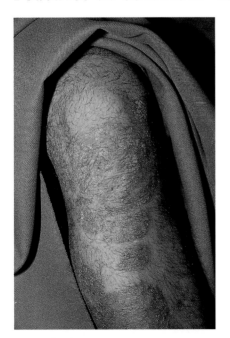

Figure 8.9.1 Psoriasis.

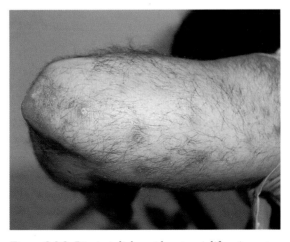

Figure 8.9.2 Pityriasis lichenoides et varioliformis acuta.

Distinguishing features

	PSORIASIS	PITYRIASIS LICHENOIDES
Physical examination	No vesicles	Papulovesicular lesions
Morphology	Silvery scale	Yellow-brown-colored micaceous-like scale
	No crust present	Crust
	Appearance of lesions monomorphous	Appearance of lesions polymorphous
	No scarring	Lesions heal with scar
Distribution	Generalized: predilection for extensor surfaces of body and scalp	Generalized: trunk, thighs, upper arms; predilection for flexural surfaces
History	Family history of psoriasis in 10%–20% of patients may be present	No family history
	No fever except in pustular variants	Occasionally fever at onset
Symptoms	Disease usually insidious, slow onset	Sudden onset of lesions in crops
	Asymptomatic to moderate pruritus	Asymptomatic
Exacerbating factors	Infections: Streptococcal, human immunodeficiency virus, and upper respiratory tract Medications: antimalarials, angiotensin-converting enzyme inhibitors, β-adrenergic blocking agents, corticosteroid withdrawal, lithium, quinidine, nonsteroidal anti-inflammatory drugs	None known
Associated findings	No associated malignancies	Rarely associated with lymphomatoid papulosis or cutaneous T-cell lymphoma
	Arthritis	No arthritis
	Onychodystrophy	No onychodystrophy
Epidemiology	Any age	More common in children
Biopsy	Usually not necessary Psoriasiform epidermal hyperplasia with neutrophil microabscesses in epidermis and stratum corneum	Yes Wedge-shaped lichenoid infiltrate with epidermal necrosis, scale crust, extravasated erythrocytes in epidermis and upper dermis
Laboratory	None	None
Treatment	Topical therapy: corticosteroids, tars, anthralin, calcipotriene, and retinoids	No optimal therapy Topical therapy: corticosteroids Oral antibiotics occasionally are helpful: erythromycin or tetracycline
	Light: ultraviolet B, PUVA	Light: PUVA
	Systemic therapy: retinoids, methotrexate, cyclosporine	Systemic therapy: rarely methotrexate
Outcome	Chronic	Acute to chronic

Abbreviation: PUVA, psoralen plus ultraviolet A light.

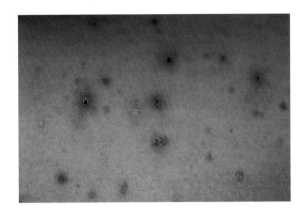

Figure 8.9.3 Pityriasis lichenoides.
Clue to diagnosis: Crusted chickenpox-
like papules.

Discussion

CUTANEOUS T-CELL LYMPHOMA

Definition and etiology: Cutaneous T-cell lymphoma (mycosis fungoides) is a slowly progressive malignancy of helper T lymphocytes that have an affinity for the skin.

Clinical features: Although mycosis fungoides is not an inflammatory dermatosis, most affected individuals have scaling plaques that resemble dermatitis. The disease is often misclassified as a dermatitis for approximately 5 to 6 years before an accurate diagnosis is made. Early on, the clinical and pathologic findings are nondiagnostic. Three clinical stages of cutaneous T-cell lymphoma (mycosis fungoides) are recognized, which correspond with progressive evolution of the lymphoma: patch, plaque, and nodular stages. In the patch stage, slightly scaly, well-demarcated patches of varying sizes occur on the trunk and extremities. Lesions resemble dermatitis or psoriasis. Unlike in dermatitis or psoriasis, scaling is slight, but erythema may be prominent. There is a predilection for the chest and buttocks. Biopsy at this stage is most often nondiagnostic. On closer inspection of the skin, slight atrophy (manifested as telangiectasia and wrinkling) is present. Patches become progressively thicker, redder, and more indurated as the transition to the plaque stage occurs. Plaques frequently have a somewhat annular and serpiginous appearance. Over several years, nodules develop. Some of the nodules may ulcerate. The development of nodular lesions correlates with genetic transformation of the lymphoma to a more aggressive state.

The major diseases in the differential diagnosis include dermatitis, psoriasis, and drug eruption. Atrophy is typically a feature of at least some of the lesions of mycosis fungoides. Other lesions may be serpiginous, and scaling is on the average less than that encountered in dermatoses. When an adult has generalized dermatitis that cannot be classified as contact dermatitis, atopic dermatitis, nummular dermatitis, dermatitis medicamentosa, or seborrheic dermatitis, mycosis fungoides should be suspected. Biopsy of the lesions should be done periodically to establish a diagnosis of mycosis fungoides. Serial biopsies over time are often necessary because the histologic findings in the first few years may be nonspecific. Some pathologists have a relatively high index of suspicion for mycosis fungoides and may diagnose it with a high frequency but with false positive findings; other pathologists may diagnose mycosis fungoides with less sensitivity but with a higher rate of specificity. A biopsy diagnostic for cutaneous T-cell lymphoma will reveal a bandlike infiltrate within the dermis with extension of lymphocytes into the epidermis (epidermotropism). In psoriasis, silver-colored scaling plaques involve the scalp, elbows, and knees. Nodules do not occur. Certain drugs, especially seizure medications such as phenytoin (Dilantin), can also produce a mycosis-fungoides-like rash. Biopsy may reveal an increased number of lymphocytes trafficking in the skin, closely mimicking results seen in mycosis fungoides. A drug eruption should be suspected if the eruption starts a few weeks after a new medication is taken.

Treatment: Many different treatment options exist, but unfortunately no universally proven cure is available. For patch-stage lesions, topical treatment with nitrogen mustard (mechlorethamine) cream, ointment, or solution; psolaren plus ultraviolet A light (PUVA); or topical steroids can be used. In our experience, photochemotherapy with psoralen and ultraviolet A light is most helpful. Total-body electron-beam therapy, oral retinoids, ultraviolet B light, and combinations thereof are also effective. For advanced disease, systemic interferon therapy and conventional chemotherapy can be used. Cutaneous T-cell lymphoma is a chronic disease with a long-term survival of greater than 10 years for patients with patch- or plaque-stage disease. Approximately 50% of patients die of unrelated causes. The rest may die of sepsis or tumor burden.

LICHEN NITIDUS

Definition and etiology: Lichen nitidus is an uncommon, usually self-limited, inflammatory dermatosis of unknown cause characterized by flesh-colored discrete papules.

Clinical features: Pinhead-sized (1 to 2 mm) papules are seen, predominantly overlying the forearms, abdomen, chest, genitalia, and buttocks. A relationship between lichen planus and lichen nitidus has been considered, but lesions of lichen nitidus are skin colored and asymptomatic, unlike those of lichen planus. Mucosal involvement in lichen nitidus is extremely rare; when it occurs, it consists of papules and not the white reticulated patches characteristic of lichen planus. Pitting of the nails may occur but not the onychodystrophy seen in lichen planus. Occasionally, lesions of both lichen planus and lichen nitidus can be found in the same patient.

The differential diagnosis includes lichen scrofulosorum, which is a now uncommon manifestation of tuberculosis infection; keratosis pilaris; phrynoderma; and lichen spinulosus. In lichen scrofulosorum, small grouped lichenoid papules develop as a hypersensitivity response to *Mycobacterium tuberculosis*. Lesions of lichen scrofulosorum are yellow to reddish-brown in color and occur predominantly on the trunk. Lesions of keratosis pilaris are follicular based and rough to palpation. Skin-colored horny papules are located on the extensor surfaces of thighs and arms. Lichen spinulosus is a variant of keratosis pilaris. The horny papules in lichen spinulosus are distributed in clusters that form plaques several centimeters in diameter. Rare diseases to be considered in the differential diagnosis include phrynoderma (vitamin A deficiency), drug eruptions, lichenoid sarcoidosis, and secondary syphilis. Biopsy findings in lichen nitidus reveal focal lymphohistiocytic infiltrate in the papillary dermis surrounded by a collarette of epidermis. This configuration is often referred to as a "ball and claw" pattern.

Treatment: The natural course of lichen nitidus is variable, with disease lasting a few weeks to several years. A short course of several months is typical. Topical steroids may be of some help.

LICHEN PLANUS

Definition and etiology: Lichen planus is an idiopathic inflammatory disease characterized by a generalized eruption of purple papules that occurs on both glabrous and mucosal skin. Certain drugs such as methyldopa, β-blockers, thiazide diuretics, gold, penicillamine, and nonsteroidal anti-inflammatory agents can occasionally produce an eruption indistinguishable from classic idiopathic lichen planus.

Clinical features: Lesions of lichen planus most commonly occur on the flexural surface of the forearms near the wrists and on the extensor surfaces of the legs near the shin and ankle. Lichen planus can involve any glabrous skin surface. Nail and mucosal involvement is common (see Chs. 3 and 4). Diagnosis is usually possible on clinical inspection of characteristic purple polygonal papules. Lesions are most often very pruritic and covered with a fine white scale called Wickham's striae. Like psoriasis, lesions of lichen planus spread to areas of trauma (Koebner's phenomenon). Other morphologic variants of lichen planus include linear, annular, actinic, atrophic, hypertrophic, erythematous, follicular, exfoliative, and bullous types.

The major diseases in the differential diagnosis include lichen nitidus, psoriasis, lichen simplex chronicus, and lichen striatus. Lichen-planus-like lesions can be seen in patients with chronic graft-vs.-host disease and in overlap syndromes (lichen planus with lupus erythematosus, or lichen planus with bullous pemphigoid). In lichen nitidus, lesions are small pinpoint-sized papules that are skin colored and nonpruritic. The distribution of psoriasis is different than that of lichen planus, with prominent extensor surface involvement, the absence of oral lesions, and the presence of a white silvery scale. Lesions of lichen simplex chronicus are secondary to chronic rubbing. They are few and are usually located above the ankles or on the posterior neck. Examination of lichen simplex chronicus reveals thick red papules or plaques with prominent skin lines. In lichen striatus, the eruption is usually limited to a single elongated lesion composed of coalescing papules. Unlike in lichen planus, the papules and plaques are more pink than violaceous, and Wickham's striae are not present. Biopsy of lichen planus reveals irregular epidermal acanthosis with elongated and jagged rete ridges that resemble the teeth of a saw. Wedge-shaped hypergranulosis, compact orthokeratosis, colloid bodies, and a lymphocytic infiltrate that obscures the dermal-epidermal junction are all characteristic findings on biopsy of typical lesions.

Treatment: Lichen planus is difficult to treat. Use of topical corticosteroids leads to some improvement. In patients with extensive disease, a short course of oral prednisone or intramuscular corticosteroids is beneficial. Psoralen plus ultraviolet A light (PUVA) and retinoids are helpful. Griseofulvin, other oral antifungal agents, and antibiotics have been reported to be helpful, but these findings have not been confirmed by results of larger trials.

NUMMULAR DERMATITIS

Definition and etiology: Nummular dermatitis is characterized by coin-shaped eczematous plaques. Precipitating factors include dry skin, irritation due to topical agents such as soaps, diuretics, forced air heating, and secondary bacterial colonization.

Clinical features: Nummular dermatitis occurs most commonly in adult men but can also occur in children and women. The sites of predilection include the trunk, hands, forearms, and areas with the least number of sebaceous glands. The hallmark of nummular dermatitis is oval pruritic plaques. Individual plaques are discrete and well marginated. They are erythematous, scaling, and edematous; may weep serous fluid; and have overlying crust. Vesicles may be present on the surface of the plaques along with areas of oozing and crust.

The differential diagnosis includes psoriasis, pityriasis lichenoides, discoid lupus erythematosus, and other papulosquamous diseases. Isolated lesions can be confused with basal cell carcinoma or squamous cell carcinoma (see Ch. 13). Lesions of psoriasis are bright red and not dusky red in color. They are covered with silvery scale. Scalp and nail involvement does not occur in nummular dermatitis. Pityriasis lichenoides affects children most commonly and also young adults. Lesions develop in sudden crops, and papules predominate rather than plaques. The lesions have central necrosis with scale crust formation and may scar. Although lesions of discoid lupus erythematosus may also be coin shaped, lesions of cutaneous lupus have foci of atrophy, follicular plugging, hyper- and hypopigmentation, and telangectasias. In addition, when scales are gently lifted from the skin, they have the appearance of carpet tacks.

Treatment: The mainstay of therapy for nummular dermatitis is topical steroids and emollients. In impetiginized lesions, antibiotics may also be helpful.

PITYRIASIS LICHENOIDES

Definition and etiology: Pityriasis lichenoides (guttate parapsoriasis) is an idiopathic papulosquamous disease with both an acute and a chronic form. The acute variant, pityriasis lichenoides et varioliformis acuta, has also been called Mucha-Habermann disease, while pityriasis lichenoides chronica has been called guttate parapsoriasis.

Clinical features: Pityriasis lichenoides occurs mainly in adolescents and young adults. A slight male predominance has been reported. Pityriasis lichenoides acuta is characterized by the sudden onset of papules on the trunk, thigh, and upper arms. Some individuals have primarily truncal lesions, others have acral lesions, and some have a combination of both. Papules frequently have small central vesicles. With time, central necrosis and crust develop. Lesions may be purpuric. Crops of lesions develop, as in varicella. Papules in different stages of evolution are characteristic. The polymorphous appearance and persistence of the eruption are clues to diagnosis. Scarring may occur. Patients with pityriasis lichenoides may closely resemble individuals with varicella (chickenpox). Pityriasis lichenoides chronica may develop from the acute form or

de novo. Papulosquamous lesions predominate instead of vesicles or necrotic lesions. Unlike in the acute form, vesicular necrotic papules are not present. The papules and plaques are covered with a micaceous (thin-layered) platelike scale.

The differential diagnosis of pityriasis lichenoides acuta includes varicella (chickenpox), insect bites, and scabies infection. The eruption of varicella is self limited and vesicular, and fever is present. The lesions in scabies are concentrated on the hands, axilla, umbilicus, and genitalia, and burrows are present. Insect bites predominate in exposed skin sites and may be asymmetric. Pityriasis lichenoides chronica is most commonly confused with pityriasis rosea or guttate psoriasis. No herald patch is present in pityriasis lichenoides chronica. Scale is thicker, and the disease is chronic rather than self limiting. Pityriasis rosea does not last longer than 20 weeks. If a case of pityriasis lasts longer than 20 weeks, a biopsy should be performed, which will usually show the changes of pityriasis lichenoides chronica. Histologic changes in pityriasis lichenoides include dyskeratotic keratinocytes, bandlike lymphocytic infiltrate, scale crust, and extravasated erythrocytes.

Treatment: Pityriasis lichenoides acuta and chronica can last months to years. The acute form frequently heals after treatment with erythromycin or tetracycline. Ultraviolet light is helpful in severe cases.

PITYRIASIS ROSEA

Definition and etiology: Pityriasis rosea is an acute self-limiting dermatosis characterized by papulosquamous lesions on the trunk and proximal extremities. The cause is still unknown, although a virus is suspected.

Clinical features: Papules rapidly enlarge into a scaly plaque that is often several centimeters in diameter. Because this patch marks the onset of disease, it is called a herald patch. The herald patch is often misdiagnosed as tinea corporis. One to two weeks after the onset of the herald patch, additional patches and plaques develop on the trunk and proximal extremities. Plaques are oval, have a pink color, and are covered with a fine scale. An erythematous rim is present in many cases, and a brown discoloration may be seen in the center. The long axis of lesions follows skin lines. When truncal lesions are examined from a distance, one can imagine the silhouette of a Christmas tree. Pityriasis rosea resolves over a period of 6 to 10 weeks but may last as long as 20 weeks. Recurrences rarely occur.

The differential diagnosis includes other papulosquamous diseases such as psoriasis, nummular dermatitis, tinea versicolor, tinea corporis, secondary syphilis, and pityriasis lichenoides. Psoriasis can be diagnosed when its characteristic lesions occur on extensor surfaces and the scalp. Nail involvement with oil spots, pits, and onycholysis is a feature of psoriasis, not of pityriasis rosea. The chronic nature of psoriasis and the characteristic white-silvery scale also aid in diagnosis. Nummular dermatitis primarily affects elderly men with dry skin in the wintertime. Lesions are coin-shaped rather than oval. Vesicles may be present in nummular dermatitis but not in psoriasis. Potassium hydroxide test results will be positive in tinea versicolor and tinea corporis. The lesions of tinea versicolor usually are poorly demarcated and slightly scaly, as opposed to the well-demarcated lesions of pityriasis rosea. Hypopigmentation and hyperpigmentation occur in tinea versicolor on the upper back and chest. Plaques of tinea corporis are serpiginous and exhibit central clearing and peripheral scaling. Secondary syphilis may be morphologically identical to pityriasis rosea. A rapid plasma reagin or other serologic test should be performed to exclude a diagnosis of syphilis. Individuals with secondary syphilis usually have palmar and plantar involvement, generalized malaise, and lymphadenopathy, features not seen in pityriasis rosea. Presence of a primary genital chancre or condyloma latum establishes a diagnosis of syphilis. Pityriasis lichenoides (guttate parapsoriasis) is chronic, unlike pityriasis rosea, which is self limited. Polymorphous lesions develop in crops. Papulovesicular lesions with central hemorrhagic crusts are present, mimicking varicella. Unlike in pityriasis rosea, some lesions heal with scarring. Biopsy is not required to make a diagnosis of pityriasis rosea. The histologic findings are those of dermatitis, and correct pathologic diagnosis requires clinical correlation.

Treatment: Pityriasis rosea is a self-limited eruption, and treatment is not necessary. Topical steroids and antihistamines may be used if pruritus is prominent. Ultraviolet phototherapy has been shown to hasten resolution of lesions.

PITYRIASIS RUBRA PILARIS

Definition and etiology: Pityriasis rubra pilaris encompasses a group of diseases with the common features of follicular papules, palmar-plantar keratoderma (thick, hyperkeratotic palms and soles), and psoriasiform plaques. Pityriasis rubra pilaris is idiopathic, but some cases can be inherited in an autosomal dominant manner. The different forms of pityriasis rubra pilaris include classic adult onset, atypical adult onset, classic juvenile onset, circumscribed juvenile, and atypical juvenile onset disease.

Clinical features: The rash of classic adult pityriasis rubra pilaris frequently starts in the head and neck area as erythematous, salmon-colored, scaly psoriasiform plaques and follicular papules. The rash becomes generalized over a few weeks, and patients often present with erythroderma. Thick yellow palmar-plantar keratoderma is a universal finding and is said to resemble carnauba wax.

The major disease in the differential diagnosis is psoriasis. Lesions of pityriasis rubra pilaris are often orange-red, whereas those of psoriasis are red. The keratoderma has a distinctive yellow hue, and follicular-based papules are present. The face is frequently involved in pityriasis rubra pilaris but is rarely involved in psoriasis. In patients with erythroderma, a clue to the diagnosis of pityriasis rubra pilaris is the finding of small islands of uninvolved skin in the center of erythematous skin. A diagnosis of pityriasis rubra pilaris may be confirmed by skin biopsy, which reveals epidermal acanthosis with broad-based rete ridges, follicular plugging, and alternating vertical and horizontal parakeratosis. Because of the follicular-based papules, pityriasis rubra pilaris can also be confused with lichen spinulosus and keratosis pilaris. In these diseases, psoriasiform plaques and keratoderma do not occur.

Treatment: Adult-onset pityriasis rubra pilaris may last a few years. The most effective treatment includes systemic retinoids. Oral methotrexate has also been beneficial in a select group of patients. Topical emollients and antihistamines may relieve pruritus.

PSORIASIS

Definition and etiology: Psoriasis is an inflammatory disease characterized by increased epidermal proliferation. The cause of psoriasis is unknown, but abnormal epidermal kinetics as well as the activation of the immune system within the skin must be taken into account.

Clinical features: Approximately one-third of patients have a family history positive for psoriasis. Psoriasis is relatively common and affects about 2% of the population of the United States. The most common age of onset is the third decade of life, but psoriasis can present at any time. Major precipitating factors include infections such as streptococcal pharyngitis or human immunodeficiency virus infection. Trauma to the skin, emotional stress, and use of drugs such as β-blocking agents, angiotensin-converting enzyme inhibitors, fluoxetine, and lithium may aggravate psoriasis.

Examination reveals bright red erythematous plaques covered with white-silvery scales. Areas of predilection include the elbows, knees, scalp, and sacrum. Pitting of the nails, oil spots, and onychodystrophy are frequently seen. Although the majority of patients with psoriasis have only a few lesions, generalized disease and even erythroderma can occur. Clinical variants of psoriasis include generalized pustular psoriasis of Von Zumbusch (see Ch. 11), palmar plantar psoriasis (see Ch. 4), guttate psoriasis, and inverse psoriasis. In guttate psoriasis, the lesions are small (teardrop-sized) and are commonly related to streptococcal infections. In inverse psoriasis, lesions are localized to the flexural areas of the axilla and groin instead of the extensor surfaces.

The differential diagnosis includes other papulosquamous eruptions such as nummular dermatitis, pityriasis rosea, lichen planus, pityriasis rubra pilaris, and secondary syphilis. Psoriasis is easily diagnosed if the classic symmetric distribution of red plaques with silvery-white-colored scales is present. In pityriasis rubra pilaris, follicular-based papules are present, and islands of normal skin are noted within large plaques. Plaques are salmon-orange, and palmar-plantar hyperkeratosis is more marked. Patients with secondary syphilis have lymphadenopathy, may have residual primary lesions, complain of malaise, and may have moth-eaten alopecia. Lesions are predominantly truncal and pityriasis-rosea-like. In pityriasis rosea, the presence of a herald patch, the truncal and proximal extremity disease distribution, the fine rose color, the fine peripheral scale, and the distribution of lesions along skin lines allow for a correct diagnosis. Lesions of lichen planus are distributed on flexural surfaces and have a purple color. Papules predominate and are very pruritic. Mucosal lesions may be present. Skin biopsy helps clarify the diagnosis if clinical findings are equivocal. In psoriasis, there is regular epidermal acanthosis, loss of the granular cell layer, subcorneal and intraepidermal micropustules, and tortuous blood vessels in the dermal papillae.

Treatment: The treatment of psoriasis depends on the severity of disease. For limited involvement, topical tar preparations, calcipotriene (vitamin D$_3$), anthralin, and topical corticosteroids may be used. For more generalized disease, ultraviolet B light or PUVA therapy is highly effective. Oral retinoids, methotrexate, and cyclosporine are helpful in refractory disease. Systemic corticosteroids should generally be avoided because they may lead to a pustular flare-up or destabilization of psoriasis upon withdrawal.

SECONDARY SYPHILIS

Diagnosis and etiology: Syphilis (except for congenital syphilis) is a sexually transmitted disease caused by the spirochete *Treponema pallidum*. Syphilis is one of the great imitators and can present with a wide variety of cutaneous and systemic manifestations.

Clinical features: The clinical features of syphilis can be subdivided into four different stages: primary, secondary, latent, and tertiary syphilis. The primary stage occurs 9 to 90 days after inoculation, when a painless firm ulcer, the "syphilitic chancre," develops in the genital region. Secondary syphilis occurs 8 weeks to approximately 2 years after inoculation and has protean manifestations, such as a truncal papular rash, moth-eaten alopecia (see Ch. 1), and white wartlike lesions in the genitalia known as condylomata lata. Without treatment, the lesions of secondary syphilis resolve, and the disease evolves into a latent stage, only to erupt many years later in some patients as ter-

tiary syphilis. The cutaneous manifestations of tertiary syphilis include nodular and psoriasiform serpiginous plaques and gummas. Gummas are painless necrotic ulcerating nodules.

The scaling patches and plaques of secondary syphilis can be confused with those of any other papulosquamous disease. Like pityriasis rosea, the rash is symmetric and occurs on the trunk, and lesions follow skin lines. The rash starts out as asymptomatic nonscaly red macules and develops into slightly scaly papules and patches. Older lesions have an annular appearance that mimics tinea or granuloma annulare. Clues to the diagnosis of secondary syphilis include the presence of malaise, generalized nontender lymphadenopathy, patchy moth-eaten alopecia, and condyloma latum, and involvement of the palmar-plantar surfaces with copper or ham-covered macules. The diagnosis should be confirmed with serologic testing (Venereal Disease Research Laboratory, rapid plasma reagin, and fluorescent treponemal antibody absorption tests) or biopsy. Biopsy tissue should be stained with Warthin-Starry, Steiner, or Deiterle's stains to highlight spirochetes. Mobile spirochetes can be identified on darkfield examination of tissue smears.

Treatment: Intramuscular penicillin (2.4 million units) weekly for 2 weeks cures primary or secondary syphilis. Oral tetracycline or erythromycin tablets are effective in patients allergic to penicillin. Occasionally, patients with human immunodeficiency virus infection may not respond to the usual therapeutic regimens, and their serologic studies may have false-positive or false-negative results.

TINEA CORPORIS

Definition and etiology: Tinea corporis is an infection of the skin caused by a dermatophyte.

Clinical features: Patients present with irregularly shaped scaly patches and plaques. A characteristic finding is the presence of central clearing and a peripheral rim of scaling. Although tinea corporis is known as ringworm, frequently misdiagnosis can be avoided by realizing that lesions start as round symmetric papules and plaques and may over a period of weeks exhibit an irregular serpiginous or annular appearance.

The differential diagnosis includes other dermatoses such as psoriasis and pityriasis rosea. If the old dictum, "If a lesion is scaly, a KOH should be performed" is followed, an incorrect diagnosis of tinea will not be made. Psoriatic and dermatitic lesions are not serpiginous and do not usually exhibit central clearing. The herald patch of pityriasis rosea is frequently misdiagnosed as tinea. This mistake would not occur if a KOH test were performed. A diagnosis of tinea corporis should not be made without identifying a possible source of disease, such as contact with another person with a dermatophyte infection (children playing with each other, wrestlers) or with a pet. Tinea corporis is more likely in an individual with onychomycosis or tinea pedis.

Treatment: For localized disease, topical therapy is usually effective in clearing the eruption. The most effective agent currently available is terbinafine, because it has fungistatic and fungicidal activity. Also effective are numerous imidazole agents. Oral griseofulvin, itraconazole, or terbinafine can be used in cases of generalized or refractory disease.

Suggested Readings

CUTANEOUS T-CELL LYMPHOMA
Bunn PA, Jr., Hoffman SJ, Norris D et al., Systemic therapy of cutaneous T-cell lymphomas (mycosis fungoides and the Sézary syndrome) (review). Ann Intern Med 1994;121:592–602.

Lorincz AL. Cutaneous T-cell lymphoma (mycosis fungoides) (review). Lancet 1996;347:871–76.

Patterson JW. Lymphomas (review). Dermatol Clin 1992; 10:235–51.

Souteyrand P, d'Incan M. Drug-induced mycosis fungoides-like lesions (review). Curr Prob Dermatol 1990; 19:176–82.

LICHEN PLANUS
Bleicher PA, Dover JS, Arndt KA. Lichenoid dermatoses and related disorders. II. Lichen nitidus, lichen sclerosus et atrophicus, benign lichenoid keratoses, lichen aureus, pityriasis lichenoides, and keratosis lichenoides chronica. J Am Acad Dermatol 1990;22:671–75.

Camisa C. Lichen planus and related conditions. Adv Dermatol 1987;2:47–70.

Dabski C. Lichen planus. Am Fam Physician 1989;39: 120–26.

Halevy S, Shai A. Lichenoid drug eruptions. J Am Acad Dermatol 1993;29:249–55.

Helm TN, Camisa C, Liu AY et al. Lichen planus associated with neoplasia: a cell-mediated immune response to tumor antigens? J Am Acad Dermatol 1994;30: 219–24.

Oliver GF, Winkelmann RK. Treatment of lichen planus. Drugs 1993;45:56–65.

Thompson DF, Skaehill PA. Drug-induced lichen planus. Pharmacotherapy 1994;14:561–71.

LICHEN NITIDUS
Lapins NA, Willoughby C, Helwig EB. Lichen nitidus. A study of forty-three cases. Cutis 1978;21:634–37.

Samman PD, Porter DI. Lichen nitidus. Br J Dermatol 1970;82:424.

NUMMULAR DERMATITIS
Buxton PK. ABC of dermatology. Eczema and dermatitis. Br Med J Clin Res Ed 1987;295:1048–51.

Kleinsmith DM, Perricone NV. Common skin problems in the elderly. Dermatol Clin 1986;4:485–99.

Kulp KR, Kaplan RJ. The diagnosis and treatment of dermatitis. J Tenn Med Assoc 1978;71:815–30.

Rollins TG. From xerosis to nummular dermatitis. The dehydration dermatosis. JAMA 1968;206:637.

Sternbach G, Callen JP. Dermatitis. Emerg Med Clin North Am 1985;3:677–92.

PITYRIASIS LICHENOIDES
Rogers M. Pityriasis lichenoides and lymphomatoid papulosis (review). Semin Dermatol 1992;11:73–79.

PITYRIASIS ROSEA
Allen RA, Janniger CK, Schwartz RA. Pityriasis rosea (review). Cutis 1995;56:198–202.

Horn T, Kazakis A. Pityriasis rosea and the need for a serologic test for syphilis. Cutis 1987;39:81–82.

Leenutaphong V, Jiamton S. UVB phototherapy for pityriasis rosea: a bilateral comparison study. J Am Acad Dermatol 1995;33:996–99.

Parsons JM, Pityriasis rosea update: 1986 (review). J Am Acad Dermatol 1986;15:159–67.

PITYRIASIS RUBRA PILARIS
Cohen PR, Prystowsky JH. Pityriasis rubra pilaris: a review of diagnosis and treatment (see comments). J Am Acad Dermatol 1989;20:801–7.

Fox BJ, Odom RB. Papulosquamous diseases: a review. J Am Acad Dermatol 1985;12:597–624.

PSORIASIS
Farber EM. Therapeutic perspectives in psoriasis (review). Int J Dermat 1995;34:456–60.

Greaves MW, Weinstein GD. Treatment of psoriasis (see comments) (review). N Engl J Med 1995;332:581–88.

Lebwohl M, Abel E, Zanolli M et al. Topical therapy for psoriasis (review). Int J Dermatol 1995;34:673–84.

Naldi L. Psoriasis (review). Dermatol Clin 1995;13: 635–47.

Phillips TJ. Current treatment options in psoriasis (review). Hosp Prac 1996;31:155–57.

SYPHILIS
Johnson PC, Farnie MA. Testing for syphilis (review). Dermatol Clin 1994;12:9–17.

Pandhi RK, Singh N, Ramam M. Secondary syphilis: a clinicopathologic study. Int J Dermat 1995;34:240–43.

Sanchez MR. Infectious syphilis (review). Semin Dermatol 1994;13:234–42.

TINEA CORPORIS

Aly R. Ecology and epidemiology of dermatophyte infections (review). J Am Acad Dermat 1994;31:S21–25.

Cohn MS. Superficial fungal infections. Topical and oral treatment of common types (review). Postgrad Med 1992;91:239–44.

Odom R. Pathophysiology of dermatophyte infections (review). J Am Acad Dermatol 1993;28:S2–S7.

Rezabek GH, Friedman AD. Superficial fungal infections of the skin. Diagnosis and current treatment recommendations (review). Drugs 1992;43:674–82.

Smith EB. Topical antifungal drugs in the treatment of tinea pedis, tinea cruris, and tinea corporis. J Am Acad Dermatol 1993;28:S24–S28.

9 *Excoriations*

ALGORITHM FOR EXCORIATIONS

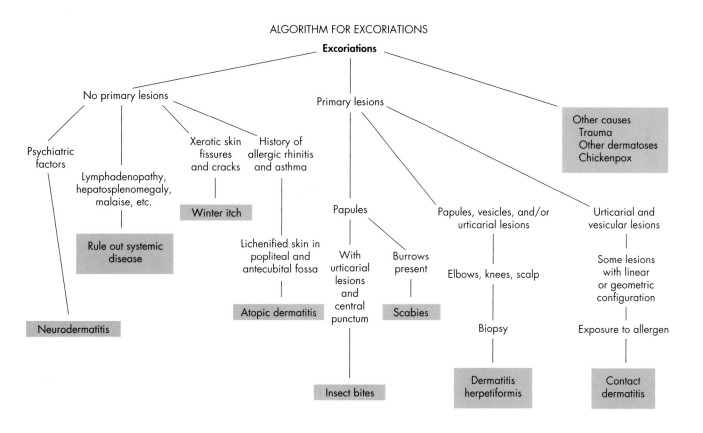

Introduction

An excoriation is an area of scratched skin. A variety of different triggers may lead to excoriations. In many cases, affected individuals already know the precipitating cause because the excoriations were due to an external factor such as contact with a pet, another person, an insect, or a prickly plant. Individuals presenting to the office for help with excoriated skin have been scratching because of severe pruritus. In some patients, the cause of the pruritus may be obvious (e.g., acute allergic contact dermatitis). Other patients who have "sensitive skin" or atopic dermatitis are in search of relief, not a diagnosis. For patients in whom the diagnosis is not obvious, a more careful examination is necessary to rule out a systemic disease or to find the characteristic burrow and mite of scabies. Finally, excoriations may be a manifestation of a psychiatric problem or unresolved emotional conflicts or may be a response to stress.

1. SCABIES
VERSUS
NEURODERMATITIS

Features in common: Excoriations.

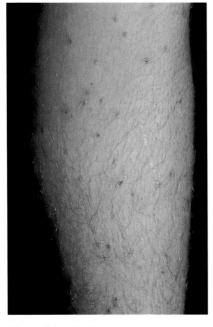

Figure 9.1.1 Scabies.

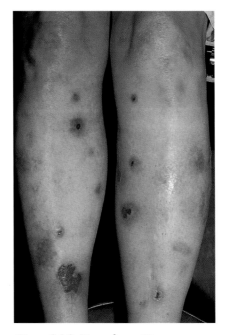

Figure 9.1.2 Neurodermatitis.

Distinguishing features

	SCABIES	NEURODERMATITIS
Physical examination	Papules	No papules
Morphology	Burrows	No burrows
Distribution	Generalized: lesions most prominent in finger webs, skin creases in palm and wrist, axilla, umbilicus, genitalia	Most prominent on upper extremities and upper back
History	Severe pruritus	Severe pruritus
Symptoms	Family members or friends may be itching too No psychiatric factors or stresses	Other family members uninvolved Psychiatric factors and/or stresses present
Exacerbating factors	Immunosuppression	Stress Delusions of parasitosis
Associated findings	None	Nail biting occasionally Nails buffed owing to chronic scratching
Epidemiology	Any age; may be sexually transmitted in adults, usually transmitted through close intimate contact	Usually adults; female predominance
Biopsy	No Insect bite reaction: epidermal spongiosis and eosinophils; only rarely are mites, feces, or eggs seen in the stratum corneum	No Compact stratum corneum and focal superficial epidermal necrosis, minimal dermal inflammation
Laboratory	Scabies scraping positive for mites, eggs, or feces	Scabies preparation negative
Treatment	Topical lindane lotion or permethrin cream	Antianxiolytic agents (e.g., buspirone), protective bandages, and psychologic counseling; fingernails should be cut short to minimize damage
Outcome	Curable with treatment; postscabietic dermatitis may be present 1–2 weeks	Variable; usually chronic

Differential diagnosis of excoriations

Atopic dermatitis
Dermatitis herpetiformis
Insect bites
  Scabies

Neurodermatitis
Pruritus of systemic disease
Trauma
Winter itch/eczema craquelé

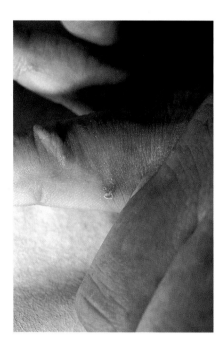

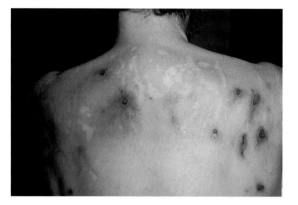

Figure 9.1.4 Neurodermatitis. *Clue to diagnosis:* Excoriations only in easily accessible areas.

Figure 9.1.3 Scabies. *Clue to diagnosis:* Burrow on finger. Scabies mites measure less than 0.3 mm.

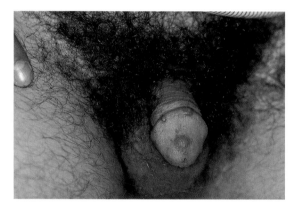

Figure 9.1.5 Scabies. *Clue to diagnosis:* Papules in genital area.

2. DERMATITIS HERPETIFORMIS
VERSUS
ATOPIC DERMATITIS

Features in common: Eczematous itchy rash and excoriations.

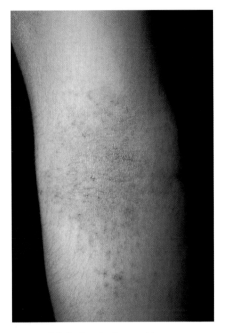

Figure 9.2.1 Atopic dermatitis.

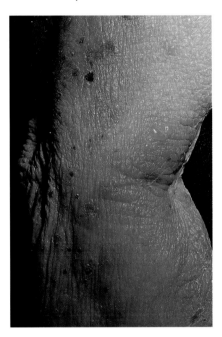

Figure 9.2.2 Dermatitis herpetiformis.

Distinguishing features

	DERMATITIS HERPETIFORMIS	**ATOPIC DERMATITIS**
Physical examination	Primary lesion: papules, vesicles, or urticarial macules	No primary lesions—only manifestations of chronic rubbing or scratching
Morphology	Grouped vesicles occasionally No lichenified skin	No vesicles Lichenified skin
Distribution	Predilection for extensor surfaces: elbows, knees, buttocks, scalp	Predilection for flexural surfaces: antecubital and popliteal fossae
History Symptoms	"Burning" more than itching in some cases	Severe itching
Exacerbating factors	Gluten-rich diet Iodine in diet	Stress, secondary infections
Associated findings	Gluten-sensitive enteropathy	Asthma and allergies Dry skin, Dennie-Morgan folds, white dermatographism

Continues

Distinguishing features (Continued)

	DERMATITIS HERPETIFORMIS	ATOPIC DERMATITIS
Associated findings *(continued)*	No family history	Family history of atopic dermatitis, asthma, or allergies frequently encountered
	Associated with gastrointestinal lymphoma	No associated lymphoma
Epidemiology	Most common in young adults	Most common in children
Biopsy	Yes Subepidermal blister with stuffing of the dermal papillae with neutrophils	No Epidermal acanthosis, slight spongiosis, compact stratum corneum, and superficial perivascular lymphocytic infiltrate
Laboratory	Circulating antiendomysial antibodies in 80% to 100% of patients Direct immunofluorescence: granular deposition of IgA along the dermal-epidermal junction	Increased IgE levels in approximately 80% of patients Skin culture frequently positive for *Staphylococcus aureus*
Treatment	Gluten-free diet Oral dapsone	Topical steroids, emollients, antihistamines, ultraviolet phototherapy, antibiotics if impetiginized
Outcome	Chronic disease	Chronic disease in adults; children may outgrow

Differential diagnosis of eczematous rashes

Asteatotic dermatitis
Atopic dermatitis
Contact dermatitis
Cutaneous T-cell lymphoma
Dermatophytid
Dyshidrotic dermatitis
Lichen simplex chronicus
Neurodermatitis
Nummular dermatitis
Psoriasis
Scabies
Seborrheic dermatitis

In children:

Acrodermatitis enteropathica
Genodermatosis
    Ichthyosis
    Hartnup disease
    Phenylketonuria
    Ectodermal dysplasia
Immunodeficiency disease
    Severe combined immunodeficiency
    Ommen's syndrome
    Job (hyper-IgE) syndrome
    X-linked agammaglobulinemia
    Wiskott-Aldrich syndrome
Langerhans cell granulomatosis

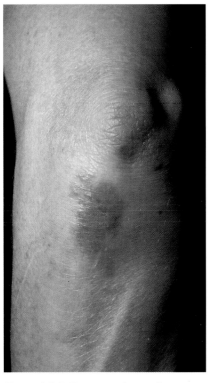

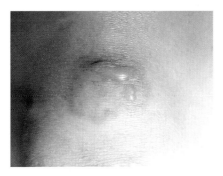

Figure 9.2.4 Dermatitis herpetiformis. *Clue to diagnosis:* Grouped blisters.

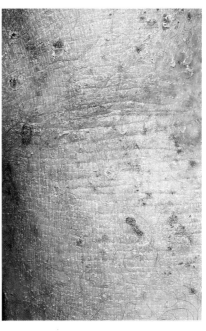

Figure 9.2.5 Atopic dermatitis. *Clue to diagnosis:* Lichenified skin.

Figure 9.2.3 Dermatitis herpetiformis. *Clue to diagnosis:* Lesions over elbows, knees, and buttocks.

3. ATOPIC DERMATITIS

VERSUS

CONTACT DERMATITIS

Features in common: Red, scaly, itchy skin.

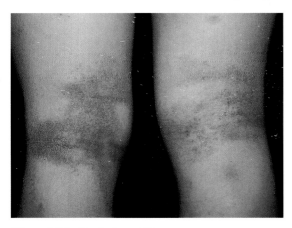

Figure 9.3.1 Atopic dermatitis.

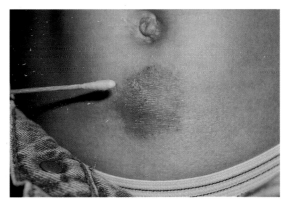

Figure 9.3.2 Allergic contact dermatitis due to nickel in belt buckle.

Distinguishing features

	ATOPIC DERMATITIS	CONTACT DERMATITIS
Physical examination	No primary lesion—rash entirely manifestation of chronic rubbing or scratching	Primary lesion vesicle or urticarial plaque
Morphology	No linear vesicles/plaques	Linear and geometric-shaped plaques/vesicles
	Excoriations common	Few excoriations but not prominent feature
	Lichenified skin common	No lichenified skin unless chronic and undiagnosed
Distribution	Predilection for flexural surfaces: antecubital and popliteal fossae	Areas of contact
History		
Symptoms	Severe itching	Severe itching
Exacerbating factors	Stress, secondary infections, dry skin	Reexposure to allergen or exposure to additional allergens
Associated findings	Asthma and allergies Dry skin, Dennie-Morgan folds, white dermatographism	None
Epidemiology	Most common in children	Can occur at any age
Biopsy	No Nonspecific dermatitis	No Spongiotic dermatitis with eosinophils
Laboratory	Increased IgE levels in approximately 80% of patients Skin culture frequently positive for *Staphylococcus aureus*	Positive patch test
Treatment	Topical steroids, emollients, antihistamines Oral antibiotics if impetiginized	Resolves after exposure to allergen terminated Topical steroids or oral prednisone in severe cases
Outcome	Chronic disease in adults; children may outgrow	Excellent

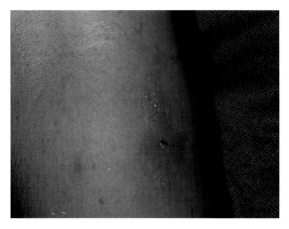

Figure 9.3.3 Contact dermatitis. *Clue to diagnosis:* Linear vesicles.

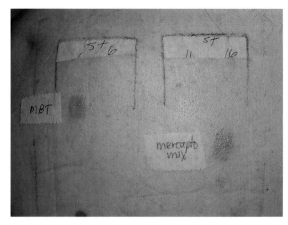

Figure 9.3.4 Contact dermatitis. *Clue to diagnosis:* Positive patch tests.

4. PRURITUS OF SYSTEMIC DISEASE
VERSUS
WINTER ITCH

Features in common: Itchy excoriated skin with minimal rash, usually in older adults.

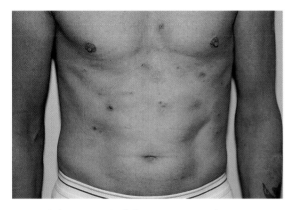

Figure 9.4.1 Excoriated skin in patient with non-Hodgkin's lymphoma.

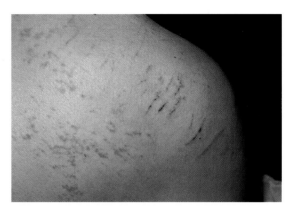

Figure 9.4.2 Excoriated skin in patient with dry skin.

Distinguishing features

	WINTER ITCH	PRURITUS OF SYSTEMIC DISEASE
Physical examination		
Morphology	Skin dry and flaky Skin in dry areas cracked and fissured with "dried riverbed" appearance	No dry skin No fissures or cracks unless patient also has acquired ichthyosis secondary to systemic disease
Distribution	Most prominent on lower extremities and exposed surfaces	Generalized
History		
Symptoms	Pruritus relieved by scratching	Pruritus unrelieved by scratching Patients may feel that the itching is coming from below the skin
Exacerbating factors	Atopic dermatitis Frequent bathing Harsh soaps	Not applicable
Associated findings	Lichenified skin secondary to chronic rubbing, eczematous changes	Dependent on systemic disease Lymphoma: fever, night sweats, weight loss, lymphadenopathy Metabolic: hair loss in thyroid disease Liver: jaundice
Epidemiology	Any age, but more prevalent in elderly	Increases with age

Continues

Distinguishing features (Continued)

	WINTER ITCH	PRURITUS OF SYSTEMIC DISEASE
Biopsy	No Normal skin; epidermal necrosis due to scratching	No Normal skin; epidermal necrosis due to scratching
Laboratory	Normal	Chest x-ray, liver function tests, complete blood count with differential, renal and thyroid function tests Other tests as per clinical suspicion
Treatment	Emollients, mild topical steroids, mild soaps	Treat underlying disease and use soothing emollients
Outcome	Resolves with therapy	Variable; depends on underlying disease

Systemic causes of pruritus

Iatrogenic: drug allergy, opiates
Renal disease
Hepatic disease
Hematologic: anemia, polycythemia vera, paraproteinemia
Malignancies: most commonly lymphoma
Infections: parasites
Metabolic: diabetes, thyroid disease, carcinoid
Miscellaneous: pregnancy
Psychiatric: stress, delusions of parasitosis

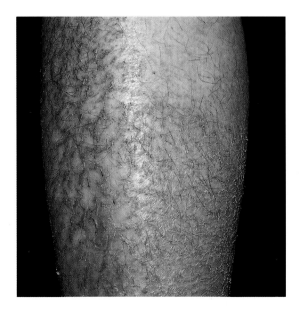

Figure 9.4.3 Winter itch. *Clue to diagnosis:* Cracked fissured skin with a riverbed-like appearance.

Discussion

ATOPIC DERMATITIS

Definition and etiology: Atopic dermatitis is a form of chronic dermatitis (usually starting in childhood) in patients with a familial predisposition for dermatitis, hay fever, and asthma. Patients with atopic dermatitis are born with "sensitive skin."

Clinical features: Early on, a slight amount of macular erythema may be present, but the primary skin manifestations are the result of chronic rubbing and excoriation of skin. Examination reveals lichenified erythematous scaly patches and plaques, with the rash most prominent in the antecubital area and popliteal fossa. In adults, the primary manifestation of atopic dermatitis may be hand dermatitis. Because of the morphologic similarity between atopic dermatitis and other dermatoses, guidelines for diagnosis have been established. Three of the major features and three or more minor features must be present for the diagnosis to be made.

Major features

Pruritus

Eczematous rash

Chronic rash

Flexural distribution in adults, facial
   and extensor involvement in infants

Personal or family history of atopy
   (dermatitis, asthma, allergic rhinitis)

Minor features

Xerosis

Ichthyosis

Keratosis pilaris

Childhood onset

Intolerance of wool cloths

Dennie-Morgan infraorbital fold

Food intolerance

White dermatographism

Susceptibility to cutaneous infections

Elevated serum IgE level

Early-onset cataracts

Itch-aggravated sweating

Pityriasis alba

Using these criteria, it is usually possible to make an accurate diagnosis of atopic dermatitis. The major differential diagnostic considerations would be other dermatoses,

such as scabies, and neurodermatitis. In acute contact dermatitis, vesicles are present. In chronic contact dermatitis, the distribution, history, and results of patch testing will lead to an accurate diagnosis. In scabies, papules and burrows are present, and the rash has a predilection for the finger webs, wrists, axillae, umbilicus, and genitalia. Other family members or friends may also be itching. Neurodermatitis primarily affects adults, and excoriations and scarring occur predominantly on the arms and upper back, areas easily accessible to scratching. Psychologic stresses are also usually readily apparent. In babies and infants, atopic-like dermatoses can also be associated with a variety of immunodeficiency states. The signs of immunodeficiency are usually readily apparent (e.g., frequent infections, failure to thrive, and diarrhea). A skin biopsy is not necessary to make the diagnosis of atopic dermatitis. Biopsy results would be identical to those in any other chronic dermatosis, revealing epidermal acanthosis, slight spongiosis, parakeratosis, and a superficial perivascular lymphocytic infiltrate.

Treatment: The mainstay of treatment of atopic dermatitis includes avoidance of irritants, moisturization of the skin, and judicious use of topical steroids as well as antihistamines. Oral antibiotics effective against *Staphylococcus aureus* are helpful when evidence of secondary infection is present, such as pustules, fissures, and yellow crusting. In exceptional cases, ultraviolet phototherapy, systemic steroids, and immunomodulators may be necessary.

CONTACT DERMATITIS

Definition and etiology: Contact dermatitis is inflammation of the skin resulting from the interaction between the skin and chemicals. Contact dermatitis can be either an irritant type or an allergic type. Irritant contact dermatitis is a nonimmunologic reaction to a chemical that irritates the skin and causes inflammation. Conversely, allergic contact dermatitis is an individualized immunologic response to the chemical (i.e., the person who is allergic to the chemical will develop a rash when the chemical is absorbed through the skin, whereas another person who is not allergic to the chemical will not develop a rash upon contact). Irritant contact dermatitis is most frequently seen on the hands, whereas allergic contact dermatitis can occur in any part of the body in contact with the allergen.

Clinical features: In acute cases, erythema, scaling, vesicles, and swelling can be found. In patients with persistent disease, the erythema and scaling persist but vesicles can no longer be found and the skin becomes lichenified. The rash is severely pruritic, and patients may present with numerous excoriations. The most common cause of acute allergic contact dermatitis is contact with poison ivy, poison oak, or poison sumac. The first exposure to the allergen requires sensitization by the immune system, and the eruption does not appear until 7 to 10 days later. Upon subsequent exposures, however, the rash will develop within 12 to 72 hours. The area of greatest contact with the offending allergen will develop vesicular and urticarial lesions first, with other lesions developing within the next week. A characteristic finding in allergic contact dermatitis secondary to exposure to plants is linear vesicles in spots where the skin brushed against the plant. Common allergens other than plants include nickel, rubber components, chromates, fragrances, and preservatives (e.g., ethylenediamine, formaldehyde, quarternium 15, and bronopol).

The differential diagnosis of contact dermatitis depends on the location of the rash (see Chs. 2 and 4). In cases of generalized eruption with prominent excoriations, the differential diagnosis could include neurodermatitis, scabies, pruritus of systemic disease, atopic dermatitis, and winter itch. To make the correct diagnosis, a high index of suspicion is required. Individuals must be asked about possible antigen exposure and patch testing performed. In none of these other diseases are vesicles routinely found (see discussion on atopic dermatitis). The diagnosis of contact dermatitis can be made clinically or by patch testing. A biopsy, usually not necessary, would show only epidermal spongiosis, and a superficial perivascular infiltrate as in other dermatoses.

Treatment: Reexposure to the allergen or irritant should be avoided. In severe cases, 2 weeks of systemic steroids may be helpful. Shorter courses of steroids should generally be avoided, since patients may suffer from a rebound rash if the steroid is tapered too quickly. In milder cases, strong topical steroids can be used. Oral antihistamines are helpful for itching. Topical antihistamines should be avoided, since they occasionally can also produce an allergic contact type of dermatitis. Topical doxepin cream has found to be a frequent sensitizer.

DERMATITIS HERPETIFORMIS

Definition and etiology: Dermatitis herpetiformis is a chronic, intensely pruritic autoimmune blistering disease. The pathogenesis of dermatitis herpetiformis involves deposition of IgA immune complexes in dermal papillae. The IgA deposition may be triggered by gluten, since approximately three-fourths of patients with dermatitis herpetiformis have asymptomatic gluten-sensitive enteropathy. If patients with dermatitis herpetiformis avoid all gluten, a ubiquitous protein found in wheat products, IgA complexes eventually will no longer be detected in the skin, and the disease will remit.

Clinical features: An intensely pruritic burning sensation is the hallmark of dermatitis herpetiformis. The glutern-sensitive enteropathy is usually asymptomatic. The disease most often begins in adulthood and may be misdiag-

nosed for years as a form of dermatitis. Sometimes patients will note a flare-up of disease activity after eating foods containing a high amount of gluten.

Symmetrically distributed grouped vesicles typically occur on the elbows, knees, buttocks, low back, and shoulders and are typical of dermatitis herpetiformis. Because of intense itching, however, crusts and excoriations may be the only signs of previous blisters. In most patients, the vesicles are hard to detect. Dermatitis-like changes or excoriations may be the predominant feature. In such patients, dermatitis herpetiformis can be confused with scabies, neurodermatitis, or pruritus of systemic disease. In scabies, burrows are seen, and other family members often are also infested. Neurodermatitis primarily involves the extremities and upper back. In pruritus of systemic disease, no primary lesions or blisters are seen. In suspected cases of dermatitis herpetiformis, the diagnosis should always be confirmed or excluded based skin biopsy of lesions. Biopsy results reveal subepidermal blistering with neutrophilic infiltrates, and immunofluorescence reveals granular deposition of IgA along the basement membrane in perilesional normal skin. Indirect immunofluorescence reveals circulating antibodies to endomysium in a sizable proportion of cases.

Treatment: The skin lesions of dermatitis herpetiformis clear and patients characteristically become asymptomatic quite rapidly after the institution of oral dapsone therapy. Although difficult to maintain, a gluten-free diet should be followed if possible. The beneficial effects of a gluten-free diet are unfortunately not seen for months after institution of the diet; however, the diet is helpful in bringing dermatitis herpetiformis under long-term control.

NEURODERMATITIS

Definition and etiology: Neurodermatitis is a term used to describe dermatitis in individuals who present with pruritic excoriated skin but in whom no underlying cause (except for psychologic factors and stress) can be found.

Clinical features: The predominant features are numerous excoriations and scars in areas easily accessible to scratching. Primary lesions are not found. Owing to chronic rubbing, the skin may become thickened (lichenified) with prominent skin markings. Patients may have other associated habits such as nail biting or trichotillomania (pulling out of hairs). The differential diagnosis includes other dermatoses such as atopic dermatitis, scabies infection, winter itch, and pruritus of systemic disease. Usually, patients with neurodermatitis will readily admit to scratching their skin and to underlying psychologic stresses. In scabies, burrows and papules should be found. Primary lesions are also not seen in pruritus of systemic disease, atopic dermatitis, and winter itch. In winter itch, patients have very dry skin, and the rash is usually worse in the lower extremity. Atopic dermatitis usually starts in childhood. Patients have a history of atopy, and the lesions are more prominent in the flexural and popliteal fossae. The pruritus of systemic disease is a generalized unrelenting process.

Treatment: Treatment is difficult. Counseling or psychiatric help to relieve underlying stress may be helpful. Patients should be instructed to cut their nails short to minimize possible damage to the skin due to scratching. If the lesions have become impetiginized, a short course of oral antibiotics may be helpful. Other helpful therapies include topical steroids, neuroleptics, antipruritic medications, and covering of lesions with occlusive bandages or dressings that expedite the natural healing process and protect affected areas from manipulation.

PRURITUS OF SYSTEMIC DISEASE

Definition and etiology: A variety of systemic diseases can produce pruritus by a wide range of mechanisms.

Clinical features: Occasionally, patients present with a chief complaint of pruritic skin. Sometimes no clinical lesions can be seen. Other patients have pruritus with generalized excoriations. If no apparent dermatologic disease is causing the pruritus, a variety of systemic diseases should be excluded. Patients with liver disease, renal disease, blood diseases, internal malignancies, endocrine diseases, allergies, or parasitic infections all may suffer from pruritus. In our experience, patients with pruritus secondary to an underlying lymphoma may state that the pruritus seems to be coming from underneath the skin and, unlike in other causes of pruritus, is not relieved by scratching. Our routine work-up includes a complete blood count with differential to exclude iron deficiency anemia, polycythemia, and leukemia. Liver and renal function tests are done to exclude liver and renal disease. Thyroid function is tested to exclude hyper- or hypothyroidism. Fasting blood glucose testing is ordered to exclude diabetes. Stool is checked for ova and parasites. In elderly patients, an erythrocyte sedimentation rate, chest x-ray, mammogram, and stool guaiac test should be obtained to help exclude malignancies. A thorough drug and allergy history should be undertaken.

Treatment: The underlying disease should be treated. If this is not possible, symptomatic treatments include antihistamines, topical or oral doxepin, topical steroids, psoralen plus ultraviolet A light (PUVA) and activated charcoal.

HUMAN SCABIES INFECTION

Definition and etiology: Scabies is a mite infestation affecting mammals. Human scabies is caused by *Sarcoptes scabiei var. hominis.* The mite lives, reproduces, and feeds in the stratum corneum layer of human skin, thereby producing an extremely pruritic rash.

Clinical features: Patients with scabies complain of a very itchy rash that frequently is worse at night, preventing sleep. The infection is contagious through direct contact, and other family members, close friends, roommates, and playmates may also complain of an itchy rash. The characteristic lesion of scabies is the burrow, a linear papule with a small black punctum at one end where the mite is located. Burrows can be found in the finger webs, the skin creases of the wrists, the axillae, the periumbilical areas, the genitalia, and the feet. Burrows can be overshadowed by generalized excoriations, urticarial papules, and eczematous plaques. The latter two lesions result from a generalized hypersensitivity response to the mite.

Whenever scabies infection is suspected, the burrows and papules should be scraped, and the scrapings should be examined under the microscope for mite parts or scybala (feces and eggs). Burrows are not seen in any other disease. Although animal mites can infest humans, they do not produce burrows. In children, scabies infection can be mistaken for atopic dermatitis, but the latter is a chronic disease characterized by lichenified plaques with prominent involvement of the flexural surfaces. Unlike atopic dermatitis, scabies infection does not involve the face and scalp. In adults, the differential diagnosis also includes winter itch and pruritus of systemic disease. If a patient has a "scabieslike" rash that persists a number of weeks, and no one else who has been in close contact is itching, a systemic disease, not scabies, should be suspected, since scabies infection is contagious.

Treatment: The patient and any close contacts are treated with topical lindane or permethrin cream from the neck downward. The entire body, especially under the fingernails, is treated. Patients treated with lindane should be retreated in 1 week to ensure that any mites that may have hatched from eggs are killed, since lindane is less effective as an ovicidal agent than permethrin. All recently used clothing and linen should be washed to kill any mites that have fallen off the skin.

WINTER ITCH

Definition and etiology: Winter itch (asteatotic dermatitis) is a pruritic eruption most commonly seen in the elderly. It is caused by dryness of the skin.

Clinical features: With age, the skin becomes thinner, contains less collagen and less ground substance, and functions as a less effective barrier. It also becomes dryer. These factors make the skin more susceptible to environmental insults. In the winter, the dry skin can be very pruritic and inflamed. Patients complain most frequently of itchy skin rather than skin changes. If the skin is very dry, it can be fissured and cracked and can develop some eczematous changes. These findings are termed "eczema craquelé." Usually, the dryness is most accentuated in the lower legs. Exacerbating factors include dry weather, harsh soaps, and forced air heating. The diagnosis can be readily made by palpating the patient's skin and noting its dry, rough feel. Unlike in pruritus of systemic disease, the patient's symptoms are relatively mild and respond well to simple therapy.

Treatment: Patients should avoid harsh soaps. The length of baths or showers should be less than 15 minutes, and a moisturizer should be applied immediately after the skin has been patted dry. Creams are generally more effective than lotions. Some of the newer moisturizers containing lactic acid or glycolic acids not only may prevent evaporation of water from the skin but also can draw water into the skin from the blood. A short course of antihistamines may also help with the itching.

Suggested Readings

ATOPIC DERMATITIS
De Prost Y. Atopic dermatitis: recent therapeutic advances (review). Pediatr Dermatol 1992;9:386–89.
Frank LA. Atopic dermatitis (review). Clin Dermatol 1994;12:565–71.
Friedmann PS, Tann BB, Musaba E et al. Pathogenesis and management of atopic dermatitis (review). Clin Exp Allergy 1995;25:799–806.
Morren MA, Przybilla B, Bamelis M et al. Atopic dermatitis: triggering factors (review). J Am Acad Dermatol 1994;31:467–73.
Sehgal VN, Jain S. Atopic dermatitis: clinical criteria (review). Int J Dermatol 1993;32:628–37.

CONTACT DERMATITIS
Klaus MV, Wieselthier JS. Contact dermatitis (review). Am Fam Physician 1993;48:629–32.
Krasteva M. Contact dermatitis (review). Int J Dermatol 1993;32:547–60.

DERMATITIS HERPETIFORMIS
Andersson H, Mobacken H. Dietary treatment of dermatitis herpetiformis (review). Eur J Clin Nutr 1992; 46:309–15.
Hall RPD. Dermatitis herpetiformis (review). J Invest Dermatol 1992;99:873–81.
Smith EP, Zone JJ. Dermatitis herpetiformis and linear IgA bullous dermatosis (review). Dermatol Clin 1993;11:511–26.

NEURODERMATITIS
Borrek S. Neurodermatitis (German). Kinderkrankenschwester 1995;14:144–45.
Laihinen A. Psychosomatic aspects in dermatoses. Ann Clin Res 1987;19:147–49.
Tupker RA, Coenraads PJ, van der Meer JB. Treatment of prurigo nodularis, chronic prurigo and neurodermatitis circumscripta with topical capsaicin (letter). Acta Derm Venereol 1992;72:463.

PRURITUS OF SYSTEMIC DISEASE
Greco PJ, Ende J. Pruritus: a practical approach (review). J Gen Intern Med 1992;7:340–49.
Klecz RJ, Schwartz RA. Pruritus (review). Am Fam Physician 1992;45:2681–86.
Lober CW. Pruritus and malignancy (review). Clin Dermatol 1993;11:125–28.

SCABIES
Angarano DW, Parish LC. Comparative dermatology: parasitic disorders (review). Clin Dermatol 1994;12:543–50.
Orkin M. Scabies in AIDS (review). Semin Dermatol 1993;12:9–14.
Orkin M. Scabies: what's new? (review). Curr Prob Dermatol 1995;22:105–11.
Orkin M, Maibach HI. Scabies therapy—1993 (review). Semin Dermatol 1993;12:22–25.
Rasmussen JE. Scabies (review). Pediatr Rev 1994;15:110–14.

WINTER ITCH
Fleischer AB Jr. Pruritus in the elderly (review). Adv Dermatol 1995;10:41–59.
Levine N. "Winter itch"; what's causing this rash? Geriatrics 1996;51:20.

10

Generalized Vesicular and Bullous Diseases

ALGORITHM FOR GENERALIZED VESICULAR AND BULLOUS DISEASES

Generalized vesicular and bullous diseases

Primarily vesicles

Localized pattern — Diffuse pattern

Ungrouped — Grouped — Vesicles, pustules, crusts

Geometric, linear, sharp outlines — Eczematous Favors extensor, elbows and knees, lower back — Tzanck +

Areas of contact — Marked pruritus — Intraepidermal vesicle

Irritant or allergen (patch test +) — Dermatome + — Subepidermal vesicle — IF or culture +

Tzanck + — **Varicella**

Intraepidermal vesicle

Contact dermatitis

IF or culture + — IF + Dermal papillae

Herpes zoster

Dermatitis herpetiformis

Other causes
Linear IgA disease
Epidermolysis bullosa
  acquisita and inherited forms
Bullous impetigo
Drug eruption
Eczema herpeticum
Rickettsiapox
Epidermolytic hyperkeratosis
Incontentia pigmenti
Burn
Phototoxic
Congenital syphilis
Porphyria
Diabetic bullae

Bullae + vesicles

No target lesions — Target lesions — No mucosal involvement

Usually involves mouth — Subepidermal bullae

Tense subepidermal bullae — **Erythema multiforme** — Widespread sloughing skin and superficial erosions

Flaccid intraepidermal bullae — Severe blistering with mucous membrane involvement — Intraepidermal blister

IF + at dermoepidermal junction — **Steven-Johnson syndrome** — Focus of *S. aureus* infection

IF + at intercellular epidermis — **Toxic epidermal necrolysis** — **Staphylococcal scalded skin syndrome**

Bullous pemphigoid

Pemphigus vulgaris

IF = Immunofluorescence

Introduction

Vesicles and bullae are easily recognized primary lesions that when ruptured produce erosions, crusting, and weeping. A number of diseases are characterized by the presence of blisters. The clinician should rule out common diseases such as contact dermatitis or varicella before considering rare diseases such as bullous pemphigoid or pemphigus vulgaris. If the physical examination is not distinctive (e.g., target lesions diagnostic of erythema multiforme), then laboratory tests such as the Tzanck smear or skin biopsy are quite helpful in differentiating these diseases. Depending on the disease, blister formation characteristically occurs within the epidermis or subepidermis. For example, herpes infections, contact dermatitis, and pemphigus vulgaris occur intraepidermally. Bullous pemphigoid, dermatitis herpetiformis, and erythema multiforme occur beneath the epidermis. The autoimmune diseases have characteristic immunofluorescence findings that are distinctive and important in making the diagnosis. Thus, the clinical features plus the pathologic findings allow the clinician to formulate a definite diagnosis and appropriate therapy.

1. CONTACT DERMATITIS
VERSUS
BULLOUS PEMPHIGOID

Features in common: Scattered vesicles and bullae.

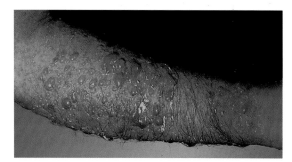

Figure 10.1.1 Contact dermatitis.

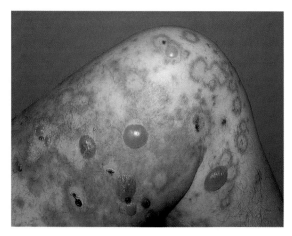

Figure 10.1.2 Bullous pemphigoid.

Distinguishing features

	CONTACT DERMATITIS	BULLOUS PEMPHIGOID
Physical examination		
Morphology	Vesicles predominate, bullae occasionally Lichenified plaques	Tense bullae No lichenified plaques
Distribution	Asymmetric Areas of contact—geometric, linear configuration	Symmetric Groin, axillae, flexor extremities
History		
Symptoms	Pruritus	Pruritus
Exacerbating factors	Exposure to allergen or irritant	No exposure to allergen or irritant Medications: furosemide
Associated findings	No oral involvement	Oral involvement in 1/3
Epidemiology	Common All ages	Rare Elderly
Biopsy	Intraepidermal blister Spongiosis	Subepidermal blister with eosinophils
Laboratory	Immunofluorescence negative Patch test positive	Direct and indirect immunofluorescence positive Patch test negative
Treatment	Steroids	Steroids Immunosuppressives Tetracycline, niacinamide
Outcome	Curable; remove contactant	Chronic; low mortality

Differential diagnosis of scattered vesicles and bullae

Dermatitis herpetiformis
Erythema multiforme
Disseminated herpes simplex
  and herpes zoster
Impetigo

Varicella
Linear IgA disease
Epidermolysis bullosa
Drug eruption

Bullous insect bite eruption
Burn
Contact dermatitis
Bullous pemphigoid

Common allergens

Plants
  Poison ivy and oak
  Primrose
Metals
  Nickel
  Chromate

Cosmetics
  Fragrances
  Preservatives
  Paraphenylenediamine
  Lanolin
Gloves/shoes
  Rubber chemicals

Medicaments
  Benzocaine
  Neomycin
  Bacitracin
Resins
  Epoxy
  Colophony

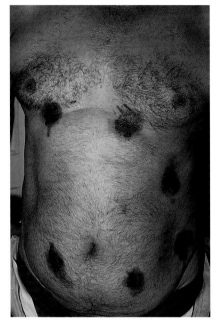

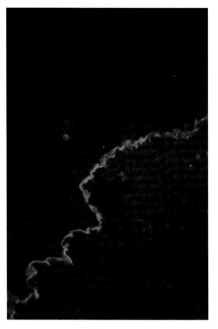

Figure 10.1.3 Contact dermatitis. *Clue to diagnosis:* Geometric outlines where there is contact.

Figure 10.1.4 Bullous pemphigoid. *Clue to diagnosis:* Positive immunofluorescent staining shows linear deposit at dermal-epidermal junction.

2. BULLOUS PEMPHIGOID

VERSUS

PEMPHIGUS VULGARIS

Features in common: Generalized bullae.

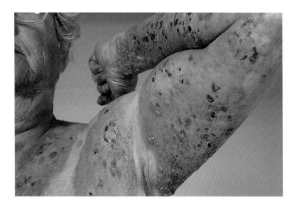

Figure 10.2.1 Bullous pemphigoid.

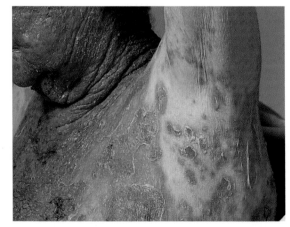

Figure 10.2.2 Pemphigus vulgaris.

Distinguishing features

	BULLOUS PEMPHIGOID	PEMPHIGUS VULGARIS
Physical examination		
Morphology	Tense bullae Harder to rupture Smaller erosions Nikolsky's sign negative	Flaccid bullae Easily ruptured Large erosions Nikolsky's sign positive
Distribution	Generalized, flexural areas	Generalized, no flexural attenuation
History		
Symptoms	Pruritus	Pain
Exacerbating factors	Medications: furosemide	Medications: penicillamine, captopril
Associated findings	Oral involvement in 33%	Oral involvement in 95%
Epidemiology	Rare Elderly	Rare Middle-aged
Biopsy	Subepidermal blister No acantholysis	Intraepidermal blister Acantholysis
Laboratory	Immunofluorescence: linear stain at dermal-epidermal junction	Immunofluorescence: intercellular staining of epidermis
Treatment	Immunosuppressives	Immunosuppressives
Outcome	Chronic; low mortality	Chronic; high mortality if untreated

Differential diagnosis of generalized bullae

Contact dermatitis
Dermatitis herpetiformis
Erythema multiforme
Impetigo
Varicella
Disseminated zoster

Kaposi's varioliform eruption
Rickettsialpox
Staphylococcal scalded skin syndrome
Pemphigoid
Pemphigus
Epidermolysis bullosa acquisita

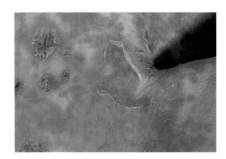

Figure 10.2.3 Pemphigus vulgaris. *Clue to diagnosis:* Nikolsky's sign.

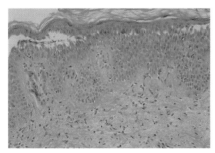

Figure 10.2.4 Pemphigus vulgaris. *Clue to diagnosis:* Biopsy reveals intraepidermal blister with acantholysis.

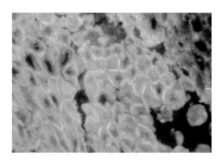

Figure 10.2.5 Pemphigus vulgaris. *Clue to diagnosis:* Immunofluorescence shows intercellular staining in the epidermis.

3. ERYTHEMA MULTIFORME
VERSUS
BULLOUS PEMPHIGOID

Features in common: Generalized bullae with vesicles.

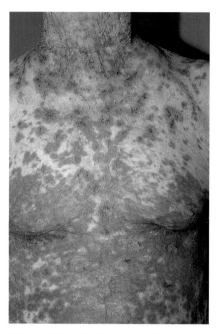

Figure 10.3.1 Erythema multiforme.

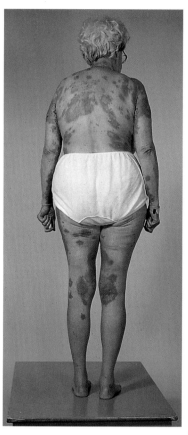

Figure 10.3.2 Bullous pemphigoid.

Distinguishing features

	ERYTHEMA MULTIFORME	**BULLOUS PEMPHIGOID**
Physical examination		
Morphology	Target lesions	No target lesions
	Tense bullae	Tense bullae
	Urticarial papules and plaques	Few urticarial papules and plaques
Distribution	Symmetric, favors extremities	Groin, axillae, flexor extremities
History		
Symptoms	Systemically ill	Not systemically ill
	Little pruritus	Pruritus

Continues

Distinguishing features (Continued)

	ERYTHEMA MULTIFORME	BULLOUS PEMPHIGOID
History (continued)		
Exacerbating factors	Drugs; antibiotics, anticonvulsants, nonsteroidal anti-inflammatory drugs Infections: viral, bacterial, fungal	Drugs: furosemide No infection
Associated findings	Mucous membranes of mouth, eyes, nose, genitalia involved	Oral involvement in 33%
Epidemiology	Uncommon All ages	Rare Elderly
Biopsy	Epidermal necrosis Subepidermal blister with lymphocytes	No necrosis Subepidermal blister with eosinophils
Laboratory	Immunofluorescence negative	Direct and indirect immunofluorescence positive
Treatment	Supportive Role of steroids debated	Steroids Immunosuppressives Tetracycline, niacinamide
Outcome	Acute Minor: spontaneously resolves in a couple weeks Major: Stevens-Johnson syndrome and toxic epidermal necrolysis; may be fatal	Chronic; low mortality

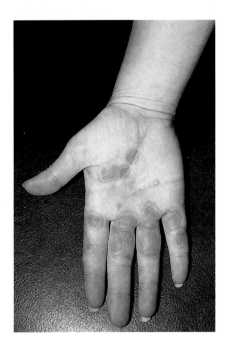

Figure 10.3.3 Erythema multiforme.
Clue to diagnosis: Target lesion.

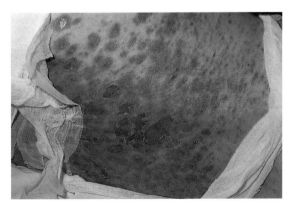

Figure 10.3.4 Erythema multiforme major/Stevens-Johnson syndrome.

4. TOXIC EPIDERMAL NECROLYSIS
VERSUS
STAPHYLOCOCCAL SCALDED SKIN SYNDROME

Features in common: Generalized bullae.

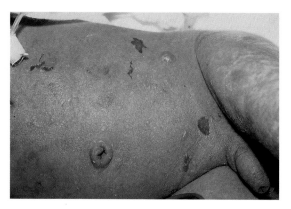

Figure 10.4.1 Toxic epidermal necrolysis.

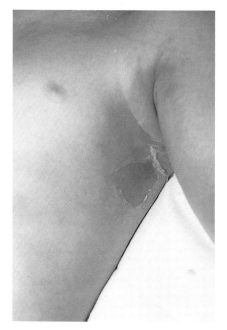

Figure 10.4.2 Staphylococcal scalded skin syndrome.

Distinguishing features

	TOXIC EPIDERMAL NECROLYSIS	STAPHYLOCOCCAL SCALDED SKIN SYNDROME
Physical examination		
Morphology	Tense bullae Deeper erosions	Flaccid bullae Superficial erosions
Distribution	Generalized	Face, neck, groin, axillae
History		
Symptoms	Extremely ill	Mildly ill
Exacerbating factors	Drugs No *Staphylococcus aureus* infection	No drugs *Staphylococcus aureus* infection
Associated findings	Mucous membranes affected	Mucous membranes not affected
Epidemiology	Rare; adults or children	Rare; children, adults with renal failure

Continues

Distinguishing features (Continued)

	TOXIC EPIDERMAL NECROLYSIS	STAPHYLOCOCCAL SCALDED SKIN SYNDROME
Biopsy	Subepidermal blister Necrotic epidermis	Subcorneal blister No necrosis
Laboratory	Culture negative	Culture positive for *Staphylococcus aureus*
Treatment	Supportive, burn care	Supportive No evidence that antibiotics (*Staphylococcus* coverage) help
Outcome	Frequently fatal (20%–50%)	Not fatal

Drugs causing toxic epidermal necrolysis

Sulfonamides   Nonsteroidal anti-inflammatory drugs
Anticonvulsants   Allopurinol

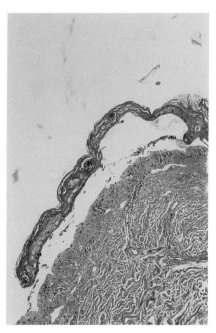

Figure 10.4.3 Toxic epidermal necrolysis.
Clue to diagnosis: Subepidermal blister
and necrotic epidermis.

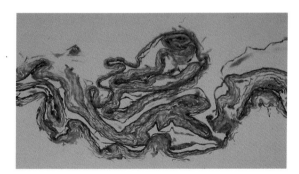

Figure 10.4.4 Staphylococcal scalded skin syndrome.
Clue to diagnosis: Intraepidermal blister.

5. DERMATITIS HERPETIFORMIS
VERSUS
VARICELLA

Features in common: Generalized vesicles.

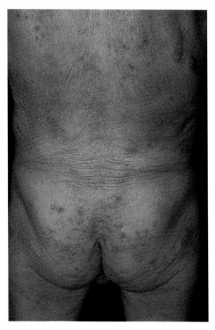

Figure 10.5.1 Dermatitis herpetiformis.

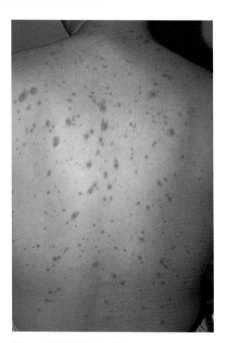

Figure 10.5.2 Varicella.

Distinguishing features

	DERMATITIS HERPETIFORMIS	**VARICELLA**
Physical examination		
Morphology	Vesicles rare, secondary to excoriations	Vesicles common
	Grouped vesicles	Individual vesicles
	Eczematous plaques	Lesions in different stages: vesicles, papules, pustules, crusts
		No eczematous lesions
Distribution	Localized: elbows, knees, buttocks, low back, shoulders	Generalized
History		
Symptoms	No fever	Fever
	No systemic symptoms	Systemic symptoms
Exacerbating factors	Gluten	Adulthood, pregnancy,
	Iodine	immunosuppression

Continues

Distinguishing features (Continued)

	DERMATITIS HERPETIFORMIS	VARICELLA
Associated findings	Gluten-sensitive enteropathy No pneumonia, hepatitis, encephalitis	No enteropathy Pneumonia, hepatitis, encephalitis occasionally
Epidemiology	Rare Young adults, male predominance 2:1	Common Children
Biopsy	Subepidermal blister with neutrophils Tzanck negative	Intraepidermal blister, ballooning degeneration Multinucleated giant cells Tzanck positive
Laboratory	Culture negative Immunofluorescence: granular IgA in dermal papillae Circulating antiendomysial antibody	Culture often negative Immunofluorescence: herpes, varicella-zoster
Treatment	Dapsone Gluten-free diet	Acyclovir (immunosuppressed and adults) Antipruritics
Outcome	Chronic	Acute

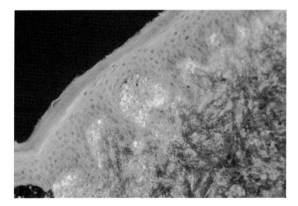

Figure 10.5.3 Dermatitis herpetiformis. *Clue to diagnosis:* IgA in dermal papillae on immunofluorescence.

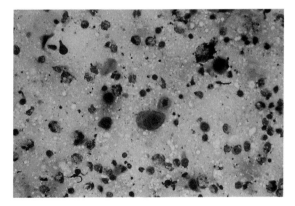

Figure 10.5.4 Varicella. *Clue to diagnosis:* Positive Tzanck test results showing multinucleated giant cells.

6. VARICELLA
VERSUS
DISSEMINATED HERPES ZOSTER

Features in common: Generalized vesicles.

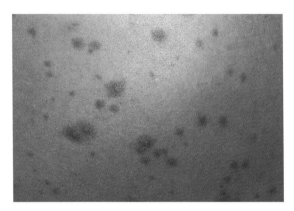

Figure 10.6.1 Varicella.

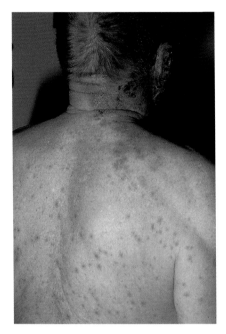

Figure 10.6.2 Herpes zoster.

Distinguishing features

	VARICELLA	HERPES ZOSTER DISSEMINATED
Physical examination		
Morphology	Lesions not grouped	Lesions grouped
	Lesions in different stages: vesicles, papules, pustules, crusts	Lesions in different stages: vesicles, papules, pustules, crusts
Distribution	Not dermatomal	Dermatomal initially
	Generalized	Generalized
History		
Symptoms	No pain	Pain
	Marked pruritus	Little pruritus
	Fever	Little fever
	Systemic symptoms	Few systemic symptoms
Exacerbating factors	Adulthood	
	Immunosuppression, pregnancy	Immunosuppression, pregnancy
Associated findings	Pneumonia, hepatitis, encephalitis occasionally	Pneumonia, hepatitis, encephalitis occasionally
	No cancer, AIDS	Cancer, AIDS

Continues

Distinguishing features (*Continued*)

	VARICELLA	HERPES ZOSTER DISSEMINATED
Epidemiology	Common Children	Common Adults
Biopsy	Intraepidermal blister Ballooning degeneration Multinucleated giant cells Tzanck results positive	Intraepidermal blister Ballooning degeneration Multinucleated giant cells Tzanck results positive
Laboratory	Culture often negative Immunofluorescence: herpes, varicella-zoster	Culture often negative Immunofluorescence: herpes, varicella-zoster
Treatment	Acyclovir (immunosuppressed and adults) Antipruritics	Acyclovir, valacyclovir, famciclovir
Outcome	Acute Rarely fatal No residual pain	Acute Rarely fatal Postherpetic neuralgia

Abbreviation: AIDS, acquired immunodeficiency syndrome.

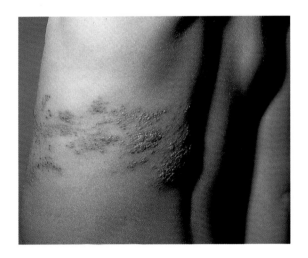

Figure 10.6.3 Herpes zoster. *Clue to diagnosis:* Initial dermatomal involvement.

Discussion

BULLOUS PEMPHIGOID

Definition and etiology: Bullous pemphigoid is an autoimmune disease characterized by tense subepidermal bullae.

Clinical features: Bullous pemphigoid occurs predominantly in the elderly. Pruritus is a significant symp-

tom, as is the discomfort caused by oozing and weeping blisters. Immunoglobulin G autoantibodies directed against the bullous pemphigoid antigen found in the basement membrane zone cause the blistering process. These antibodies can be detected along with C3 antigen in direct and indirect immunofluorescence studies.

The large tense blisters of bullous pemphigoid occur on normal or erythematous appearing skin. They can occur anywhere on the head, trunk, and extremities but have a preferred distribution in the groin, axilla, and antecubital and popliteal fossae. The blisters of bullous pemphigoid are usually not fragile and heal without scarring. About one-third of patients have oral mucous membrane involvement.

The differential diagnosis of bullous pemphigoid includes any of the chronic blistering diseases, particularly pemphigus vulgaris, dermatitis herpetiformis, erythema multiforme, and contact dermatitis. Before immunofluorescence studies, pemphigus and bullous pemphigoid were considered to be the same disease; therefore, differentiation based on morphology alone can be very difficult. In contact dermatitis, possible exposure to allergens should be present, and the lesions have symmetric, linear, and geometric patterns. In erythema multiforme, blisters are less prominent, and target lesions are present.

Treatment: Because the blistering skin of bullous pemphigoid has a tendency to heal, the prognosis is excellent with a low mortality rate. Bullous pemphigoid, however, may last months or years, and the morbidity caused by widespread blistering usually requires treatment with immunosuppressive agents such as systemic steroids. The use of immunosuppressive agents, however, has been debated. In limited cases, tetracycline and niacinamide have been effective.

CONTACT DERMATITIS

Definition and etiology: Contact dermatitis is an inflammatory reaction to an exogenous chemical, irritant, or allergen that comes in contact with the skin. Irritant contact dermatitis is precipitated by a substance that has direct toxic properties, whereas allergic contact dermatitis is triggered by a delayed-type hypersensitivity reaction. Irritating chemicals include acids, alkalies, solvents, and detergents. There are numerous allergens, including plants (poison ivy and oak), metals (nickel), rubber chemicals, cosmetic ingredients (fragrances and preservatives), and topical medicines (neomycin and bacitracin).

Clinical features: Contact dermatitis varies from acute to chronic, which results in varying appearances. Acute contact dermatitis has marked epidermal edema, or spongiosis. This causes vesicles and bullae to rupture, resulting in oozing and crusting. The hallmark of chronic contact dermatitis is lichenification or thickening of the epidermis associated with scaling and fissuring. The distribution of contact dermatitis corresponds with the area of contact. Streaks, geometric outlines, and sharp margins typically occur where there has been application of the contactant or brushing by the leaf or stem of poison ivy or oak. The diagnosis of acute contact dermatitis is usually straightforward. In the case of an irritant, patients develop symptoms quite quickly and know they have come in contact with a caustic material. For an allergen, this may not be so obvious, since it takes one or two days after exposure for the blistering to develop. A history of outdoor activity,

however, and finding of a typical configuration make the diagnosis of allergic contact dermatitis to poison ivy or oak easy to establish. For other allergens, patch testing is often required to identify the cause. Results of a skin biopsy, if needed, reveal an intraepidermal spongiotic blister.

Treatment: The management of contact dermatitis should emphasize prevention and complete avoidance of the offending irritants or allergens. This may require a change in occupation or lifestyle. The principal treatment is topical steroids; for those individuals with severe or widespread contact dermatitis, a short course of systemic steroids is indicated. Colloidal oatmeal baths reduce inflammation and itching. Antihistamines are also used to reduce itching.

DERMATITIS HERPETIFORMIS

Definition and etiology: Dermatitis herpetiformis is a chronic, intensely pruritic autoimmune vesicular disease. The pathogenesis of dermatitis herpetiformis is related to IgA immune complex deposition in the dermal papillae. The IgA deposition may be related to gluten, since approximately three-fourths of patients with dermatitis herpetiformis have asymptomatic gluten-sensitive enteropathy. When patients with dermatitis herpetiformis avoid gluten, IgA complexes are not detected in the skin, and the blistering remits.

Clinical features: Intense pruritus and burning are the hallmarks of dermatitis herpetiformis. Although gluten-sensitive enteropathy typically occurs in these patients, it is usually asymptomatic. Disease activity usually begins in early adulthood, and often years elapse before a definitive diagnosis is made. Sometimes, patients will note a flare-up of disease activity after eating foods containing a high amount of gluten.

Symmetrically distributed grouped vesicles, typically occur on the elbows, knees, buttocks, low back, and shoulders. Because of intense itching, crusting and excoriation may be the only sign of the previous vesicle. In many patients, the vesicles are hard to detect, and, as the name implies, dermatitic changes are prominent.

The differential diagnosis of dermatitis herpetiformis initially includes a number of other blistering disorders such as varicella or dermatitis. The skin biopsy, which reveals a subepidermal blister with collections of neutrophils in the papillary dermis, along with immunofluorescence findings revealing granular IgA deposits in the dermal papilla, confirms the diagnosis of dermatitis herpetiformis. Eighty percent of patients also have antiendomysial antibody in their serum.

Treatment: Characteristically, dermatitis herpetiformis clears and becomes asymptomatic quite rapidly after the institution of dapsone or sulfapyridine therapy.

Although difficult to maintain, a gluten-free diet should be initiated. The beneficial effects of a gluten-free diet, however, are not seen for months.

ERYTHEMA MULTIFORME

Definition and etiology: Erythema multiforme is a characteristic inflammatory reaction in the skin secondary to a wide variety of causes. The most common are medications and infections such as herpes simplex virus or *Mycoplasma pneumoniae* infection. Other causes include neoplasms, connective tissue diseases, physical agents, foods, and topical agents.

Clinical features: Erythema multiforme ranges in severity from the self-limited minor form, which spontaneously resolves in a couple of weeks, to a severe major form, which may be fatal. Recurrent erythema multiforme minor is usually secondary to herpes labialis or herpes genitalis. The Stevens-Johnson syndrome may be considered the most severe form of erythema multiforme major. Whether toxic epidermal necrolysis is a form of erythema multiforme is still being debated. The more severe forms of erythema multiforme are usually caused by drugs: sulfonamides, penicillins, nonsteroidal anti-inflammatory agents, barbiturates, and dilantin, among others.

The examination of the skin reveals a characteristically symmetric eruption that favors the extremities. The lesions, being multiform, vary from urticarial papules and plaques to large bullae. The target or iris lesion is diagnostic of erythema multiforme and has three zones of color: (1) a central dark erythematous area or blister, (2) a surrounding pale erythematous zone, and (3) a peripheral erythematous ring. Widespread blistering and erosions of the skin and mucous membranes occur in erythema multiforme major, Stevens-Johnson syndrome, and toxic epidermal necrolysis. These patients are systemically ill with fever, arthralgias, and severe malaise. Death can occur owing to secondary infection or electrolyte imbalance.

The differential diagnosis of erythema multiforme is usually not difficult if characteristic target lesions are present. The acute onset usually differentiates it from other widespread blistering diseases such as bullous pemphigoid and pemphigus vulgaris. Contact dermatitis, with its asymmetric distribution and geometric and linear configuration, should be relatively easy to distinguish from erythema multiforme. If a skin biopsy is needed, findings will show the characteristic signs of necrotic keratinocytes, interface lymphocytic inflammation, and a subepidermal blister.

Treatment: Erythema multiforme usually resolves spontaneously after the precipitating factor has been eliminated. Within the first few days of disease onset, systemic steroids have been used, but their efficacy has been controversial. Prolonged steroid use is not advised because of the possibility of their masking the signs of infection. An oph-

thalmologist should be consulted if there is eye involvement to prevent scarring. Topical dressings may help heal the erosions. In severe cases, the patient should be treated in a burn unit, where infection and electrolyte and fluid balance can be closely monitored.

DISSEMINATED HERPES ZOSTER

Definition and etiology: Herpes zoster is caused by the recrudescence of latent varicella-zoster virus in individuals who have had varicella. The vesicular dermatomal eruption is distinctive, and on occasion cutaneous dissemination occurs.

Clinical features: Herpes zoster occurs in both normal and immunosuppressed individuals. It may be the presenting sign of acquired immunodeficiency syndrome or lymphoma, particularly if there is dissemination. Typically, the eruption is preceded by a painful prodrome, which may be confused with a migraine, pleurisy, myocardial infarction, or appendicitis.

The examination characteristically reveals grouped vesicles on an erythematous base distributed unilaterally along a dermatome. When cutaneous dissemination occurs, individual papules, vesicles, and pustules are found widely scattered on the trunk, extremities, and head.

The dermatomal distribution of herpes zoster is diagnostic and rarely causes confusion. Varicella is not characterized by this distinctive dermatomal focus of vesicles. Herpes simplex virus infection may rarely occur in a dermatomal fashion but would be recurrent, in contrast to herpes zoster, which does not recur. Since varicella and herpes zoster are caused by the same virus, the Tzanck preparation results, immunofluorescence findings, and culture results are identical.

Treatment: Herpes zoster in the immunocompetent patient who is younger than 50 years of age need not be treated. For those older than 50 years of age, immunocompromised patients, and patients with disseminated herpes zoster, antiviral therapy with acyclovir, valacyclovir, or famciclovir should be instituted to lessen the amount of postherpetic neuralgia and prevent further disease progression or dissemination.

PEMPHIGUS VULGARIS

Definition and etiology: Pemphigus vulgaris is an autoimmune blistering disease that affects the skin and mucous membranes. The bullae occur intraepidermally, where autoantibodies against a normal component of the keratinocyte cell membrane are deposited. This results in loss of adhesion between keratinocytes with the formation of acantholysis and blisters.

Clinical features: Pemphigus vulgaris is a rare blistering disease occurring in approximately 1 of 100,000 people. The oral mucosa is almost always involved and frequently is the presenting site.

The examination reveals generalized blistering of the skin. The bullae are flaccid and superficial, range in size from 1 centimeter to several centimeters, and are fragile, leaving large denuded, bleeding, weeping, and crusted erosions. Extension of the bulla laterally with application of peripheral pressure is characteristic of pemphigus vulgaris; this is called *Nikolsky's sign.* Involvement of the oral cavity is frequent and may be severe with widespread erosions (see Ch. 3).

The differential diagnosis of pemphigus vulgaris mainly includes autoimmune chronic blistering diseases such as bullous pemphigoid, dermatitis herpetiformis, epidermolysis bullosa acquisita, linear IgA bullous dermatosis, and the other forms of pemphigus (vegetans, foliaceus, and erythematosus). A skin biopsy and immunofluorescence studies help separate pemphigus from the other autoimmune diseases. The blister occurs intraepidermally just above the basal layer with loss of cohesion between epidermal cells (acantholysis). Results of direct and indirect immunofluorescence studies are positive, showing deposits of immunoglobulins (usually IgG) and complement in the intracellular spaces between keratinocytes.

Treatment: The treatment of choice for pemphigus vulgaris is systemic steroids. Once blistering has subsided and disease activity has been controlled, other immunosuppressive agents such as azathioprine may be added for their steroid-sparing effect. Before systemic corticosteroids were available, pemphigus vulgaris had a high mortality rate because of widespread blistering with resultant fluid and electrolyte imbalance and infection. Other therapies include topical steroids, cyclosporin, dapsone, parenteral gold, cyclophosphamide, and methotrexate.

STAPHYLOCOCCAL SCALDED SKIN SYNDROME

Definition and etiology: Staphylococcal scalded skin syndrome is a widespread superficial blistering disease caused by an exfoliative toxin produced by certain strains of *Staphylococcus aureus,* usually group II.

Clinical features: Staphylococcal scalded skin syndrome occurs predominantly in young children but may also affect immunosuppressed adults with renal failure. Although febrile and irritable, the patient is usually not very ill. Characteristically, the skin is tender and erythematous. Superficial vesicles and bullae occur on the face, neck, axilla, and groin. This leads to widespread sloughing of the skin, leaving a red, slightly weeping, moist base and a scalded appearance.

The diagnosis of staphylococcal scalded skin syndrome is usually straightforward, since it has the characteristic appearance of scalded skin. At one time, it was thought to be a form of toxic epidermal necrolysis, but the clinical features, skin biopsy results, and etiologic factors clearly separate these two entities. Although a biopsy is not usually necessary, biopsy findings reveal an intraepidermal blister just below the stratum corneum. The infection is not within the bullae, as in bullous impetigo, but is found in a distant focus such as the nasal mucosa or is localized. Culture results from the widespread blisters will be negative, since blisters are a result of the exfoliative toxin.

Treatment: Antistaphylococcal antibiotics that eradicate the toxin-producing organisms are commonly used but have not been shown to affect the outcome of the skin rash. Topical antibiotics and dressings can be used, as in routine wound care.

TOXIC EPIDERMAL NECROLYSIS

Definition and etiology: Toxic epidermal necrolysis (TEN) is considered by many to be the most severe form of erythema multiforme. However, since target lesions may not be present, others feel that TEN is a distinct disease. It is usually secondary to drug use.

Clinical features: The sudden onset of widespread blistering of the skin and mucous membranes in a gravely ill patient makes this disease a dermatologic emergency. Fortunately, it is relatively rare.

The examination shows widespread blistering and sloughing of the epidermis and mucous membranes of the mouth, nose, eyes, and genitalia. Large erosions leaving raw red dermis develop in patients who are severely ill.

Toxic epidermal necrolysis should be easily distinguished from staphylococcal scalded skin syndrome. Results of a skin biopsy reveal full-thickness epidermal necrosis with subepidermal blister formation.

Treatment: Discontinuation of the precipitating drug is paramount. Although controversial, systemic steroids are frequently used. Most important are supportive measures, which require specialized nursing care in a burn unit to avoid sepsis and fluid and electrolyte imbalances. Death may occur in up to 50% of patients with toxic epidermal necrolysis.

VARICELLA

Definition and etiology: Varicella, or chickenpox, is an acute highly contagious infection caused by the varicella-zoster virus.

Clinical features: Varicella is predominantly a childhood disease. A 2- to 3-week incubation period occurs after exposure. The first signs and symptoms of the disease are a 2- to 3-day prodrome of chills, fever, malaise, headache, sore throat, anorexia, and dry cough. The characteristically pruritic vesicular eruptions then occur. The patient is infectious for approximately 1 week, from a couple of days before the rash develops until all the vesicles have become crusted.

Varicella is a markedly pruritic vesicular eruption affecting all regions of the body, including the mucous membranes of the mouth and the conjunctiva. Characteristically, there are crops of rapidly progressive lesions beginning with macules, which evolve into papules, vesicles, and pustules. Crusting and necrosis follow. A typical lesion has been described as a "dew drop on a rose petal." Typically, all these types of lesions are present at the same time.

The differential diagnosis of varicella once included smallpox before eradication of that disease. The acute onset, limited duration, and occurrence in childhood separate varicella from dermatitis herpetiformis. Disseminated herpes zoster and varicella are caused by the same virus. Disseminated herpes zoster, however, has distinctive dermatomal involvement. Other diseases that might be considered in the differential diagnosis are disseminated herpes simplex, coxsackievirus, echovirus, and rickettsialpox. The diagnosis of varicella is usually straightforward. A Tzanck preparation reveals multinucleated giant cells typical of a herpesvirus infection. Direct immunofluorescence is the most sensitive and specific way of confirming the diagnosis.

Treatment: Treatment of chickenpox in the normal child is largely symptomatic, with use of antihistamines and topical agents to reduce itching. In adults and immunosuppressed patients, acyclovir reduces disease length, severity, and complications such as pneumonia, encephalitis, and hepatitis. The live attenuated varicella vaccine appears to be safe and moderately effective and is recommended for those in good health who have no history of clinical varicella and who are older than 1 year of age. Immunodeficient patients who are exposed to varicella may be immunized with varicella-zoster immune globulin (VZIG) prophylactically, but not for active disease.

Suggested Readings

BULLOUS PEMPHIGOID, DERMATITIS HERPETIFORMIS, PEMPHIGUS VULGARIS
Bystryn JC. The adjuvant therapy of pemphigus. An update. Arch Dermatol 1996;132:203–12.

Fine JD. Management of acquired bullous skin diseases. N Engl J Med 1995;333:1475–84.

Hall RP. Dermatitis herpetiformis. J Invest Dermatol 1992; 99:873–81.

Helm KF, Peters MS. Immunodermatology update: the immunologically mediated vesiculobullous diseases. Mayo Clin Proc 1991;66:187–202.

ERYTHEMA MULTIFORME
Huff JC, Weston WL, Tonnesen MG. Erythema multiforme: a critical review of characteristics, diagnostic criteria, and causes. J Am Acad Dermatol 1983;8:763–75.

Rasmussen JE. Erythema multiforme. Should anyone care about the standards of care? Arch Dermatol 1995;131: 726–29.

STAPHYLOCOCCAL SCALDED SKIN SYNDROME
Elias PM, Fritsch P, Epstein EH. Staphylococcal scalded skin syndrome. Arch Dermatol 1977;113:207–19.

VARICELLA
Dunkle LM, Arvin AM, Whitley RJ et al. A controlled trial of acyclovir for chickenpox in normal children. N Engl J Med 1991;325:1539–44.

Famciclovir for herpes zoster. Med Lett 1994;36:97–98.

Feder HM. Treatment of adult chickenpox with oral acyclovir. Arch Intern Med 1990;150:2061–65.

Krause PR, Klinman DM. Efficacy, immunogenicity, safety, and use of live attenuated chickenpox vaccine. J Pediatr 1995;127:518–25.

Straus SE. Shingles. Sorrows, salves, and solutions. JAMA 1993;269:1836–39.

Straus SE, Ostrove JM, Inchauspe G et al. Varicella-zoster virus infections. Biology, natural history, treatment, and prevention. Ann Intern Med 1988;108:221–37.

Valacyclovir. Med Lett 1996;38:3–4.

Wood MJ, Johnson RW, McKendrick MW et al. A randomized trial of acyclovir for 7 days or 21 days with and without prednisolone for treatment of acute herpes zoster. N Engl J Med 1994;330:896–900.

11
Macular and Urticarial Rashes

ALGORITHM FOR MACULAR AND URTICARIAL RASHES

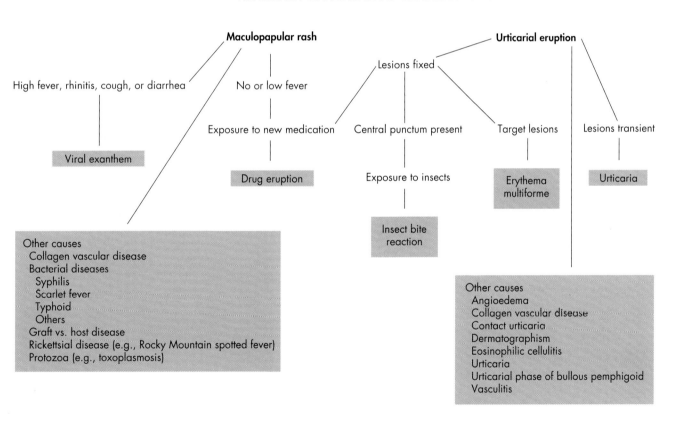

Introduction

Maculopapular and urticarial rashes are perhaps morphologically the most easily recognizable type of skin rash. Unfortunately, recognition of the eruption does not immediately unveil its cause. A maculopapular drug rash is morphologically indistinguishable from a maculopapular viral exanthem. Correct diagnosis is made possible only by taking a careful history, looking for ancillary findings, observing symptoms, and obtaining blood tests. Ultimately, the clinical course will confirm a correct diagnosis. Urticarial eruptions can be seen in patients with urticaria or erythema multiforme and after insect bites. In these eruptions, a careful history, a skin biopsy, and careful inspection of the skin will result in the correct diagnosis.

1. MACULOPAPULAR DRUG ERUPTION
VERSUS
VIRAL EXANTHEM

Features in common: Symmetric red macules and papules on the trunk and extremities.

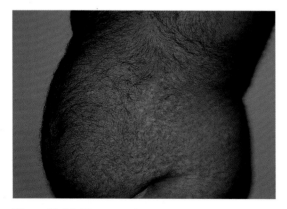

Figure 11.1.1 Drug eruption.

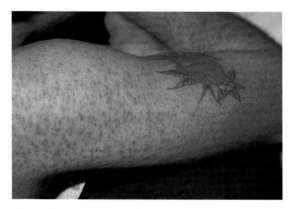

Figure 11.1.2 Viral exanthem.

Distinguishing features

	MACULOPAPULAR DRUG ERUPTION	VIRAL EXANTHEM
Physical examination Morphology	May be identical: symmetric and confluent macules and papules on trunk No Koplik's spots or slapped-cheek appearance	May be identical: symmetric and confluent macules and papules on the trunk Koplik's spots in measles (white grainy papules on a red base, usually on buccal mucosa) Slapped-cheek appearance in erythema infectiosum
Distribution	Trunk and extremities	Trunk and extremities
History Symptoms	No or low-grade fever Starts 1 to 10 days after starting medication No other patients with similar complaints Pruritus	Low- to high-grade fever No new medication Other patients with similar symptoms in community Minimal or no pruritus
Exacerbating factors	None	Immunosuppression
Associated findings	No systemic symptoms	Systemic symptoms usually present (malaise, myalgia, rhinorrhea, diarrhea, risk of miscarriage in erythema infectiosum)
Epidemiology	Any age	Most common in children
Biopsy	No, nonspecific Superficial nonspecific lymphocytic infiltrate	No, nonspecific Superficial nonspecific lymphocytic infiltrate
Laboratory	Occasionally peripheral eosinophilia	Lymphocytosis or lymphopenia may be present
Treatment	Stop medication Antipruritic	None necessary
Outcome	Resolves	Resolves

Differential diagnosis of maculopapular eruptions

Viral exanthem
 Measles (rubeola) (paramyxovirus)
 German measles (rubella)
 Erythema infectiosum (parvovirus)
 Roseola infantum (herpesvirus 6)
 Infectious mononucleosis (Epstein-Barr virus)

Viral exanthem (*continued*)
 Hepatitis
 Human immunodeficiency virus (retrovirus)
 Miscellaneous viruses: echovirus, adenovirus, dengue
Drug eruption
Urticaria
Collagen vascular diseases
 Still's disease

Syphilis
Toxoplasmosis
Bacterial diseases
 Brucellosis
 Scarlet Fever
 Typhoid
Rickettsial diseases
 Rocky Mountain spotted fever
 Typhus
Kawasaki's disease

2. URTICARIA

VERSUS

ERYTHEMA MULTIFORME

Features in common: Urticarial plaques.

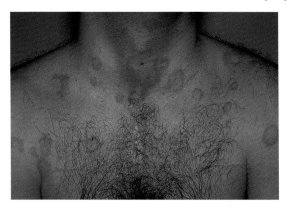

Figure 11.2.1 Urticaria.

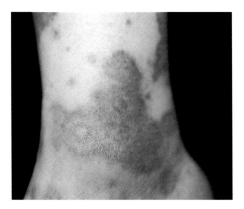

Figure 11.2.2 Erythema multiforme.

Distinguishing features

		ACUTE URTICARIA	ERYTHEMA MULTIFORME
Physical examination			
	Morphology	No target lesions	Target lesions
		Lesions transient and move around	Lesions fixed
		No mucous membrane lesions	Mucous membrane lesions
	Distribution	Generalized, no acral predominance; lesions rarely on hands and feet	Generalized, but acral predominance with lesions on hands and feet
History			
	Symptoms	Occasional prodromal upper respiratory tract infection	Occasional prodromal upper respiratory tract infection
		Ingestion of new medication	Ingestion of new medication
		No fevers	Fever rarely presents, more common in prodrome, malaise
		No problem eating or drinking	Can't eat or drink
		No pain and discomfort	Pain and discomfort
		Severe pruritus	No pruritus
	Exacerbating factors	Aspirin, salicylates, and nonsteroidal anti-inflammatory agents	None
Associated findings		Occasionally angioedema	No angioedema
		Usually idiopathic	Rarely idiopathic
		Numerous associations	Numerous associations
		Infections: streptococcal, sinus, urinary tract, viral, parasitic	Infections: *Mycoplasma pneumoniae*, herpes simplex

Continues

Distinguishing features (Continued)

	ACUTE URTICARIA	ERYTHEMA MULTIFORME
Associated findings *(con't)*	Most medications	Most common medications: nonsteroidal anti-inflammatory agents, antibiotics, barbiturates
	Rarely associated with neoplasm or connective tissue disease	Rarely associated with neoplasm or connective tissue disease
	Occasionally associated with physical factors: cold, sunlight, vibration, pressure, exercise, water	Not associated with physical factors
Epidemiology	Young adults	Young adults
Biopsy	No	Yes
	No epidermal necrosis; sparse perivascular mixed inflammatory infiltrate composed of lymphocytes, neutrophils, and eosinophils	Epidermal necrosis with underlying lymphocytic infiltrate
Laboratory	Work-up usually not necessary except as directed by symptoms or if urticaria becomes chronic	Work-up usually required for underlying cause
Treatment	Antihistamines	Treat underlying cause. Role of systemic steroids debated
Outcome	Good	Good; usually resolves over 4–6 weeks
	Usually resolves spontaneously by 6 to 8 weeks	Rarely fatal if sepsis occurs

Differential diagnosis of urticarial lesions

Angioedema (acquired and inherited C1 esterase inhibitor deficiency)
Collagen vascular disease
Contact urticaria
Dermatographism
Drug eruption
Eosinophilic cellulitis

Insect bite reaction
Urticaria
   Cold
   Pressure
   Heat
   Cholinergic
   Exercise
   Aquagenic

Urticaria *(continued)*
   Vibratory
   Solar
   Familial
Urticarial phase of bullous pemphigoid
Vasculitis

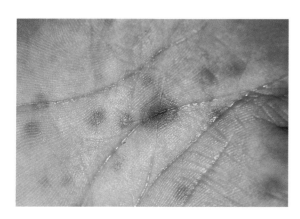

Figure 11.2.3 Erythema multiforme.
Clue to diagnosis: Target lesion.

3. URTICARIA
VERSUS
INSECT BITE REACTION

Features in common: Urticarial plaques or papules.

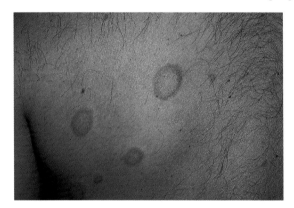

Figure 11.3.1 Urticaria.

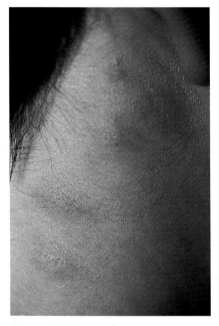

Figure 11.3.2 Insect bite reaction.

Distinguishing features

	URTICARIA	INSECT BITE REACTION
Physical examination		
Morphology	Lesion transient	Lesions fixed
	No vesicles	Vesicles may be present
	No central punctum	Central punctum or necrosis may be present
Distribution	Generalized	Localized, usually to exposed surfaces
	Lesions not grouped	Lesions may be grouped (breakfast, lunch, and dinner)
History		
Symptoms	Occasional prodromal upper respiratory tract infection	No prodromal symptoms
	Occasionally new medication	No new medication
	Pruritus	Pruritus
Exacerbatiing factors	Aspirin, salicylates, and nonsteroidal anti-inflammatory agents	None

Continues

Distinguishing features (*Continued*)

	URTICARIA	INSECT BITE REACTION
Associated findings/causes	No angioedema except in patients with acquired or inherited C1 esterase inhibitor deficiency Usually idiopathic Numerous associations Infections: streptococcal, sinus, urinary tract, viral, parasitic Medications Rarely associated with neoplasm or connective tissue disease Occasionally associated with physical factors: cold, sunlight, vibration, pressure, exercise, water	In highly allergic patients, angioedema and shock may occur Source of insects usually outdoor exposure or pets Numerous possible insects: fleas, mites, spiders, mosquitoes No history of medication intake No associated diseases May be associated with outdoor activities
Epidemiology	Young adults	Any age
Biopsy	No Sparse perivascular mixed inflammatory infiltrate composed of lymphocytes, neutrophils, and eosinophils	Occasionally Wedge-shaped mixed inflammatory infiltrate usually composed of lymphocytes and eosinophils
Laboratory	Work-up usually not necessary except as directed by symptoms or if urticaria becomes chronic	None necessary
Treatment	Antihistamines Topical therapy is of minimal benefit	Topical corticosteroids and antihistamines
Outcome	Good; usually resolves spontaneously by 6 to 8 weeks	Good; resolves spontaneously within 1–3 weeks

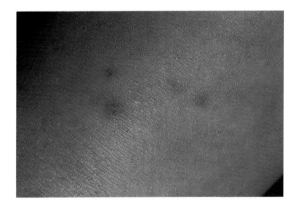

Figure 11.3.3 Insect bite reaction.
Clue to diagnosis: Central punctum.

Discussion

ACUTE URTICARIA

Definition and etiology: Urticaria is commonly known as hives. Urticaria is a transient pruritic swelling of the skin due to histamine and other vasoactive substances released in the skin. Histamine release can be mediated by immunoglobulin E (IgE) or complement or effected through a direct mast-cell-releasing agent. Acute urticaria most commonly is idiopathic but can have a number of causes, including infections and medications.

Clinical features: Urticaria is easily recognized because of the characteristic transient, pink, edematous, nonscaling swelling of the skin. Lesions are not fixed; they disappear and reappear in different locations throughout the day. Urticaria can be subdivided into acute and chronic cases. Episodes lasting less than 6 weeks are considered acute. In both acute and chronic cases of urticaria, an underlying cause is found in only a minority of patients. In acute cases of urticaria, work-up is rarely indicated, and diagnosis should be based on history and symptoms. Some causes include foods, salicylates, medications (e.g., penicillin, sulfonamides, morphine, codeine), and infections such as streptococcal sore throat, viruses, sinusitis, and urinary tract infection. Patients should also be asked if the urticaria can be induced by physical factors such as exercise, sunlight, cold, heat, vibration, pressure, and water.

The differential diagnosis includes insect bites, erythema multiforme, urticarial vasculitis, and the urticarial phase of bullous pemphigoid. In these diseases, lesions are not transient. Target lesions, mucosal lesions, and lesions on the hands and feet are common in erythema multiforme. The lesions of insect bites are usually papular and asymmetric and may be vesicular or have a central punctum or necrotic area. Urticaria is predominantly a disease of young individuals, whereas bullous pemphigoid occurs in elderly adults. The lesions of bullous pemphigoid ultimately will blister and are more prominent on flexural surfaces. In urticarial vasculitis, a variant of leukocytoclastic vasculitis, the lesions stay in one area longer than 24 to 48 hours and frequently are purpuric. A biopsy will also distinguish between the two. In urticaria, a sparse mixed perivascular infiltrate is present, whereas in urticarial vasculitis, vasculitis involving postcapillary venules is present.

Treatment: Any possible underlying causes should be eliminated. Since most cases of urticaria are acute and therefore self limited, overly aggressive therapy and work-up should be minimized. The mainstay of therapy is antihistamines. Oral prednisone is occasionally necessary; however, it should be avoided if possible in cases of chronic urticaria because of its side effects.

DRUG ERUPTION

Definition and etiology: Drug eruptions are produced after parenteral or percutaneous absorption of a medication. They may be an allergic or a toxic reaction to virtually any medication.

Clinical features: Medications can produce a wide variety of cutaneous eruptions. Almost any cutaneous reaction pattern can be produced by medications. Eruptions that are exanthematous, urticarial, psoriasiform, pityriasis-rosea-like, blistering, lichenoid, vasculitic, lymphomatoid, photosensitive, or granulomatous can be produced by medications. Other possibilities include alopecia, pigmentary abnormalities, and nail dystrophy. One of the most common types of rash is the exanthematous or maculopapular eruption. This eruption may start 1 to 2 days after onset of medication administration if the patient has had prior exposure; it may begin in 7 to 10 days if the medication is taken for the first time. The most common drugs producing exanthematous eruptions are antibiotics in the penicillin, cephalosporin, and sulfonamide families. However, almost any drug can be the culprit.

The major differential diagnostic consideration is viral exanthem. Viral exanthems usually occur in children and are uncommon in adults. The timing of onset of the rash (after starting a new medication) and the lack of systemic symptoms such as myalgia, high fever, rhinorrhea, and diarrhea (which could be caused by a viral infection) help clarify the diagnosis. In some of the childhood exanthems, ancillary physical findings (such as Koplik's spots in measles or a slapped-cheek appearance in erythema infectiosum) help in establishing a precise diagnosis.

Treatment: Drug eruptions clear within a couple of days to 2 weeks after discontinuing the medication. Occasionally, the rash can resolve even if the drug is continued owing to desensitization of the immune system by continued exposure. Antihistamines and topical steroids are helpful for pruritus.

ERYTHEMA MULTIFORME

Definition and etiology: Erythema multiforme is a reactive inflammatory skin disease secondary to a wide variety of stimuli. Common causes include medications and infections, most commonly caused by *Mycoplasma pneumoniae* or herpes simplex. Other possibilities include infections (viral, bacterial, mycobacterial, fungal, protozoal), medications (sulfonamides, penicillins, nonsteroidal anti-inflammatory agents, barbiturates, phenytoin), neoplasms (especially lymphoma), connective tissue diseases, physical agents (radiation therapy), foods, topical agents, and miscellaneous causes (pregnancy, sarcoidosis, inflammatory bowel disease).

Clinical features: Erythema multiforme commonly involves both mucosal and glabrous skin. In the mucosa, generalized erosions with pseudomembrane and crust formation are seen. Sometimes mucosal involvement can precede skin findings, which include symmetric urticarial macules and papules. Rarely, mucosal involvement is the only manifestation of erythema multiforme. Within the first few days, some of the lesions develop concentric color changes owing to necrosis, producing the characteristic "target" or "iris" lesions. Blisters may also develop. The lesions appear first on extremities and then extend onto the trunk. Patients complain of pain due to the mucosal involvement along with mild malaise or itching. In the severe form (erythema multiforme major), fever, arthralgia, severe malaise, and even death due to secondary infection can occur. Erythema multiforme major characteristically has mucous membrane involvement (oral, nasal, ocular) as well as severe and widespread skin disease (Stevens-Johnson syndrome). The relationship between erythema multiforme and toxic epidermal necrolysis (TEN), a disease with widespread tissue desquamation, continues to be debated. In TEN, target lesions are not present. In addition to TEN, the major disease in the differential diagnosis is urticaria. Unlike in urticaria, the lesions of erythema multiforme are fixed and have a tendency to involve the hands and feet. Also, oral lesions, blisters, and necrotic lesions are not seen in urticaria. For cases without target lesions, a biopsy may be necessary to establish the diagnosis of erythema multiforme. Typical pathologic findings in erythema multiforme include scattered dyskeratotic keratinocytes, dermal edema, and an interface lymphocytic infiltrate.

Treatment: Erythema multiforme usually resolves spontaneously with supportive care if the precipitating factor has been eliminated. Some physicians advocate the use of systemic steroids in the first few days of involvement, but their efficacy has been controversial. Prolonged steroid use is not advised, since signs of underlying infection may be missed. Ophthalmologic consultation should be obtained if eye involvement is suspected to prevent synechia formation or scarring. Topical dressings may help lesions to heal. In severe cases, patients should be treated in a burn unit, and electrolyte and fluid balance should be closely monitored.

INSECT BITE REACTION

Definition and etiology: Arthropods include both carnivorous spiders and eight-legged insects. Arthropods frequently bite humans, which produces a variety of cutaneous reactions ranging from necrotic ulcers and blisters to urticarial papules and plaques. Urticarial lesions, the most common insect bite reaction, are commonly seen after bee, black fly, and mosquito bites. Papular urticarial lesions can be produced after flea, mite, and bedbug bites.

Clinical features: Arthropod bite reactions can be very difficult to diagnose, since the insect usually goes unnoticed. A clue to the diagnosis of an insect bite is the finding of pruritic lesions distributed haphazardly on exposed sites. Often, in the center of the urticarial papules or plaques, a small punctum from the bite can be found. Unlike in idiopathic urticaria, lesions are fixed and not transitory, lasting a few weeks.

Treatment: The patient needs to avoid the source of exposure to the insect, or the area needs to be fumigated. Strong topical steroids can be used to minimize inflammation. If the patient has a severe reaction with systemic symptoms (hives, hypotension, and dizziness) and there is a danger of anaphylaxis, epinephrine should be given. Epinephrine kits also exist for home use (e.g., ANA-kit, epi-pen). Oral antihistamines help alleviate the pruritus.

VIRAL EXANTHEM

Definition and etiology: A variety of viruses can produce an exanthematous maculopapular morbilliform (measleslike) eruption.

Clinical features: Viral exanthems are most commonly encountered in children but can occur in adults. A viral eruption may be morphologically indistinguishable from a drug rash. Certain viral exanthems do, however, have recognizable features. Children with erythema infectiosum infection (caused by parvovirus B19) often have a "slapped-cheek" appearance because of prominent facial erythema. Patients with measles have white grainy papules on an erythematous base on the buccal mucosa, the so-called "Koplik's spots." Frequently, the diagnosis can be made only when other features such as cough and coryza are present (as in measles). Other common symptoms of viral infections include rhinorrhea, diarrhea, and myalgia. The fever of a viral infection is often higher than the fever encountered in drug reactions.

Treatment: Childhood viral exanthems are self-limited and do not require treatment. Some infections, such as those due to human immunodeficiency virus or hepatitis B, require prolonged antiviral therapy.

Suggested Readings

ACUTE URTICARIA
Davidson AE, Miller SD, Settipane G et al. Urticaria and angioedema. Cleve Clin J Med 1992;59:529–34.
Greaves MW. Chronic urticaria. N Engl J Med 1995;332:1767–72.
Mahmood T. Physical urticarias. Am Fam Physician 1994;49:1411–4.

Mahmood T, Janniger CK. Childhood urticaria. Cutis 1993;52:78–80.

DRUG ERUPTIONS
Wolkenstein P, Revuz J. Drug-induced severe skin reactions. Incidence, management and prevention. Drug Saf 1995;13:56–68.

ERYTHEMA MULTIFORME
Brice SL, Huff JC, Weston WL. Erythema multiforme minor in children. Pediatrician 1991;18:188–94.

Fabbri P, Panconesi E. Erythema multiforme ("minus" and "maius") and drug intake. Clin Dermatol 1993;11:479–89.

INSECT BITES
Janniger CK, Schutzer SE, Schwartz RA. Childhood insect bite reactions to ants, wasps, and bees (published erratum appears in Cutis 1994;54:245). Cutis 1994;54:14–16.

Muller U. Clinical aspects, diagnosis and therapy of insect bite allergy. Schweiz Med Wochenschr 1989;119:1761–68.

VIRAL EXANTHEMS
Asano Y, Yoshikawa T. Human herpesvirus-6 and parvovirus B19 infections in children (review). Curr Opin Pediatr 1993;5:14–20

Bialecki C, Feder HM Jr, Grant-Kels JM. The six classic childhood exanthems: a review and update. J Am Acad Dermatol 1989;21:891–903.

Cherry JD. Contemporary infectious exanthems. Clin Infect Dis 1993;16:199–205.

Frieden IJ. Childhood exanthems (review). Curr Opin Pediatr 1995;7:411–14.

Zalla MJ, Su WP, Fransway AF. Dermatologic manifestations of human immunodeficiency virus infection (review). Mayo Clin Proc 1992;67:1089–1108.

12

Generalized Pustular Eruptions

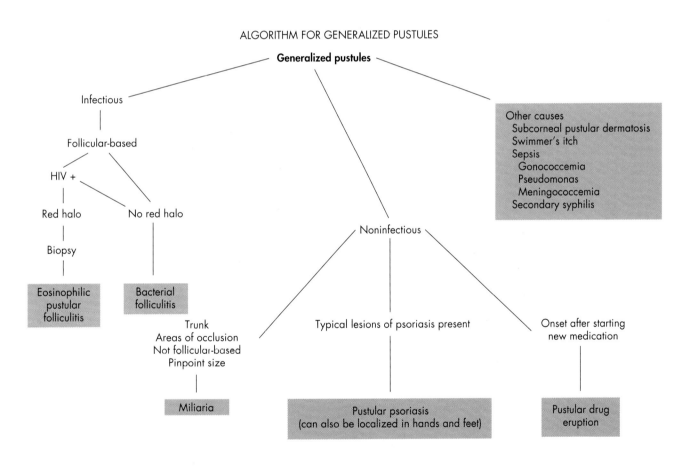

ALGORITHM FOR GENERALIZED PUSTULES

Generalized pustules

Infectious

Follicular-based

HIV +

Red halo

Biopsy

Eosinophilic
pustular
folliculitis

No red halo

Bacterial
folliculitis

Trunk
Areas of occlusion
Not follicular-based
Pinpoint size

Miliaria

Noninfectious

Typical lesions of psoriasis present

Pustular psoriasis
(can also be localized in hands and feet)

Onset after starting
new medication

Pustular drug
eruption

Other causes
  Subcorneal pustular dermatosis
  Swimmer's itch
  Sepsis
    Gonococcemia
    Pseudomonas
    Meningococcemia
  Secondary syphilis

Introduction

A pustule is a circumscribed "blister" of the skin containing pus. Microscopic evaluation reveals a focal collection of neutrophils or eosinophils. Pustular eruptions can be subdivided into either localized or generalized eruptions. Pustules can also be categorized according to cause (infectious versus noninfectious). The most common localized noninfectious form of pustular eruptions is acne, which is discussed in Chapter 2. Causes of localized infectious pustules such as impetigo and candidiasis are also discussed in Chapters 2 and 3. Generalized noninfectious pustular eruptions include pustular psoriasis, pustular drug eruptions, and miliaria. The diagnosis is usually relatively straightforward, since patients with pustular psoriasis most often have classic psoriatic lesions elsewhere. Pustular drug eruptions start after the onset of administration of a drug, and miliaria occurs in occluded areas in patients who have been sweating. Generalized infectious pustular eruptions include eosinophilic pustular folliculitis (Ofuji's disease), which is likely due to an as-yet-unidentified organism, and bacterial folliculitis.

1. EOSINOPHILIC PUSTULAR FOLLICULITIS

VERSUS

BACTERIAL FOLLICULITIS

Features in common: Follicular papules and pustules.

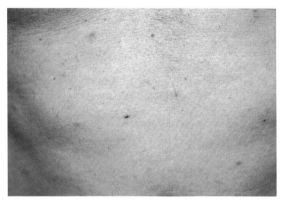

Figure 12.1.1 Eosinophilic pustular folliculitis.

Figure 12.1.2 Bacterial folliculitis.

Distinguishing features

	BACTERIAL FOLLICULITIS	EOSINOPHILIC PUSTULAR FOLLICULITIS
Physical examination		
Morphology	No surrounding halo (except in pseudomonal folliculitis, also known as hot-tub folliculitis)	Red halo surrounding pustules
	No urticarial papules	Urticarial papules
Distribution	Trunk, buttocks, and thighs	Trunk and proximal extremities favored
	Face rarely involved	Face may be involved
History		
Symptoms	Pruritus	Pruritus
Exacerbating factors	Diabetes	None known
Associated findings	None	None
Epidemiology	No age or sex predilection	Most common in patients with acquired immunodeficiency syndrome or individuals of Japanese heritage
	Most commonly seen in normal population but can also occur in patient with human immunodeficiency virus disease	Rarely can be seen in normal population
Biopsy	No	Yes
	Pustule filled with neutrophils connected to hair follicle	Pustule filled with eosinophils connected to hair follicle
Laboratory	Culture positive for *Staphylococcus aureus*	Culture negative
Treatment	Topical or systemic antibiotics	Ultraviolet light, isotretinoin (Accutane), oral metronidazole (Flagyl), antihistamines, topical steroids, itraconazole
	Antibiotic soaps	
Outcome	Good	Chronic

Differential diagnosis of folliculitis

Acne vulgaris
Bacterial folliculitis
  (*Staphylococcus, Pseudomonas*)
Dermatitis herpetiformis
Eosinophilic pustular folliculitis
Folliculitis decalvans
Grover's disease
Hidradenitis suppurativa
Insect bites
Keratosis pilaris

Lichen planus
Miliaria
Newborn
  Candidiasis
  Erythema toxicum neonatorum
  Pustular melanosis of infancy
Pseudomonas folliculitis
Scurvy
Sycosis barbae

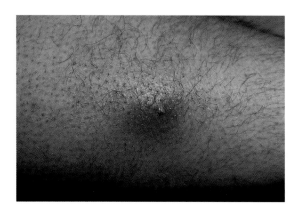

Figure 12.1.3 Bacterial folliculitis.
Clue to diagnosis: Furuncle (follicular-based abscess).

2. MILIARIA RUBRA

VERSUS

BACTERIAL FOLLICULITIS

Features in common: Generalized papules and pustules.

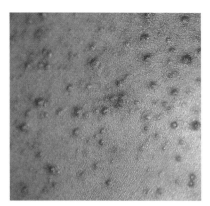

Figure 12.2.1 Miliaria.

Figure 12.2.2 Bacterial folliculitis.

Distinguishing features

	BACTERIAL FOLLICULITIS	MILIARIA RUBRA
Physical examination		
Morphology	Primary lesion: pustule, no vesicles	Primary lesion: small papules and vesicles (pustules secondary finding)
	Excoriations common	Excoriations rare
Distribution	Trunk, buttocks, and thighs	Trunk or in areas of occlusion like diaper area in children
History		
Symptoms	Use of hot tub in *Pseudomonas* folliculitis	No hot tub use
	Pruritus	No pruritus
Exacerbating factors	None	Occlusive clothing
		Hot humid climate

Continues

Distinguishing features *(Continued)*

	BACTERIAL FOLLICULITIS	MILIARIA RUBRA
Associated findings	Diabetes	Fever, profuse sweating
Epidemiology	No age or sex predilection	Most common in babies and infants
Biopsy	No Pustule filled with neutrophils connected to hair follicle	No Dilated and obstructed eccrine duct
Laboratory	Culture positive for *Staphylococcus aureus*	Culture negative
Treatment	Topical or systemic antibiotics Antibiotic soaps	Usually self limited Avoid occlusive clothing and sweating
Outcome	Good	Good

Differential diagnosis of generalized pustular eruptions

Common causes
  Folliculitis
  Impetigo
  Miliaria
  Pustular drug eruption
  Pustular psoriasis
  Transient neonatal pustular
    melanosis

Rarer causes
  Ecthyma gangrenosum
  Eosinophillic pustular folliculitis
    (Ofuji's disease)
  Erythema toxicum neonatorum
  Gonococcemia
  IgA pemphigus

Rarer causes *(continued)*
  Impetigo herpetiformis
  Pyoderma gangrenosum
  Reiter's disease
  Secondary syphilis
  Subcorneal pustular dermatosis
  Swimmer's itch

Figure 12.2.3 Bacterial folliculitis.
Clue to diagnosis: Follicular-based
pustule.

3. PUSTULAR PSORIASIS
VERSUS
PUSTULAR DRUG ERUPTION

Features in common: Generalized pustules.

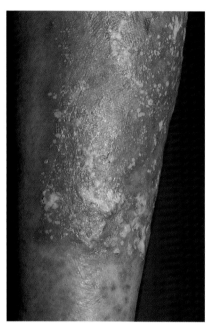

Figure 12.3.1 Pustular psoriasis.

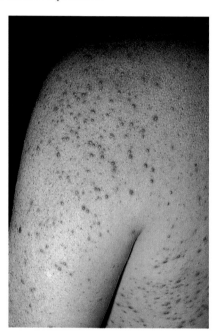

Figure 12.3.2 Pustular drug eruption.

Distinguishing features

	PUSTULAR PSORIASIS	**PUSTULAR DRUG ERUPTION**

Physical examination
  Morphology
	Red papules and plaques
	Silvery-colored scale
	Pustules not follicular based
	Annular plaques/patches with
	  peripheral pustules may be present
		No plaques
		No scale
		Pustules may be follicular based
		No annular lesions

Distribution	Scalp and predilection for extensor
	  surfaces of body
		Truncal, no predilection for
		  extensor surfaces

History Symptoms	No new drug Fever	New drug Fever rare
Exacerbating factors	Tapering of oral steroids Infections Pregnancy Medications Irritating topical medications Sunburn	None

Continues

Distinguishing features *(Continued)*

	PUSTULAR PSORIASIS	PUSTULAR DRUG ERUPTION
Associated findings	Positive family history in 10% to 20% of patients	No family history of psoriasis
	Improves with sun exposure	No relationship to sun exposure
	Arthritis in some patients	No arthritis
	Onychodystrophy	No onychodystrophy
Epidemiology	Any age, no sex predilection	Usually adults
Biopsy	Yes	Sometimes
	Psoriasiform epidermal hyperplasia with neutrophil microabscesses in epidermis and stratum corneum	Nonspecific subcorneal pustule
Laboratory	Increased erythrocyte sedimentation rate (ESR)	Slight leukocytosis
	Leukocytosis	
	Hypocalcemia	
Treatment	Etretinate most effective	Discontinuation of drug
	Ultraviolet B light, dapsone, methotrexate	Supportive topical care
Outcome	Chronic disease	Resolves after drug is discontinued

Drugs causing pustular eruption

Androgens
Corticosteroids
Isoniazid
Lithium

Halogens (iodide, bromide)
Miscellaneous: antibiotics,
   phenytoin, diltiazem,
   furosemide, carbamazepine

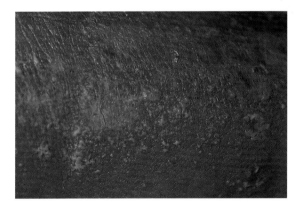

Figure 12.3.3 Pustular psoriasis.
Clue to diagnosis: Pustules within psoriasiform plaque.

Discussion

BACTERIAL FOLLICULITIS

Definition and etiology: Bacterial folliculitis is an infection of hair follicles, most often due to *Staphylococcus aureus* but also sometimes due to *Pseudomonas aeruginosa*. *Pseudomonas* folliculitis is most commonly seen in patients who have been using hot tubs.

Clinical features: Bacterial folliculitis can occur on any body site that has hair follicles. Folliculitis decalvans and dissecting cellulitis are specific variants that occur on the scalp. Sycosis barbae is a form that occurs on the beard area. The most common sites of bacterial folliculitis are the legs, thighs, and trunk. Examination reveals follicular-based papules and pustules that often have a central hair. The lesions are highly pruritic and often excoriated. Because of chronic scratching, eczematous changes may be present.

The differential diagnosis includes miliaria pustulosa, acne, dermatitis herpetiformis, *Pityrosporum* folliculitis, and Grover's disease (transient acantholytic dermatosis). Unlike in acne, comedones are not present in folliculitis, and the distribution of lesions is usually different. Miliaria pustulosa is caused by occlusion of eccrine glands. Miliaria most commonly occurs suddenly after an episode of severe sweating in sites of occlusion, such as the trunk. The lesions are usually smaller than lesions of folliculitis, and small vesicles and pustules are present. Grover's disease is a very pruritic, nondescript papular truncal eruption (pustules are usually absent) that is predominantly found in adult men. *Pityrosporum* folliculitis is morphologically identical to bacterial folliculitis but is due to *Pityrosporum orbiculare*, a commensal yeast. It occurs more commonly in immunosuppressed individuals and may uncommonly be a presenting sign of underlying disease, such as Hodgkin's disease. The diagnosis is made clinically, and positive culture results are confirmatory. In most cases of folliculitis, a biopsy is not necessary.

Treatment: Occlusive clothing should be avoided. In severe cases, oral antibiotics effective against *Staphylococcus aureus* should be used. In milder cases, topical antibiotics and antibiotic soaps are effective. In some cases, recurrence is common and the disease difficult to eradicate despite use of appropriate antibiotics and antibacterial soaps. Work-up for immune deficiency or diabetes, however, is usually still negative.

EOSINOPHILIC PUSTULAR FOLLICULITIS

Definition and etiology: Eosinophilic pustular folliculitis (Ofuji's disease) is an idiopathic disorder hypothe-

sized to be infectious. This form of folliculitis is characterized by an eosinophilic inflammatory infiltrate within and surrounding hair follicles.

Clinical features: Although eosinophilic pustular folliculitis was originally described as a form of pruritic folliculitis of the scalp in Japanese men, it most commonly presents as a chronic pruritic eruption on the trunk in individuals with human immunodeficiency virus infection. Follicular papules and pustules are seen. Unlike in bacterial folliculitis, urticarial papules are also present, and the pustules are frequently surrounded by a bright red urticarial halo. Although the diagnosis can be suspected in patients with acquired immunodeficiency syndrome, diagnosis ultimately depends on the histologic finding of an eosinophilic pustule within the follicular infundibulum. The differential diagnosis includes Grover's disease (transient acantholytic dermatosis) and miliaria pustulosa. Grover's disease primarily affects adult men and is characterized by pruritic nondescript papules that are not follicular based. A characteristic feature of Grover's disease is severe pruritus with minimal clinical findings. In miliaria, the lesions are smaller and not follicular based. They appear suddenly after severe sweating.

Treatment: Treatment is difficult. Ultraviolet light therapy, isotretinoin (Accutane), intraconazole, and oral metronidazole have been reported to help.

MILIARIA RUBRA

Definition and etiology: Miliaria is an eruption due to obstruction of eccrine glands. It can be subdivided into miliaria crystallina, rubra, or profunda depending on the site of obstruction. The sites of obstruction are the stratum corneum in miliaria crystallina, the epidermis in miliaria rubra, and within the dermis in miliaria profunda.

Clinical features: Miliaria presents as an acute pruritic eruption after an episode of severe sweating. Covered sites such as the trunk or diaper are most commonly involved. In miliaria crystallina, small pinpoint-sized vesicles are seen. In miliaria rubra, small vesicles, papules, and pustules are present. In miliaria profunda, papular lesions predominate. The major differential diagnostic considerations are folliculitis and Grover's disease. The lesions of folliculitis are predominantly pustular and not vesicular, as in miliaria. Folliculitis is centered around hair follicles. Although sweating may have a pathogenic role in producing the lesions of Grover's disease, it is typically a chronic nonpruritic eruption in elderly men that requires a biopsy for definitive diagnosis.

Treatment: The eruption of miliaria is usually self limited and does not require therapy. Wearing occlusive clothing and sweating should be minimized. Cool baths, compresses, and air conditioning may be helpful.

PUSTULAR DRUG ERUPTION

Definition and etiology: Rarely, certain medications can induce a pustular eruption.

Clinical features: There are two common types of pustular drug eruptions: generalized and acneiform. Acneiform pustular drug eruptions resemble acne except that lesions are predominantly monomorphous pustules, and comedones are rarely found. Acneiform drug eruptions are most commonly produced by androgens, oral corticosteroids, isoniazid, lithium, and halogens. Generalized pustular drug eruptions are most commonly produced by a variety of different antibiotics and can be confused with pustular psoriasis. The lesions are predominantly truncal; numerous pustules on an erythematous base are found; and the pustules are not follicular centered. As in pustular psoriasis, fever may be present. The onset of the rash after ingestion of a medication, the lack of a family history of psoriasis, and the lack of classic psoriatic lesions help distinguish pustular drug eruptions from pustular psoriasis.

Treatment: Pustular drug eruptions improve spontaneously after the medication is discontinued. Acneiform eruptions will take weeks to months to resolve, whereas generalized pustular eruptions resolve in 1 to 3 weeks. Use of a standard acne regimen including antibiotics, benzoyl peroxide, and topical retinoids can hasten the resolution of the acneiform eruptions.

PSORIASIS

Definition and etiology: Psoriasis is an inflammatory disease characterized by increased epidermal proliferation. The cause of psoriasis is unknown, but abnormal epidermal kinetics, activation of the immune system within the skin, and genetic factors must be taken into account.

Clinical features: Approximately one-third of individuals with psoriasis have a positive family history. Psoriasis is a relatively common skin disease, affecting about 2% of the population of the United States. Asians are less commonly affected. The most common age of onset is during the third decade, but psoriasis can present at any age. In most cases of psoriasis, examination reveals bright red erythematous plaques covered with white to silvery-colored scale. Areas of predilection include the elbows, knees, scalp, and sacrum. Extensor surface involvement predominates. Pitting of the nails and onychodystrophy occur frequently. Nails may appear to have an oil drop under them and small pits. Pustular psoriasis is a rare variant of psoriasis in which

pustules are found. Pustular psoriasis can be further divided into four subtypes: palmoplantar acral pustular psoriasis (see Ch. 4), acute generalized pustular psoriasis of von Zumbusch, subacute annular psoriasis, and a mixed type.

Acute generalized pustular psoriasis of the von Zumbusch type occurs in patients with a history of classic psoriasis. The generalized pustular flare-up is precipitated by a variety of factors, such as corticosteroid withdrawal, pregnancy, infection, sunlight, or irritating topical therapy (e.g., coal tar or anthralin). Patients are seriously ill with fever and have an elevated erythrocyte sedimentation rate as well as leukocytosis and arthritis. Preexisting lesions become bright red and develop pustules. Sheets of pustules spread to previously uninvolved skin to cover the entire integument. Isolated pustules, annular lesions, and plaques of pustules are found.

In the subacute annular form of pustular psoriasis, the lesions start as annular areas of erythema that become raised and edematous and have a serpiginous appearance. Eventually, pustules appear at the advancing edge of the lesions. Unlike in the acute form, lesions develop slowly, and patients are not as sick. In the mixed form, features of both the acute and the subacute annular form are seen.

The major differential diagnostic considerations include pustular drug eruption, subcorneal pustular dermatosis (Sneddon-Wilkinson, disease), bacterial folliculitis, and acrodermatitis continua (Hallopeau's acrodermatitis). Pustular drug eruption occurs 1 to 2 weeks after onset of administration of certain medications. Patients are usually not as sick as patients with pustular psoriasis, do not have high fever, have minimal leukocytosis, and do not have a history of preceding psoriatic lesions. In subcorneal pustular dermatosis, the lesions are mostly localized to flexural areas such as the axilla and groin. A characteristic finding is pustules with a meniscus of clear overlying fluid. In acrodermatitis continua, which may also be a variant of pustular psoriasis, the pustules predominantly start around fingernails and cause confusion with paronychia infection.

Treatment: The treatment of choice for generalized pustular psoriasis is oral etretinate. Alternative therapies include methotrexate, oral dapsone, and hospitalization.

Suggested Readings

BACTERIAL FOLLICULITIS
Berger RS, Seifert MR. Whirlpool folliculitis: a review of its cause, treatment, and prevention (review). Cutis 1990;45:97–98.

Feingold DS. Staphylococcal and streptococcal pyodermas (review). Semin Dermatol 1993;12:331–35.

Herman LE, Haraw SJ, Glossein RA, Kurban AK. Folliculitis. A clinicopathologic (review). Pathol Annu 1991;2: 201–46.

EOSINOPHILIC PUSTULAR FOLLICULITIS

Camacho-Martinez F. Eosinophilic pustular folliculitis (review). J Am Acad Dermatol 1987;17:686–88.

Dupond AS, Aubin F, Bourezane Y et al. Eosinophilic pustular folliculitis in infancy: report of two affected brothers. (review). Br J Dermatol 1995;132:296–99.

MILIARIA RUBRA

Feng E, Janniger CK. Miliaria (review). Cutis 1995;55: 213–26.

PUSTULAR DRUG ERUPTION

Burrows NP, Russell Jones RR. Pustular drug eruptions: a histopathological spectrum. Histopathology 1993;22: 569–73.

Spencer JM, Silvers DN, Grossman ME. Pustular eruption after drug exposure: is it pustular psoriasis or a pustular drug eruption? Br J Dermatol 1994;130:514–19.

Webster GF. Pustular drug reactions (review). Clin Dermatol 1993;11:541–43.

PSORIASIS

Abel EA et al. Drugs in exacerbation of psoriasis (review). J Am Acad Dermatol 1986;15:1007–22.

Farber EM, Nall L. Pustular psoriasis (review). Cutis 1993; 51:29–32.

Zelickson BD, Muller SA. Generalized pustular psoriasis. A review of 63 cases. Arch Dermatol 1991;127:1339–45.

Zelickson BD, Muller SA. Generalized pustular psoriasis in childhood. Report of thirteen cases. J Am Acad Dermatol 1991;24:186–94.

III

Neoplasms

13 *Epidermal Growths*

ALGORITHM FOR EPIDERMAL GROWTHS

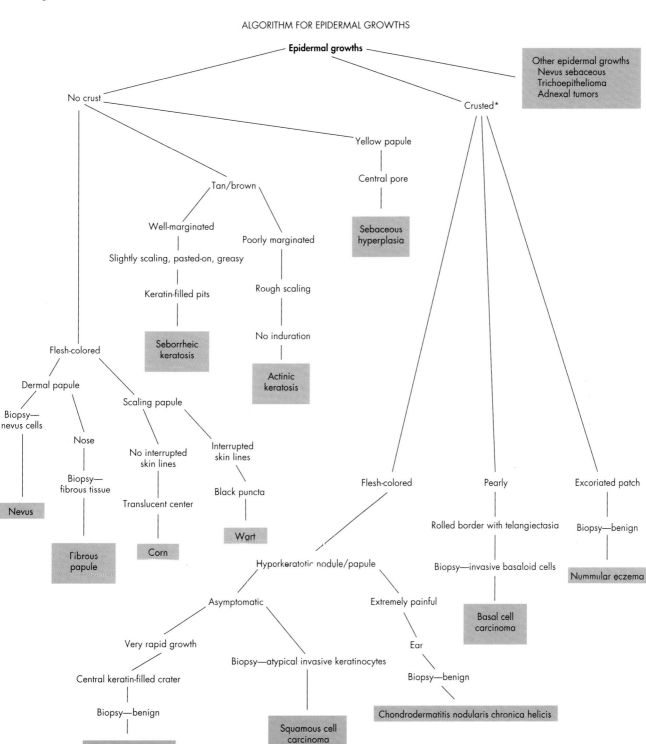

*Basal cell and squamous cell carcinoma may not be crusted when small.

DIFFERENTIAL DIAGNOSIS

DISEASE DISCUSSION

Introduction

Epidermal growths are caused by a proliferation of basal cells, or keratinocytes. They can be recognized by superficial thickening of the skin, which is often accompanied by increased production of keratin (manifested as scaling). It is important to differentiate scale (keratin) from crust (dried-up blood), since a crusting growth suggests a malignant process. For all growths that are crusted or ulcerated, a *biopsy* is mandatory unless there is a clear-cut history of preceding injury or irritation. A couple of the diseases discussed in this chapter are not epidermal growths. Sebaceous hyperplasia, flesh-colored nevi, and fibrous papule of the nose are included because they so closely resemble basal cell carcinoma. Likewise, nummular eczema, an inflammatory process, can mimic superficial basal cell carcinoma clinically.

1. PLANTAR WART

VERSUS

CORN

Features in common: Scaling papule or plaque of the feet.

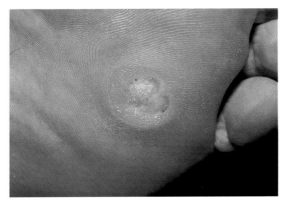

Figure 13.1.1 Wart.

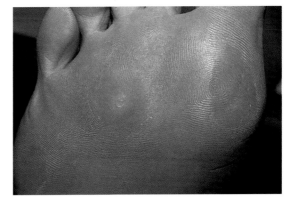

Figure 13.1.2 Corn.

Distinguishing features

	PLANTAR WART	CORN
Physical examination		
Morphology	Interrupted skin lines	No interrupted skin lines
	Black puncta	No black puncta
	No translucent center	Translucent center
	Koebner's phenomenon present	No Koebner's phenomenon
Distribution	Feet, not related to pressure points	Feet sites of pressure
	Elsewhere	Rarely hands
History		
Symptoms	Usually not painful	Painful
	More painful upon pinching	More pain upon pressure
Exacerbating factors	Immunosuppression	Ill-fitting shoes
		Bone projections
		Not immunosuppressed
Associated findings	Rarely squamous cell carcinoma	None
Epidemiology	Children predominate	Adults predominate
Biopsy	Usually not done	Not done
	Epidermal papillomatosis and koilocytosis	Keratin-filled epidermal invagination
Laboratory	None	None
Treatment	Acids, cryotherapy, surgery	New shoes, paring, pads, surgery
Outcome	Resolves spontaneously or with destructive treatment	Resolves when pressure and friction removed

Differential diagnosis of scaling papules of feet

Squamous cell carcinoma   Adnexal tumor   Seborrheic keratosis

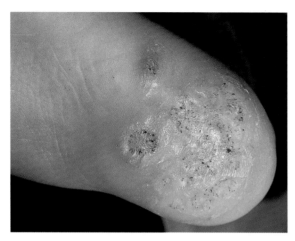

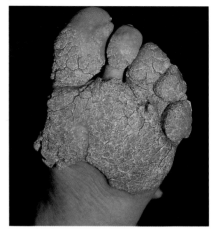

Figure 13.1.3 Wart. *Clue to diagnosis:* Interrupted skin lines, black puncta.

Figure 13.1.4 Warts in a cardiac transplant patient.

2. SEBORRHEIC KERATOSIS
VERSUS
ACTINIC KERATOSIS

Features in common: Scaling tan or brown papules.

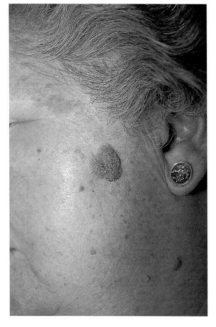

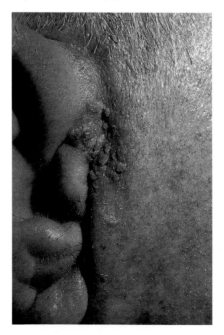

Figure 13.2.1 Seborrheic keratosis.

Figure 13.2.2 Actinic keratosis.

Distinguishing features

	SEBORRHEIC KERATOSIS	ACTINIC KERATOSIS
Physical examination		
Morphology	Well-demarcated Smooth greasy scale Pasted-on look	Poorly demarcated Rough scale Not pasted-on
Distribution	Generalized	Sun-exposed skin
History		
Symptoms	None	None
Exacerbating factors	None	Sunlight exposure Immunosuppression
Associated findings	None	Sun-damaged skin Skin cancer
Epidemiology	Common Middle-aged and elderly All skin types No relation to sun exposure	Common Adults Fair-complected skin A lot of sun exposure
Biopsy	Usually not necessary Biopsy required for irritated or atypical lesions Uniform benign keratinocytes, horn cysts	Usually not necessary Biopsy required for thick or indurated lesions Partial-thickness atypical keratinocytes, that spare adnexal structures
Laboratory	None	None
Treatment	None required	Treat hyperkeratotic lesions (cryotherapy, 5-fluorouracil)
Outcome	Persistent No malignant potential	Spontaneously involute (20%) Malignant potential for squamous cell carcinoma (< 0.1%)

Differential diagnosis

Wart
Squamous cell carcinoma

Melanoma
Basal cell carcinoma

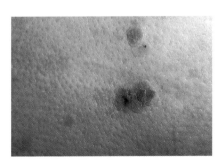

***Figure* 13.2.3** Seborrheic keratosis. *Clue to diagnosis:* Well-demarcated, pasted-on appearance.

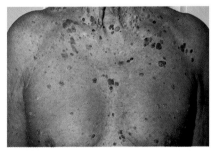

***Figure* 13.2.4** Seborrheic keratosis that is tan and brown.

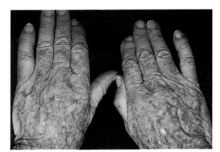

***Figure* 13.2.5** Actinic keratosis. *Clue to diagnosis:* Ill-marginated, rough scale.

3. ACTINIC KERATOSIS
VERSUS
SQUAMOUS CELL CARCINOMA

Features in common: Scaling papule or nodule.

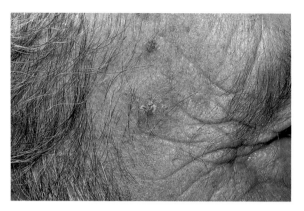

Figure 13.3.1 Actinic keratosis.

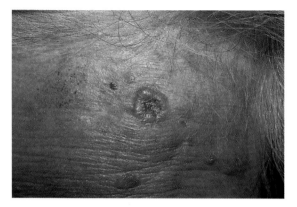

Figure 13.3.2 Squamous cell cancer.

Distinguishing features

	ACTINIC KERATOSIS	SQUAMOUS CELL CARCINOMA
Physical examination		
Morphology	Poorly demarcated Rough scale Not indurated No crust	Fairly well demarcated No rough scale Indurated May crust
Distribution	Sun-exposed skin	Usually sun-exposed
History		
Symptoms	No bleeding	May bleed
Exacerbating factors	Sunlight exposure Immunosuppression	Sunlight exposure Immunosuppression

Associated findings	Sun-damaged skin
	Skin cancer
	No chronic injury
	
	Cutaneous horn
		Sun-damaged skin
		Actinic keratosis
		Chronic injury: burn scar,
		  irradiation site, draining sinus,
		  erosive discoid lupus erythematosus
		Cutaneous horn

Epidemiology	Common	Less common

Biopsy	Usually not necessary; biopsy for
	  thick or indurated lesions
	Partial-thickness atypical keratinocytes
	  that spare adnexal structures
		Yes
		
		Full-thickness atypia and invasive
		  atypical keratinocytes

Continues

Distinguishing features (*Continued*)

	ACTINIC KERATOSIS	**SQUAMOUS CELL CARCINOMA**
Laboratory	None	None
Treatment	Treat hyperkeratotic lesions (cryotherapy, 5-fluorouracil)	Excision
Outcome	Spontaneously involute (20%) Do not metastasize Malignant potential for squamous cell cancer (< 0.1%)	Do not involute Usually do not metastasize except for lesions in scars, on lips, and in chronic ulcers

Differential diagnosis of scaling isolated papules or nodules

Basal cell carcinoma

Chondrodermatitis nodularis chronica helicis (ear)

Keratoacanthoma

Wart

Adnexal tumor

Seborrheic keratosis

Epidermal nevus

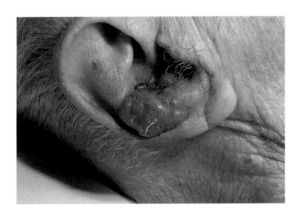

Figure 13.3.3 Squamous cell carcinoma. *Clue to diagnosis:* Crusted, indurated nodule.

4. SQUAMOUS CELL CARCINOMA
VERSUS
WART

Features in common: Scaling papule or nodule.

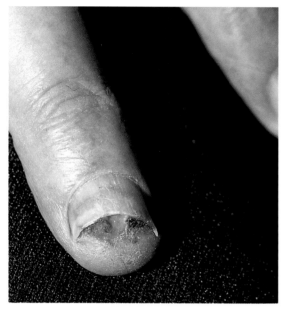

Figure 13.4.1 Squamous cell carcinoma.

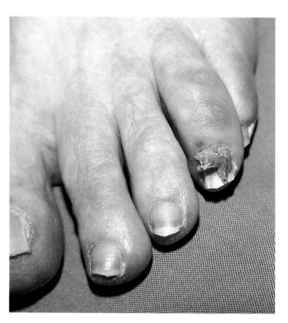

Figure 13.4.2 Wart.

Distinguishing features

	SQUAMOUS CELL CARCINOMA	WART
Physical examination		
Morphology	Not papillomatous	Papillomatous
	May crust	No crust
	Endophytic	Exophytic
	No Koebner's phenomenon	Koebner's phenomenon
	No black puncta	Black puncta
	Single lesion	Multiple lesions
Distribution	Usually sun-exposed skin	Predominantly hands, feet
History		
Symptoms	May bleed	No bleeding
Exacerbating factors	Sunlight exposure	
	Immunosuppression	Immunosuppression
Associated findings	Sun-damaged skin	No sun-damaged skin
	Actinic keratoses	No actinic keratoses

Continues

Distinguishing features (Continued)

	SQUAMOUS CELL CARCINOMA	WART
Associated findings (continued)	Chronic injury (burn scar, irradiation site, draining sinus, erosive discoid lupus erythematosus) Cutaneous horn	No chronic injury Cutaneous horn
Epidemiology	Less common Adults Fair skin A lot of sun exposure	Common Children and adults All skin types No relation to sunlight
Biopsy	Yes Full-thickness atypia and invasive atypical keratinocytes	Usually not done Epidermal papillomatosis and koilocytosis
Laboratory	None	None
Treatment	Excision	Acids, cryotherapy, surgery
Outcome	Do not involute Usually do not metastasize except for lesions in scars, on lips, and in chronic ulcers	Spontaneously involute Do not metastasize

Different types of squamous cell carcinoma

Actinic-induced
Chemical-induced
Thermal-induced (kangri cancer)
Radiation-induced
Chronic ulcer (Marjolin's ulcer)

Squamous cell carcinoma in situ (Bowen's disease, erythroplasia of Queyrat)
Verrucous carcinoma (erythroplasia of Queyrat, giant condyloma of Buschke-Löwenstein, epithelioma cuniculatum, and oral florid papillomatosis)

5. KERATOACANTHOMA
VERSUS
SQUAMOUS CELL CARCINOMA

Features in common: Flesh-colored nodule.

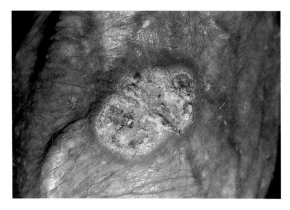

Figure 13.5.1 Keratoacanthoma.

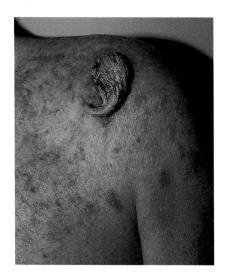

Figure 13.5.2 Squamous cell carcinoma.

Distinguishing features

	KERATOACANTHOMA	SQUAMOUS CELL CARCINOMA
Physical examination		
Morphology	Central keratin-filled crater	Rare crater
	No crust	May crust
Distribution	Usually sun-exposed skin	Usually sun-exposed skin
History		
Symptoms	No bleeding	May bleed
	Rapid growth	Not rapid growth
Exacerbating factors	None	Sunlight exposure
		Immunosuppression
Associated findings	Muir-Torre syndrome (sebaceous tumors, keratoacanthomas, low-grade internal malignancies)	No syndrome
	Sun-damaged skin	Sun-damaged skin
	Contact with tar	Actinic keratosis
	Rarely acute injury	Chronic injury (burn scar, irradiation site, draining sinus, erosive discoid lupus erythematosus)
Epidemiology	Uncommon	Less common
	Familial multiple keratoacanthoma	Not familial

Continues

Distinguishing features *(Continued)*

	KERATOACANTHOMA	SQUAMOUS CELL CARCINOMA
Biopsy	Yes: keratin core, buttress of pseudoepitheliomatous hyperplasia, eosinophilic keratinocytes	Yes: full-thickness atypia and invasive atypical keratinocytes
Laboratory	None	None
Treatment	Excision, intralesional bleomycin, 5-fluorouracil	Excision
Outcome	May spontaneously involute Rarely metastasizes	Does not involute Usually do not metastasize except for lesions in scars, on lip, and in chronic ulcers

Types of keratoacanthoma

Solitary   Giant
Subungual   Multiple

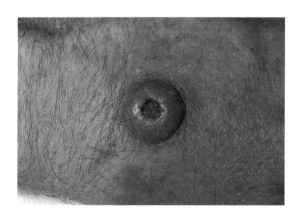

Figure 13.5.3 Keratoacanthoma. *Clue to diagnosis:* Keratin-filled central crater.

6. CHONDRODERMATITIS NODULARIS CHRONICA HELICIS VERSUS SQUAMOUS CELL CARCINOMA

Features in common: Flesh-colored nodule.

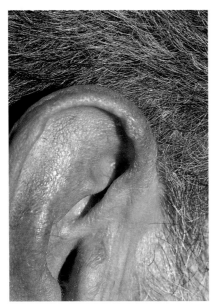

Figure 13.6.1 Chondrodermatitis nodularis chronica helicis.

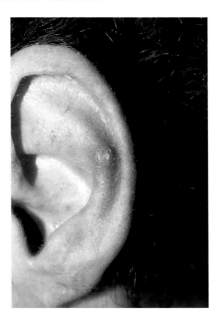

Figure 13.6.2 Squamous cell carcinoma.

Distinguishing features

	CHONDRODERMATITIS NODULARIS CHRONICA HELICIS	SQUAMOUS CELL CARCINOMA
Physical examination		
Morphology	Scale	Scale
	Crust	May crust
Distribution	Ear (helix, anthelix)	Usually sun-exposed skin
History		
Symptoms	Painful	Not painful
Exacerbating factors	Sleeping on affected ear, trauma	Sunlight exposure, immunosuppression
Associated findings	No sun-damaged skin	Sun-damaged skin
	No actinic keratosis	Actinic keratosis
		Chronic injury (burn scar, irradiation site, draining sinus, erosive discoid lupus erythematosus)
Epidemiology	Uncommon	Less common

Continues

Distinguishing features (*Continued*)

	CHONDRODERMATITIS NODULARIS CHRONICA HELICIS	SQUAMOUS CELL CARCINOMA
Biopsy	Yes: ulcerated epidermis with adjacent acanthosis, degenerated collagen, inflammation, surrounding granulation tissue	Yes: full-thickness atypia and invasive atypical keratinocytes
Laboratory	None	None
Treatment	Steroids, cryosurgery, excision, avoiding pressure on ear	Excision
Outcome	Does not involute Does not metastasize	Does not involute Usually do not metastasize except for lesions in scars, on lips, and in chronic ulcers

Differential diagnosis of flesh-colored nodule

Basal cell carcinoma
Seborrheic keratosis
Adnexal tumor
Chondrodermatitis nodularis
  chronica helicis
Fibrous papule
Nevus

Neurofibroma
Skin tag
Dermatofibroma
Leiomyoma
Syringoma
Sebaceous hyperplasia
Squamous cell carcinoma

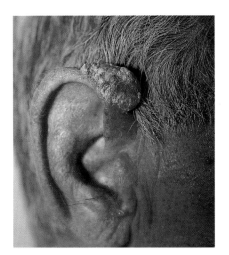

Figure 13.6.3 Squamous cell carcinoma. *Clue to diagnosis:* Scaling and crusted nodule.

7. SQUAMOUS CELL CARCINOMA
VERSUS
BASAL CELL CARCINOMA (NODULAR)

Features in common: Crusted nodule or plaque.

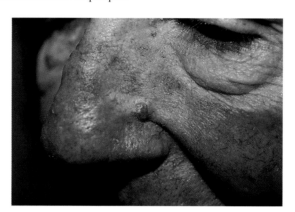

Figure 13.7.2 Basal cell carcinoma.

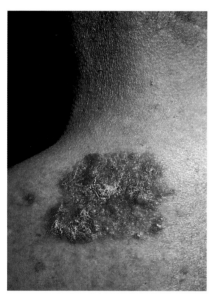

Figure 13.7.1 Squamous cell carcinoma.

Distinguishing features

	SQUAMOUS CELL CARCINOMA	BASAL CELL CARCINOMA (NODULAR)
Physical examination		
Morphology	Flesh-colored	Pearly/translucent
	Scaling	Usually no scaling
	No central depression	Central depression
	No telangiectasia	Telangiectasia
	No raised border	Raised rolled border
Distribution	Usually sun-exposed skin	Sun-exposed skin
History		
Symptoms	May bleed	May bleed
Exacerbating factors	Sunlight exposure	Sunlight exposure
	Immunosuppression	No immunosuppression
Associated findings	Sun-damaged skin	Sun-damaged skin
	Actinic keratosis	Actinic keratosis
	Chronic injury (burn scar, irradiation site, draining sinus, erosive discoid lupus erythematosus)	No injury

Continues

Distinguishing features (Continued)

	SQUAMOUS CELL CARCINOMA	BASAL CELL CARCINOMA (NODULAR)
Epidemiology	Less common	Rarely inherited (basal cell nevus syndrome) Relatively common
Biopsy	Yes: full-thickness atypia and invasive atypical keratinocytes	Yes: invasive basaloid cells with peripheral palisading and clotting clefts from stroma
Laboratory	None	None
Treatment	Excision	Excision, Mohs' surgery, electrodesiccation and curettage
Outcome	Usually do not metastasize except for lesions in scars, on lips, and in chronic ulcers	Does not metastasize

Differential diagnosis of crusted nodule

Basal cell carcinoma
Chondrodermatitis nodularis
  chronica helicis
Keratoacanthoma
Wart

Adnexal tumor
Seborrheic keratosis
Squamous cell carcinoma
Melanoma
Metastatic carcinoma

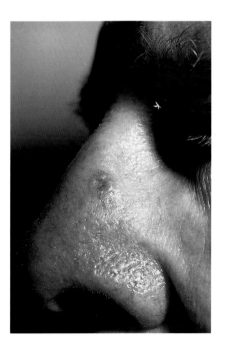

Figure 13.7.3 Basal cell carcinoma. *Clue to diagnosis:* Pearly nodule with central crust and rolled border with telangiectasia.

8. BASAL CELL CARCINOMA (NODULAR)
VERSUS
INTRADERMAL NEVUS

Features in common: Flesh-colored to pearly nodule.

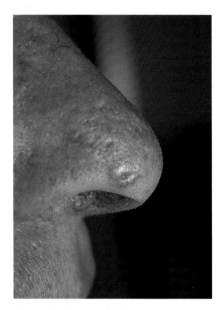

Figure 13.8.1 Basal cell carcinoma.

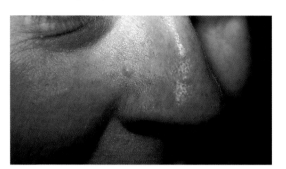

Figure 13.8.2 Nevus.

Distinguishing features

	BASAL CELL CARCINOMA (NODULAR)	INTRADERMAL NEVUS
Physical examination Morphology	Pearly/translucent	Flesh-colored, flecks of brown may be present
	May scale	No scale
	Central depression	No central depression
	May crust	No crust
	Telangiectasia	No telangiectasia
	Raised rolled border	No raised border
Distribution	Sun-exposed skin	Anywhere
History Symptoms	May bleed	Does not bleed
	Present months to a few years	Present for decades
Exacerbating factors	Sunlight exposure	None
Associated findings	Sun-damaged skin Actinic keratosis	None

Continues

Distinguishing features (Continued)

	BASAL CELL CARCINOMA (NODULAR)	INTRADERMAL NEVUS
Epidemiology	Adults Common Rarely inherited (basal cell nevus syndrome)	Children and adults Common
Biopsy	Yes: invasive basaloid cells with peripheral palisading and clefts from stroma	If uncertain: nests of nevus cells
Laboratory	None	None
Treatment	Excision, Mohs' surgery, electrodesiccation and curettage	None
Outcome	Gradually enlarges if not treated	Stable

Clinical types of basal cell carcinoma

Nodular	Fibroepitheliomatous
Superficial	Keratoid/follicular
Cystic	Morpheaform
Pigmented	

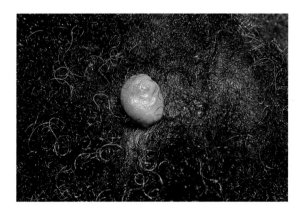

***Figure* 13.8.3** Nevus. *Clue to diagnosis:* Flesh-colored, stable, smooth nodule.

9. SEBACEOUS HYPERPLASIA
VERSUS
BASAL CELL CARCINOMA

Features in common: Pearly to yellow papule.

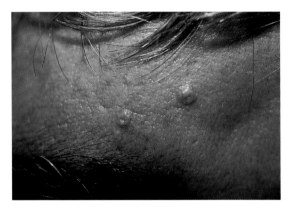

Figure 13.9.1 Sebaceous hyperplasia.

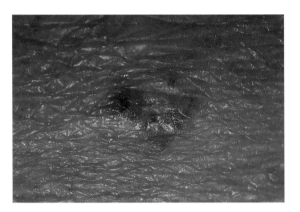

Figure 13.9.2 Basal cell carcinoma.

Distinguishing features

	SEBACEOUS HYPERPLASIA	BASAL CELL CARCINOMA
Physical examination		
Morphology	Yellow	Pearly/translucent
	No scale	May scale
	Central pore	Central depression
	No crust	May crust
	No telangiectasia	Telangiectasia
Distribution	Sun-exposed skin on face	Sun-exposed skin
History		
Symptoms	Does not bleed	May bleed
Exacerbating factors	Sunlight exposure	Sunlight exposure
	Medications (cyclosporin, anabolic steroids)	No medications
Associated findings	Sun-damaged skin	Sun-damaged skin
	Actinic keratosis	Actinic keratosis
Epidemiology	Common	Common
	Adults	Adults
		Rarely inherited (basal cell nevus syndrome)
Biopsy	If uncertain: hyperplasia of sebaceous glands	Yes: invasive basaloid cells with peripheral palisading and clefts from stroma

Continues

Distinguishing features (Continued)

	SEBACEOUS HYPERPLASIA	BASAL CELL CARCINOMA
Laboratory	None	None
Treatment	Cosmetic: acids, electrodesiccation	Excision, Mohs' surgery, electrodesiccation and curettage
Outcome	Stable	Gradually enlarges

Differential diagnosis of pearly to yellow papule or nodule

Trichoepithelioma
Syringoma
Fibrous papule
Neurofibroma

Xanthoma
Juvenile xanthogranuloma
Basal cell carcinoma
Sebaceous hyperplasia

10. FIBROUS PAPULE OF NOSE
VERSUS
BASAL CELL CARCINOMA

Features in common: Flesh-colored to pearly papule on nose.

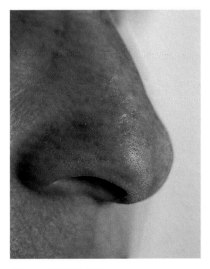

Figure 13.10.1 Fibrous papule.

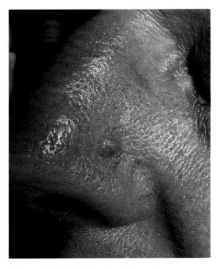

Figure 13.10.2 Basal cell carcinoma.

Distinguishing features

	FIBROUS PAPULE OF NOSE	BASAL CELL CARCINOMA
Physical examination		
Morphology	Flesh colored No scale No depression No telangiectasia No rolled border Small size	Pearly/translucent May scale Central depression Telangiectasia Raised rolled border Size small or large
Distribution	Nose, nasolabial fold	Sun-exposed skin
History		
Symptoms	Does not bleed	May bleed
Exacerbating factors	None	Sunlight exposure
Associated findings	No sun-damaged skin No actinic keratoses	Sun-damaged skin Actinic keratoses
Epidemiology	Common Adults	Common Adults Rarely inherited (basal cell nevus syndrome)
Biopsy	If uncertain: benign spindle- shaped cells	Yes: invasive basaloid cells with peripheral palisading and clefts from stroma
Laboratory	None	None
Treatment	None	Excision, Mohs' surgery, electrodesiccation and curettage
Outcome	Stable	Gradually enlarges if not treated

11. BASAL CELL CARCINOMA (SUPERFICIAL)
VERSUS
NUMMULAR ECZEMA

Features in common: Solitary scaling patch.

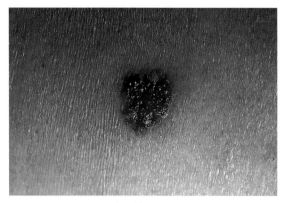

Figure 13.11.1 Superficial basal cell carcinoma.

Figure 13.11.2 Nummular eczema.

Treatment: Use of topical or intralesional steroids or cryotherapy frequently results in healing. Special pillows containing a hole are also available, which help minimize trauma to the ear while sleeping. For stubborn lesions, surgical excision of the involved cartilage is necessary.

CORN

Definition and etiology: Corns are localized thickening of the epidermis with a central keratin core secondary to chronic pressure or friction over bony prominences. They most commonly occur on the toes or feet.

Clinical features: Pain is the reason that patients with corns seek medical care. There is often a history of ill-fitting shoes or foot injury.

The examination reveals a flesh-colored to yellow, well-circumscribed, hyperkeratotic papule or nodule over a bony prominence. The center has a hyperkeratotic plug that on paring with a scalpel reveals a translucent core and preservation of the skin lines.

The differential diagnosis is usually straightforward, although confusion with a plantar wart may occur. The presence of skin lines, translucent core, and lack of black puncta identify the lesion as a corn.

Treatment: Pain due to the corn can be relieved by reducing friction and pressure. Paring down the hyperkeratotic surface provides immediate relief. Changing shoes, shielding the site with orthotic devices, and surgically removing a bony exostosis are therapeutic options.

NUMMULAR ECZEMA

Definition and etiology: Nummular eczema is idiopathic inflammation of the skin characteristically occurring in oval or coin-shaped patches.

Clinical features: The hallmark of nummular eczema is an oval pruritic patch. The individual patches are discrete, well-marginated, erythematous, scaling, edematous, slightly weeping, and crusted. Vesicles may also be present. There may be a few or many lesions on the trunk and extremities.

The differential diagnosis of a single patch of nummular eczema includes superficial basal cell carcinoma and squamous cell carcinoma in situ (Bowen's disease). Lesions of nummular dermatitis are round, whereas lesions of basal cell carcinoma or squamous cell carcinoma may be shaped irregularly. Skin biopsy findings reveal spongiosis typical of dermatitis. Any eczematous-appearing patch that is chronic and unresponsive to topical steroids should undergo biopsy to rule out carcinoma.

Treatment: Topical steroids and emollients for dry skin are the treatments of choice. Harsh soaps should be avoided.

FIBROUS PAPULE

Definition and etiology: Fibrous papule is an idiopathic flesh-colored papule that occurs on the nose of middle-aged individuals.

Clinical features: Fibrous papule is asymptomatic. Its onset in adults and history of gradual growth cause concern that this lesion may represent a basal cell carcinoma. A biopsy reveals spindle-shaped, stellate, and multinucleated fibroblasts surrounded by telangiectatic vessels as well as sclerotic collagen bundles in the superficial dermis.

Treatment: Other than for cosmetic reasons, no therapy is needed. A shave biopsy to differentiate a fibrous papule from basal cell carcinoma usually gives excellent cosmetic results.

KERATOACANTHOMA

Definition and etiology: Keratoacanthoma is a rapidly growing epidermal neoplasm with a propensity for spontaneous involution. The relationship between keratoacanthoma and squamous cell carcinoma continues to be debated. Some argue that keratoacanthoma is squamous cell carcinoma, whereas others believe that keratoacanthoma is a unique tumor.

Clinical features: Solitary acanthomas are the most common form of this neoplasm. They grow quite rapidly and usually occur on the sun-exposed skin of older individuals. Multiple familial and sporadic eruptive keratoacanthomas rarely occur. Keratoacanthomas, sebaceous tumors, and multiple low-grade visceral malignancies occur in Muir-Torre syndrome. In addition to ultraviolet light damage of the skin, pitch, tar, and human papillomavirus have been reported as possible cofactors in the development of keratoacanthoma.

Keratoacanthoma is a dome-shaped flesh-colored nodule that has rolled borders and a central crater filled with a keratin plug.

The differential diagnosis of keratoacanthoma includes other epidermal tumors, particularly squamous cell carcinoma. A skin biopsy is necessary. The pathologic changes, however, may make it difficult to differentiate keratoacanthoma from low-grade squamous cell carcinoma. Typically, keratoacanthoma has a keratin-filled central crater surrounded by pseudoepitheliomatous hyperplasia of the epidermis, which contains benign keratinocytes with an eosinophilic, glassy cytoplasm.

Treatment: Management can be guided by the results of the biopsy. If the clinicopathologic changes definitively indicate a keratoacanthoma, one may await spontaneous regression of the lesion over a 4- to 12-month period. If, however, there is any doubt whether the lesion represents low-grade squamous cell carcinoma, then a complete surgical excision should be accomplished. Other treatments for keratoacanthoma include radiotherapy, electrodesiccation and curettage, and intralesional 5-fluorouracil or bleomycin.

MELANOCYTIC NEVUS

Definition and etiology: A melanocytic nevus (mole) is a congenital or acquired benign neoplasm of melanocytes.

Clinical features: Nevi should be considered a normal skin finding. They vary in number from an average of a couple of dozen in whites to less than a dozen in blacks. Most nevi develop between the ages of 6 months and 35 years. Pregnancy and adolescence particularly influence nevi; during these times they enlarge, darken in color, and itch. Otherwise, nevi are asymptomatic and are usually brought to the attention of a physician because of irritation, change in appearance, or cosmetic reasons.

Nevi should be relatively uniform in color, surface, and border. They may be flesh-colored to darkly pigmented, nonscaling, dome-shaped papules or nodules.

The main disease in the differential diagnosis of a flesh-colored nevus, particularly on the nose or face, is nodular basal cell carcinoma. A history of the lesion having been present since childhood strongly suggests a nevus. Early nodular basal cell carcinomas may lack the typical central depression, the pearly rolled border, telangiectasia, and crusting. A skin biopsy easily differentiates these two neoplasms: a nevus reveals nests of benign nevus cells.

Treatment: Unless the nevus is irritated, cosmetically unattractive, or changing, no therapy is necessary. Depending on the situation, a punch, shave, or excisional biopsy will provide adequate tissue for pathologic examination and will also remove the lesion.

SEBACEOUS HYPERPLASIA

Definition and etiology: Sebaceous hyperplasia is a benign neoplasm of sebaceous glands.

Clinical features: Sebaceous hyperplasia is an asymptomatic growth that occurs most commonly on the sun-damaged skin of the face. It appears as a yellowish papule or a small nodule with a central pore or umbilication. It has no scale or crusting. Other than aesthetics, its only importance is its differentiation from basal cell carcinoma. When diagnosis is uncertain, biopsy findings reveal typical hypertrophied multilobulate sebaceous glands.

Treatment: No therapy is necessary. Local electrodesiccation or the application of acids can be used cautiously to destroy these benign growths.

SEBORRHEIC KERATOSIS

Definition and etiology: Seborrheic keratosis is a benign neoplasm of the epidermis that usually appears during middle age.

Clinical features: Unless irritated, seborrheic keratoses are asymptomatic. Most patients seek medical care when these benign tumors become irritated or displeasing cosmetically or when they are concerned that they may represent skin cancer.

Seborrheic keratoses typically are well-demarcated, slightly scaling, greasy-appearing, tan to dark brown *pasted-on* papules and plaques. Their surface is often verrucous or crumbly in appearance with small keratin-filled pits. They occur anywhere on the body with the exception of the palms and soles.

The well-marginated, pasted-on appearance and the finding of multiple similar-appearing papules and plaques make the diagnosis of seborrheic keratosis generally straightforward. On occasion, though, they can mimic warts, actinic keratosis, nevus, pigmented basal cell carcinoma, and malignant melanoma. When diagnosis is uncertain, biopsy findings reveal the typical uniform, well-demarcated intraepithelial proliferation of small benign squamous cells.

Treatment: No treatment is necessary for seborrheic keratoses unless they are irritated or cosmetically unacceptable. Freezing with liquid nitrogen is generally most efficient and most effective. Excisional surgery is not done unless there is concern about malignancy.

SQUAMOUS CELL CARCINOMA

Definition and etiology: Squamous cell carcinoma is a malignant neoplasm of keratinocytes that is locally invasive and has the potential to metastasize. Ultraviolet radiation, x-rays, papillomavirus infection, and chemical carcinogens such as soot and arsenic cause squamous cell carcinoma.

Clinical features: Squamous cell carcinoma is the second most common skin cancer in the United States, with more than 100,000 new cases diagnosed annually. As with other sunlight-induced skin cancers, the frequency of squamous cell carcinoma is increased in those who are fair complected or engage in many outdoor activities. The history of a bleeding growth or ulcer should arouse suspicion of squamous cell carcinoma.

Squamous cell carcinoma most often arises in sun-damaged skin. It also develops on the mucous membranes and in areas of chronic injury such as burn scars, chronic radiodermatitic lesions, chronic draining sinuses, and areas of erosive discoid lupus erythematosus.

The examination reveals a hard papule or nodule that is erythematous to flesh-colored, smooth, scaling, and crusted. Squamous cell carcinoma in situ (Bowen's disease) has a different appearance, being a well-demarcated, slightly scaling, slightly crusted, eczematous-appearing patch.

The differential diagnosis of squamous cell carcinoma includes keratoacanthoma, hypertrophic actinic keratosis, wart, basal cell carcinoma, and seborrheic keratosis. Any lesion that is crusted or ulcerated should be suspected of being squamous cell carcinoma, and biopsy must be done. This reveals a hyperkeratotic thickened epidermis containing atypical keratinocytes that invade the dermis.

Treatment: Squamous cell carcinoma should be totally excised. Follow-up to monitor for local recurrence as well as metastases is required. The squamous cell carcinomas most likely to metastasize are those that are large or histologically poorly differentiated, have deep invasion, or occur in damaged skin or the mucous membranes of the lips, glans penis, and vulva. Metastasis is generally to the regional lymph nodes, and careful attention should be given to examining them for lymphadenopathy.

WART

Definition and etiology: Warts (verruca vulgaris) are benign neoplasms of the epidermis that are caused by the papillomavirus.

Clinical features: Warts affect people of all ages but are most common in children and young adults. Anogenital warts are usually sexually transmitted by adults and are probably the most common sexually transmitted disease. In children, genital warts should raise the suspicion of sexual abuse, but is not conclusive evidence of abuse. In immunosuppressed patients, particularly transplant recipients, warts can be a difficult problem.

Warts have a somewhat different appearance depending on their type. Common and plantar warts, which occur on the hands and feet, have a flesh-colored, scaling, and corrugated surface that characteristically interupts skin lines and contains black puncta. Flat warts usually occur on the head and hand, are subtle, flesh-colored or reddish, slightly raised, flat-topped papules 2 to 5 millimeters in size. Venereal or genital warts (condyloma acuminatum) are soft, moist, often cauliflower-like, flesh- and brown-colored papules and plaques in the perineum.

A linear arrangement (Koebner phenomenon) of warts occurs from autoinulation.

The diagnosis of warts is usually straightforward from their typical clinical appearance. In adults who have a persistent lesion that crusts and is unresponsive to usual wart therapies, squamous cell carcinoma should be considered. A skin biopsy of a wart will reveal benign epidermal papillomatoses and large keratinocytes with small pyknotic nuclei (koilocytes). Plantar warts sometimes can be confused with corns or calluses. Pairing off the thick hyperkeratotic surface reveals the interruption of skin lines and black puncta of a wart. Flat warts may be confused with comedones when on the face and lichen planus when on the hands. Genital warts can appear similar to seborrheic keratoses and also the lesions of secondary syphilis, condyloma latum.

Therapy: The treatment of warts is destructive and usually painful. The goal is to eliminate the skin that is infected with the virus. The two most common methods are topical acids available over the counter and liquid nitrogen cryotherapy in the office. Overzealous treatment that results in unbearable discomfort and scarring should be avoided. Untreated, many warts, perhaps half, will spontaneously resolve in one or two years. Other treatment modalities include podophyllin (especially for genital warts), intralesionally bleomycin, cantharidin, surgical excision, electrodesiccation, and laser therapy.

Suggested Readings

ACTINIC KERATOSIS

Drake LA, Ceilley RI, Cornelison RL et al. Guidelines of care for actinic keratoses. J Am Acad Dermatol 1995; 32:95–98.

Naylor MF, Boyd A, Smith DW et al. High sun protection factor sunscreens in the suppression of actinic neoplasia. Arch Dermatol 1995;131:170–75.

Thompson SC, Jolley D, Marks R. Reduction of solar keratoses by regular sunscreen use. N Engl J Med 1993; 329:1147–51.

BASAL CELL CARCINOMA

Drake LA, Ceilley RI, Cornelison RL et al. Guidelines of care for basal cell carcinoma. J Am Acad Dermatol 1992;26:117–20.

Gallagher RP, Hill GB, Bajdik CD et al. Sunlight exposure, pigmentary factors, and risk of nonmelanocytic skin cancer. Arch Dermatol 1995;131:157–63.

Karagas MR, Stukel TA, Greenberg ER et al. Risk of subsequent basal cell carcinoma and squamous cell carcinoma of the skin among patients with prior skin cancer. JAMA 1992;267:3305–10.

Miller SJ. Biology of basal cell carcinoma (part I). J Am Acad Dermatol 1991;24:1–13.

Miller SJ. Biology of basal cell carcinoma (part II). J Am Acad Dermatol 1991;24:161–75.

Randle HW. Basal cell carcinoma. Identification and treatment of the high-risk patient. Dermatol Surg 1996; 22:255–61.

Sexton M, Jones DB, Maloney ME. Histologic pattern analysis of basal cell carcinoma. Study of a series of 1039 consecutive neoplasms. J Am Acad Dermatol 1990;23:1118–26.

Wolf DJ, Zitelli JA. Surgical margins for basal cell carcinoma. Arch Dermatol 1987;123:340–44.

CHONDRODERMATITIS NODULARIS CHRONICA HELICIS

Coldiron BM. The surgical management of chondrodermatitis nodularis chronica helicis. J Dermatol Surg Oncol 1991;17:902–4.

Lawrence CM. The treatment of chondrodermatitis nodularis with cartilage removal alone. Arch Dermatol 1991; 127:530–35.

CORN

Yale I. Podiatric Medicine. pp. 94–130. Williams & Wilkins, Baltimore, 1974

ECZEMA

See Chapter 4.

FIBROUS PAPULE

Rose LB, Suster S. Fibrous papules. A light microscopic and immunohistochemical study. Am J Dermatopathol 1988;20:109.

KERATOACANTHOMA

Schwartz RA. Keratoacanthoma. J Am Acad Dermatol 1994;30:1–19.

MELANOCYTIC NEVUS

See Chapter 13.

SEBACEOUS HYPERPLASIA

Kumar P, Marks R. Sebaceous gland hyperplasia and senile comedones: a prevalence study in elderly hospitalized patients. Br J Dermatol 1987;117:231–36.

Rosian R, Goslen JB, Brodell RT et al. The treatment of benign sebaceous hyperplasia with the topical application of bichloracetic acid. J Dermatol Surg Oncol 1991;17:876–79.

SEBORRHEIC KERATOSIS

Stern RS, Boudreaux C, Arndt KA. Diagnostic accuracy and appropriateness of care for seborrheic keratoses. A pilot study of an approach to quality assurance for cutaneous surgery. JAMA 1991;265:74–77.

SQUAMOUS CELL CARCINOMA

Bernstein SC, Lim KK, Brodland DG, Heidelberg KA. The many faces of squamous cell carcinoma. Dermatol Surg 1996;22:243–54.

Chute CG, Chuang TY, Bergstralh EJ, Su SPD. The subsequent risk of internal cancer with Bowen's disease. A population-based study. JAMA 1991;266:816–19.

Frankel DH, Hanusa BH, Zitelli JA. New primary nonmelanoma skin cancer in patients with a history of squamous cell carcinoma of the skin. Implications and recommendations for follow-up. J Am Acad Dermatol 1992;26:720–26.

Johnson TM, Rowe DE, Nelson BR, Swanson NA. Squamous cell carcinoma of the skin (excluding lip and oral mucosa). J Am Acad Dermatol 1992;26:467–84.

Kwa RE, Campana K, Moy RL. Biology of cutaneous squamous cell carcinoma. J Am Acad Dermatol 1992; 26:1–26.

Miller DL, Weinstock MA. Nonmelanoma skin cancer in the United States: incidence. J Am Acad Dermatol 1994;30:774–78.

Rowe DE, Carroll RJ, Day CL. Prognostic factors for local recurrence, metastasis, and survival rates in squamous cell carcinoma of the skin, ear, and lip. J Am Acad Dermatol 1992;26:976–90.

WART

Cobb MW. Human papillomavirus infection. J Am Acad Dermatol 1990;22:547–66.

Drake LA, Ceilley RI, Cornelison RL et al. Guidelines of care for warts: human papillomavirus. J Am Acad Dermatol 1995;32:98–103.

Quan MB, Moy RL. The role of human papillomavirus in carcinoma. J Am Acad Dermatol 1991;25:698–705.

Siegfried EC. Warts on children: an approach to therapy. Pediatr Ann 1996;25:79–90.

14 *Pigmented Growths*

ALGORITHM FOR PIGMENTED GROWTHS

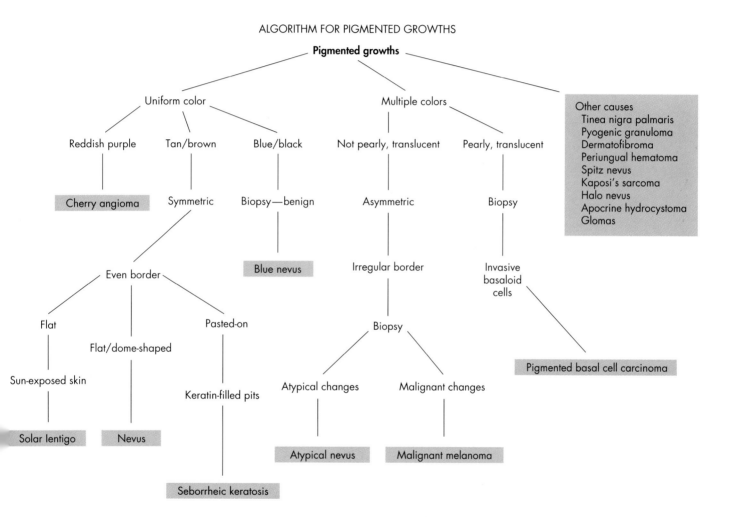

Introduction

Pigmented growths are an important group of neoplasms because their differential diagnosis includes malignant melanoma, which if recognized early is curable but if untreated is deadly. The neoplasms in this chapter are characterized by an increased amount of pigment or pigment-forming cells. For any pigmented growth in which the diagnosis is uncertain or in which malignant melanoma is a possibility, a *biopsy* is mandatory. Common pigmented lesions other than melanocytic nevus or melanoma include seborrheic keratosis, pigmented basal cell carcinoma, solar lentigines, and cherry angiomas. In seborrheic keratosis, pigmented basal cell carcinoma, and solar lentigines, the increased pigment is in keratinocytes, in contrast to cherry angiomas which only appear pigmented because of blood-filled vessels in the dermis.

1. MELANOCYTIC NEVUS
VERSUS
MALIGNANT MELANOMA

Features in common: Pigmented papule.

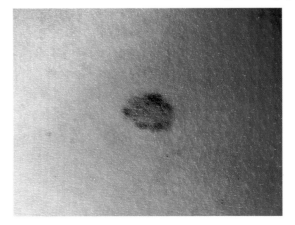

Figure 14.1.1 Nevus.

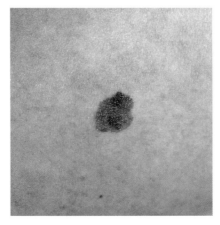

Figure 14.1.2 Malignant melanoma.

Distinguishing features

	MELANOCYTIC NEVUS	MALIGNANT MELANOMA[a]
Physical examination		
Morphology	Uniform color: tan, brown	Multiple colors: black, blue, pink, white, tan, brown
	Symmetric	Asymmetric
	Regular border	Irregular border
	< 6 mm in size (usually)	> 6 mm in size
Distribution	Generalized	Generalized
History		
Symptoms	No change in size or color	Change in size and color
	No bleeding	Bleeds
Exacerbating factors	Sunlight	Sunlight
Associated findings	None	Sun-damaged skin
		Lymphadenopathy
Epidemiology	Common	Uncommon
		Rarely familial
Biopsy	Yes, if worrisome lesion; shows melanocytes in nests	Yes; malignant melanocytes arranged in single cells and nests
	No atypia	Atypia present
Laboratory	None	Chest x-ray
Treatment	None	Wide excision
Outcome	Does not metastasize	May metastasize

[a]Large melanomas may bleed and have loss of hair follicles, but if one waits for these features to appear, the lesions will be deep and the patient's prognosis very poor.

Differential diagnosis of pigmented papules

Melanoma
Pigmented basal cell carcinoma
Seborrheic keratosis
Hemangioma, angiokeratoma
Nevi: atypical, Spitz, halo, blue
Kaposi's sarcoma
Lentigo
Tatoo
Hemorrhage (talon noir)

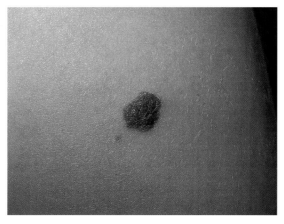

Figure 14.1.3 Nevus. *Clue to diagnosis:* Even brown color, border, surface.

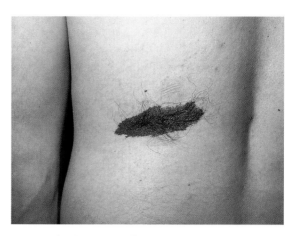

Figure 14.1.4 Congenital nevus.

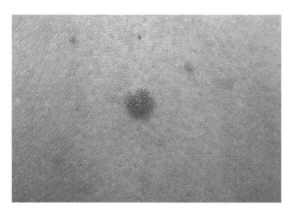

Figure 14.1.5 Compound nevus.

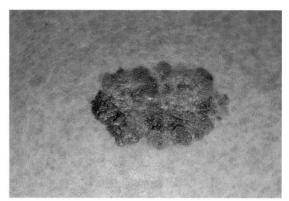

Figure 14.1.6 Malignant melanoma. *Clue to diagnosis:* Multiple colors (red, white, blue).

2. ATYPICAL NEVUS
VERSUS
MALIGNANT MELANOMA

Features in common: Pigmented papules.

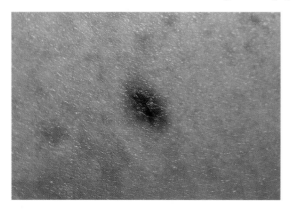

Figure 14.2.1 Atypical nevus.

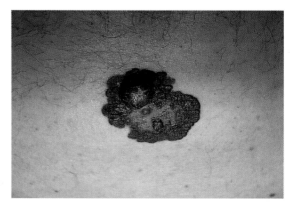

Figure 14.2.2 Malignant melanoma.

Distinguishing features

	ATYPICAL NEVUS	MALIGNANT MELANOMA[a]
Physical examination Morphology	Multiple colors: black, blue, pink, white, tan, brown Asymmetric Irregular border < 6 mm in size	Multiple colors: black, blue, pink, white, tan, brown Asymmetric Irregular border > 6 mm in size
Distribution	Generalized	Generalized
History Symptoms	Change in size or color	Change in size and color
Exacerbating factors	Sunlight	Sunlight
Associated findings	None	Sun-damaged skin Lymphadenopathy
Epidemiology	Common Rarely familial	Uncommon Rarely familial
Biopsy	Yes; melanocytes not atypical, architectural disorder	Yes; malignant melanocytes arranged in single cells and nests
Laboratory	None	Chest x-ray
Treatment	None	Wide excision
Outcome	Does not metastasize	May metastasize

[a]Large melanomas may bleed and have loss of hair follicles, but if one waits for these features to appear, the lesions will be deep and the patient's prognosis very poor.

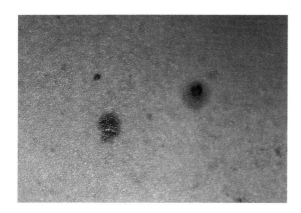

Figure 14.2.3 Atypical nevus. *Clue to diagnosis:* Variegated color, shape; border with pink hues and indistinct border in these two nevi.

3. SEBORRHEIC KERATOSIS
VERSUS
MELANOCYTIC NEVUS

Features in common: Tan or brown papule or plaque.

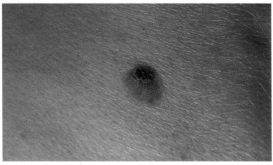

Figure 14.3.1 Seborrheic keratosis.

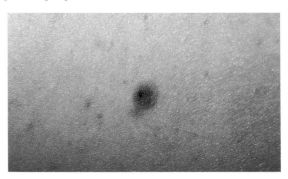

Figure 14.3.2 Nevus.

Distinguishing features

	SEBORRHEIC KERATOSIS	MELANOCYTIC NEVUS
Physical examination		
Morphology	Pasted-on appearance	Not pasted-on
	Keratin-filled pits	No pits
	Greasy	Not greasy
Distribution	Generalized	Generalized
History		
Symptoms	None	None
Exacerbating factors	None	Sunlight
Associated findings	None	None
Epidemiology	Common	Common
	Middle-aged and elderly	More common in young adults
Biopsy	No, unless worrisome or irritated	No, unless worrisome or irritated; shows nested melanocytes
Laboratory	None	None
Treatment	None; liquid nitrogen if cosmetically unacceptable or irritated	None; excision if cosmetically unacceptable or irritated
Outcome	Chronic	Chronic

Differential diagnosis of
tan or brown papule or plaque

Basal cell carcinoma   Hemangioma
Blue nevus   Malignant melanoma
                             Seborrheic keratosis

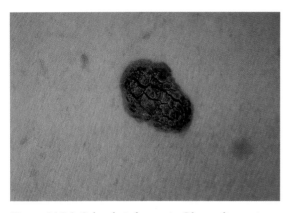

Figure 14.3.3 Seborrheic keratosis. *Clue to diagnosis:* Pasted-on well-demarcated plaque.

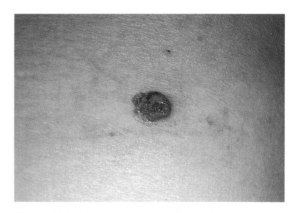

Figure 14.3.4 Irritated seborrheic keratosis.

4. MALIGNANT MELANOMA
VERSUS
PIGMENTED BASAL CELL CARCINOMA

Features in common: Pigmented papule.

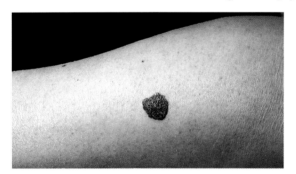

Figure 14.4.1 Malignant melanoma.

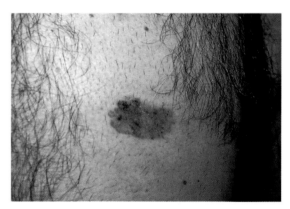

Figure 14.4.2 Pigmented basal cell carcinoma.

Distinguishing features

	MALIGNANT MELANOMA[a]	PIGMENTED BASAL CELL CARCINOMA
Physical examination		
Morphology	No telangiectasias	Telangiectasias
	Not pearly or translucent	Pearly or translucent
	Multiple colors: black, blue, pink, white, tan, brown	Multiple colors: black, blue
	No crust	Crust may be present
	Asymmetric	Asymmetric
	Irregular border	Irregular border
Distribution	Generalized	Generalized

Continues

Distinguishing features (Continued)

	MALIGNANT MELANOMA[a]	PIGMENTED BASAL CELL CARCINOMA
History Symptoms	Change in size and color	Change in size and color
Exacerbating factors	Sunlight	Sunlight
Associated findings	Sun-damaged skin Lymphadenopathy	Sun-damaged skin No lymphadenopathy
Epidemiology	Less common Rarely familial	Common Not familial
Biopsy	Yes; malignant melanocytes arranged in single cells and nests	Yes; invasive buds and lobules of basaloid cells
Laboratory	Chest x-ray	None
Treatment	Wide excision	Narrow excision
Outcome	May metastasize	Does not metastasize

[a]Large melanomas may bleed and have loss of hair follicles, but if one waits for these features to appear, the lesions will be deep and the patient's prognosis very poor.

Differential diagnosis of pigmented papules

Nevus
Seborrheic keratosis
Hemangioma
Malignant melanoma
Pigmented basal cell carcinoma

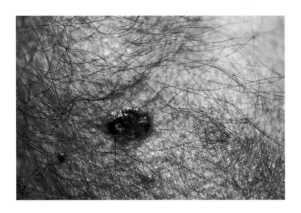

Figure 14.4.3 Pigmented basal cell carcinoma. *Clue to diagnosis:* Pearly or translucent color.

5. BLUE NEVUS
VERSUS
MALIGNANT MELANOMA

Features in common: Blue or black papule or nodule.

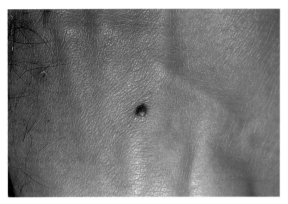

Figure 14.5.1 Blue nevus.

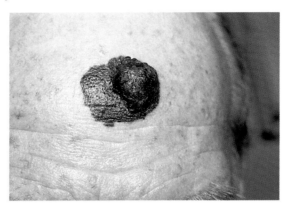

Figure 14.5.2 Malignant melanoma.

Distinguishing features

	BLUE NEVUS	MALIGNANT MELANOMA[a]
Physical examination		
Morphology	Uniform color: blue/black	Multiple colors: black, blue, pink, white, tan, brown
	Symmetric	Asymmetric
	Regular border	Irregular border
Distribution	Generalized	Generalized
History		
Symptoms	No itching	Itches
	No change in size or color	Change in size and color
	No bleeding	Bleeds
Exacerbating factors	None	Sunlight
Associated findings	None	Sun-damaged skin
		Lymphadenopathy
Epidemiology	Uncommon	Uncommon
	Not familial	Rarely familial
Biopsy	Yes, if worrisome lesion; shows melanocytes in nests	Yes; malignant melanocytes arranged in single cells and nests
	No atypia	Atypia present
Laboratory	None	Chest x-ray
Treatment	None	Wide excision
Outcome	Does not metastasize	May metastasize

[a]Large melanomas may bleed and have loss of hair follicles, but if one waits for these features to appear, the lesions will be deep and the patient's prognosis very poor.

Differential diagnosis of blue or black papule or nodule

Pigmented basal cell carcinoma
Seborrheic keratosis
Hemangioma
Angiokeratoma
Atypical nevus
Nevus
Tatoo
Hemorrhage (talon noir)
Malignant melanoma

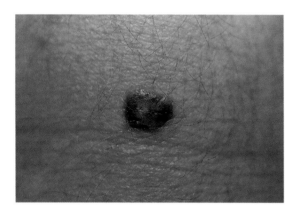

Figure 14.5.3 Blue nevus. *Clue to diagnosis:* Even color, border, surface.

6. SOLAR LENTIGO
VERSUS
LENTIGO MALIGNA MELANOMA

Features in common: Pigmented macule.

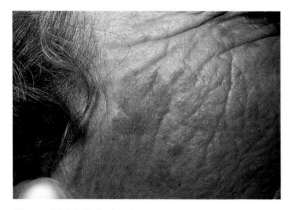

Figure 14.6.1 Solar lentigo.

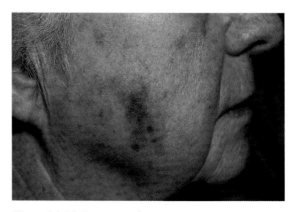

Figure 14.6.2 Lentigo maligna.

Distinguishing features

	SOLAR LENTIGO	LENTIGO MALIGNA MELANOMA[a]
Physical examination		
Morphology	Uniform color: tan, brown	Multiple colors: black, blue, pink, white, tan, brown
	Symmetric	Asymmetric
	Regular border	Irregular border
Distribution	Sun-exposed areas	Sun-exposed and nonsun-exposed areas
History		
Symptoms	No change in size or color	Change in size and color
Exacerbating factors	Sunlight	Sunlight
Associated findings	Sun-damaged skin	Sun-damaged skin
	No lymphadenopathy	Lymphadenopathy
Epidemiology	Common	Uncommon
Biopsy	Yes, if worrisom lesion; shows uniform pigmentation along basal layers of elongated rete ridges	Yes; malignant melanocytes arranged in single cells and nests
Laboratory	None	Chest x-ray
Treatment	None	Wide excision
Outcome	Does not metastasize	May metastasize

[a]Large melanomas may bleed and have loss of hair follicles, but if one waits for these features to appear, the lesions will be deep and the patient's prognosis very poor.

Differential diagnosis of pigmented macules

Common causes
- Freckle
- Simple lentigo
- Solauz lentigo
- Café au lait spot
- Becker's nevus
- Mongolian spot
- Congenital nevus
- Seborrheic keratosis
- Postinflammatory hyperpigmentation

Rarer causes
- Syndromes: leopard, Name, Peutz-Jeghers
- Degos' disease
- Confluent and reticulate papillomatosis
- Ochronosis
- Granuloma faciale
- Lichen planus
- Nevi of Ota and Ito
- Lentigo maligna melanoma

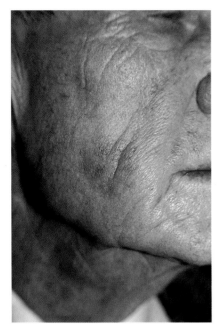

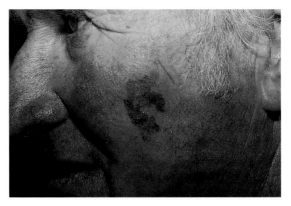

Figure 14.6.4 Lentigo maligna. *Clue to diagnosis:* Uneven blue, black, brown color.

Figure 14.6.3 Solar lentigo. *Clue to diagnosis:* Even brown or tan color.

7. CHERRY ANGIOMA

VERSUS

MALIGNANT MELANOMA

Features in common: Reddish papule or nodule.

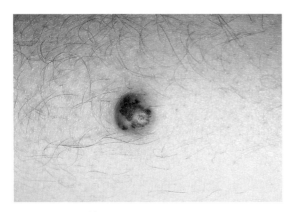

Figure 14.7.1 Cherry angioma.

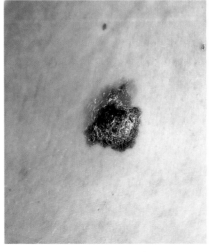

Figure 14.7.2 Malignant melanoma.

Distinguishing features

	CHERRY ANGIOMA	MALIGNANT MELANOMA[a]
Physical examination		
Morphology	Uniform color: red, violet	Multiple colors: black, blue, pink, white, tan, brown
	May blanch	Does not blanch
	Symmetric	Asymmetric
	Regular border	Irregular border
Distribution	Generalized	Generalized
History		
Symptoms	No change in size or color	Change in size and color
Exacerbating factors	None	Sunlight
Associated findings	None	Sun-damaged skin Lymphadenopathy
Epidemiology	Common Not familial	Uncommon Rarely familial
Biopsy	Yes, if worrisome lesion; shows blood vessels	Yes; malignant melanocytes arranged in single cells and nests
Laboratory	None	Chest x-ray
Treatment	None	Wide excision
Outcome	Does not metastasize	May metastasize

[a]Large melanomas may bleed and have loss of hair follicles, but if one waits for these features to appear, the lesion will be deep and the patient's prognosis very poor.

Differential diagnosis of reddish papule or nodule

Angiokeratoma

Pyogenic granuloma

Kaposi's sarcoma

Dermatofibroma

Angiolymphoid hyperplasia

Tatoo

Metastatic cancer, especially renal cell cancer

Cherry angioma

Malignant melanoma

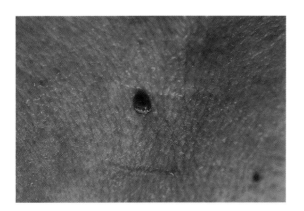

Figure 14.7.3 Cherry angioma: *Clue to diagnosis:* Red vascular appearance.

Discussion

CHERRY ANGIOMA

Definition and etiology: Cherry angioma is a benign neoplasm of blood vessels.

Clinical features: The most common form of hemangioma is the superficial cherry hemangioma that occurs in adults. Its appearance varies from a pinpoint-sized, red petechial-appearing macule to a red, blue, or purple smooth dome-shaped papule or nodule. Hemangiomas most commonly occur on the trunk, begin in early adulthood, and increase in number with age. When they are blue to purple, the differential diagnosis includes blue nevus and malignant melanoma. Blanching with pressure is a diagnostic feature of cherry angioma but may not always be found. When the diagnosis is in doubt, a biopsy should be performed and will reveal benign proliferation of small dilated blood vessels.

Treatment: Treatment of cherry angioma is usually not necessary. If removal is desired, it can be destroyed with light electrodesiccation, scalpel or scissors excision, or a laser.

MALIGNANT MELANOMA

Definition and etiology: Malignant melanoma is a cancerous proliferation of melanocytes. Although the precise cause of malignant melanoma is unknown, sunlight and heredity appear to be the most important risk factors.

Clinical features: The incidence of malignant melanoma is increasing, with more than 35,000 new cases diagnosed yearly in the United States. It is estimated that 1% of individuals in the United States will develop malignant melanoma in their lifetimes. The highest incidence of malignant melanoma in the world is in Queensland, Australia, where there is abundant equatorial sunlight and a predominantly fair-skinned population. Occasionally, there is a family history of malignant melanoma. Most individuals notice a change in the malignant melanoma prior to diagnosis, such as development of a new growth, increase in size, change in color, and rarely bleeding or itching.

The characteristic signs of a majority of malignant melanomas are referred to as the ABCDs: (1) *asymmetry*, (2) *border irregularity* (notched border), (3) *color variation* (red, white, blue), and (4) *diameter* greater than 6 mm. Four clinical types of malignant melanoma have been described: (1) superficial spreading malignant melanoma, (2) lentigo maligna melanoma, (3) nodular melanoma, and (4) acral-lentiginous melanoma. These clinical subtypes are somewhat arbitrary, since they exhibit similar fea-

tures. The superficial spreading melanoma is the most common type and demonstrates all the characteristic ABCD signs. It occurs most frequently in young and middle-aged white adults on all skin surfaces, with preference for the back and legs. Superficial spreading malignant melanoma may be present a couple of years before it metastasizes. Lentigo maligna melanoma occurs in elderly whites on sun-exposed skin, especially the head and neck. It also has the ABCD signs and can reach a diameter of 5 to 7 cm before becoming invasive and metastatic. Nodular melanoma is a rapidly growing blue, black, red, or, occasionally, flesh-colored nodule affecting young to middle-aged whites. Unfortunately, nodular melanoma often metastasizes before clinical attention is sought and the diagnosis is made. The ABCD signs do not work for nodular melanoma. Therefore, any growing or changing melanocytic neoplasm should undergo biopsy. Acral-lentiginous melanoma occurs on the palms, the soles, and the distal portion of the toes and fingers. It demonstrates the ABCD signs but unfortunately often has already metastasized before diagnosis. In contrast to other malignant melanomas, blacks and Asians most commonly have acral-lentiginous melanoma.

Atypical or suspicious pigmented lesions should undergo biopsy to rule out malignant melanoma. Watching and waiting before a diagnosis is made may result in death. The preferable method of biopsy is by excision with narrow 2- to 3-mm margins of normal skin. The biopsy findings reveal malignant melanocytes within the epidermis and dermis scattered individually and in various-sized nests, usually associated with inflammation. The differential diagnosis of malignant melanoma includes nevus, atypical nevus, blue nevus, seborrheic keratosis, cherry angioma, pigmented basal cell carcinoma, actinic lentigo, pyogenic granuloma, and dermatofibroma.

Early melanomas cannot always be distinguished from atypical nevi, since the latter can also have multiple colors and asymmetry and will be larger than 6 mm. Dermatoscopic examination may help in some lesions; however, any questionable borderline or changing lesions should undergo biopsy.

Treatment: Surgical excision is the treatment of choice and, if done early, is curative. Superficial spreading and lentigo maligna melanoma characteristically have an initial horizontal growth phase that is premetastatic and allows for early diagnosis and surgical cure. Acral-lentiginous and nodular melanoma, unfortunately, are usually already in a vertical growth phase and therefore are often metastatic before diagnosis. The prognosis for malignant melanoma is best predicted by tumor thickness, with greater depth of invasion correlated with poor 5-year survival. Patients with malignant melanoma with a thickness of less than 0.75 mm have a 5-year survival rate of 99%, whereas those with disease of more than 3 mm in thickness have a poor prognosis, with less than 50% surviving 5 years. Beliefs about the extent of surgery necessary for malignant melanoma have evolved and are still somewhat controversial. A 1-cm margin of normal skin around the melanoma is certainly adequate for thin lesions less than 1.0 mm thick, and it is probably adequate for all melanomas, no matter how deeply invasive. Elective regional lymph node dissection is controversial and is not usually recommended in thin and thick melanomas. If metastases develop, chemotherapy and immunotherapy are only palliative.

Periodic follow-up of patients is recommended. The history and physical examination of the skin, lymph nodes, liver, and spleen are the most important parameters in detecting recurrence or metastasis. A yearly chest x-ray is the only laboratory examination with significant yield in the asymptomatic patient. Certainly, extensive laboratory tests such as brain, bone, liver, and spleen scans are not indicated unless the history or physical examination suggests metastasis to these organs.

MELANOCYTIC NEVUS

Definition and etiology: A nevus or mole is a benign neoplasm of melanocytes. Nevi are so common that they can be considered a normal skin finding.

Clinical features: Nevi are congenital (occurring in 1% of newborns) or are acquired in childhood, adolescence, or early adulthood. Whites have an average of 15 to 40 nevi per person, whereas blacks have 11. Symptomatic nevi should be regarded suspiciously at any time other than during pregnancy or adolescence, when darkening in color, itching, and development of new nevi are not uncommon.

Nevi can be subdivided histologically and clinically. Junctional nevi are macular, with nevus cells confined to the basal layer of the epidermis. Intradermal nevi are papular, with nevus cells within the dermis, and compound nevi are also papular, with nevus cells in the epidermis and dermis. These different types of nevi vary in appearance and coloration but individually have a fairly symmetric configuration, a regular border, a uniform flesh to brown color, and a relatively small diameter. They may have a smooth or varicoid surface and may be sessile or polypoid. The absence or presence of skin lines or hair has no diagnostic significance.

The most important disease in the differential diagnosis of a nevus is malignant melanoma. For all suspicious lesions, a biopsy is mandatory. The histologic examination of a nevus reveals uniform cells with an epithelioid, a lymphoid, or a spindle-cell appearance; cells are arranged in nests in the basal layer of the epidermis and papillary dermis. When nevus cells extend deeper into the dermis, cord or sheetlike formations occur. Usually, melanin pigment can be found in some of the cells.

A *blue nevus* appears as a steel-blue papule or nodule. It usually appears in childhood, and its significance lies in its differentiation from nodular melanoma. The biopsy findings reveal benign cells, generally with a lot of melanin pigment.

Atypical nevus (Clark's or dysplastic nevus) is important because it resembles malignant melanoma clinically, may be a precursor of malignant melanoma in some cases, and is the characteristic finding in individuals with the rare familial atypical mole and malignant melanoma syndrome. Atypical moles can be very difficult to differentiate from malignant melanoma, since they have similar clinical features. The atypical nevus is often asymmetric, has an irregular border that blends into the normal surrounding skin, and varies in color from tan, brown, and pink to (sometimes) black. The surface is often irregular, having macular and papular portions. Atypical moles are common, with 5% of normal whites in the United States having these lesions. The risk of malignant melanoma in individuals with one or two atypical nevi is controversial but appears to be quite small. Individuals who have the familial atypical mole and melanoma syndrome will develop malignant melanoma in their lifetime, and they require close follow-up. Fortunately, this syndrome is rare. The biopsy findings in an atypical mole reveal architectural disorder of the melanocytes, dermal fibrotic response, and varying amounts of cytologic atypia.

Treatment: For a common nevus, no therapy is required unless there has been a worrisome change in color, shape, size, or amount of bleeding or itching. For suspicious lesions, an excisional biopsy with narrow margins is recommended. For clinically benign and cosmetically unsightly nevi, a shave excision with a scalpel is acceptable. However, this leaves some residual nevus cells at the biopsy site that may become darkly pigmented. All removed nevi should be examined by a pathologist to confirm their benign nature. For congenital nevi, only those that are large (greater than 20 cm in diameter) have a definitely increased potential to become malignant melanoma. Otherwise, congenital nevi can be treated similarly to acquired nevi. For an individual with atypical moles, it should be decided whether this individual has familial atypical mole and melanoma syndrome, in which case close clinical follow-up is required with periodic full-skin examinations by the physician as well as monthly patient self-examinations. Sun protection is particularly prudent for these individuals.

PIGMENTED BASAL CELL CARCINOMA

Definition and etiology: Basal cell carcinoma is a malignant neoplasm arising from the basal cells of the epidermis. Most basal cell carcinomas are caused by sunlight-induced damage to the skin. A pigmented basal cell carcinoma, as the name implies, contains blue and black pigment.

Clinical features: Basal cell carcinoma is the most frequent malignancy in the United States, with more than 750,000 new cases reported annually. Although basal cell carcinoma almost never metastasizes, its malignant nature is emphasized by the local destruction that it can cause. As with other sun-induced neoplasms of the skin, fair-complected individuals and those with a lot of sunlight exposure are most likely to develop basal cell carcinoma.

Pigmented basal cell carcinoma is a pearly, translucent, blue or black papule or nodule. Seborrheic keratosis, pigmented nevus, and, most important, malignant melanoma must be ruled out in the case of pigmented basal cell carcinoma. A skin biopsy, which reveals a thickened epidermis with invasive buds and lobules of malignant basal cells, should be accomplished to confirm the diagnosis. Seborrheic keratosis has a rough, stuck-on appearance. Nevi and malignant melanomas do not contain telangiectasias or have a pearly appearance.

Treatment: Curettage and electrodesiccation of the lesion or excision is the most common surgical modality used to treat basal cell carcinoma. Less commonly used treatments are radiation therapy, cryosurgery, and topical chemotherapy. A specialized surgical technique, Mohs' surgery, is indicated for recurrent basal cell carcinoma and for primary tumors with a high risk of recurrence.

SEBORRHEIC KERATOSIS

Definition and etiology: Seborrheic keratosis is a benign neoplasm of the epidermis that usually appears during middle age.

Clinical features: Unless irritated, seborrheic keratoses are asymptomatic. Most patients seek medical care when these benign tumors become irritated or displeasing cosmetically or when they are concerned that they may represent skin cancer, particularly malignant melanoma.

Seborrheic keratoses typically are well-demarcated, slightly scaling, greasy-appearing, tan to dark brown, pasted-on symmetric papules and plaques. Their surface is often verrucous or crumbly in appearance and has small keratin-filled pits. They occur anywhere on the body with the exception of the palms and soles.

The well-marginated (even bordered), symmetric, pasted-on appearance and the finding of multiple similar-appearing papules and plaques make the diagnosis of seborrheic keratosis generally straightforward. On occasion, though, they can mimic a wart, actinic keratosis, nevus, pigmented basal cell carcinoma, or malignant melanoma. When diagnosis is uncertain, biopsy findings reveal typical uniform well-demarcated intraepithelial proliferation of small, benign squamous cells.

Treatment: No treatment is necessary for seborrheic keratoses unless they are irritated or cosmetically unac-

ceptable. Freezing with liquid nitrogen is generally the most efficient and most effective method of treatment. Excisional surgery is not done unless there is concern about malignancy.

SOLAR LENTIGO

Definition and etiology: Solar lentigo is a brown macule induced by sunlight exposure and represents a proliferation of both keratinocytes and pigment.

Clinical features: Solar (actinic) lentigines arise in middle age and are numerous in sun-exposed skin. They are tan to brown macules ranging in size from a couple of millimeters to several centimeters. They occur on exposed areas of the body, dorsum of the hands, neck, head, and shoulders.

The main diseases in the differential diagnosis of solar lentigo are lentigo maligna melanoma and a thin seborrheic keratosis. A biopsy is mandatory for any lesion that develops an irregular border and color, particularly very dark brown or black hues. The biopsy findings in solar lentigo are characterized by hyperplastic epidermal rete ridges that contain increased amounts of melanin.

Treatment: No treatment is necessary, since solar lentigo is not a premalignant lesion. For cosmetic purposes, it may be treated with cryotherapy or with topical tretinoin.

Suggested Readings

CHERRY ANGIOMA
Sanchez JL, Ackerman AB. Cherry angioma. In, Dermatology in General Medicine, 4th Ed. Fitzpatrick TB, Freedberg IM (ed) pp. 1219–21. McGraw-Hill, New York, 1993.

MALIGNANT MELANOMA
Cohen LM. Lentigo maligna and lentigo maligna melanoma. J Am Acad Dermatol 1995;33:923–36.
Johnson TM, Smith JW, Nelson BR, Change A. Current therapy for cutaneous melanoma. J Am Acad Dermatol 1995;32:689–707.
Miller DR, Geller AC, Wyatt SW et al. Melanoma awareness and self-examination practices: results of a United States survey. J Am Acad Dermatol 1996;34:962–70.
Parker T, Zitelli J. Malignant melanoma. Dermatol Surg 1996;22:234–40.
Piepkorn M, Barnhill RL. A factual, not arbitrary, basis for choice of resection margins in melanoma. Arch Dermatol 1996;132:811–14.
Riegel DS, Friedman RJ, Kopf AW. The incidence of malignant melanoma in the United States: issues as we approach the 21st century. J Am Acad Dermatol 1996; 34:839–47.

Weiss M, Loprinzi CL, Creagan ET et al. Utility of follow-up tests for detecting recurrent disease in patients with malignant melanomas. JAMA 1995;274:1703–5.

MELANOCYTIC NEVUS
Halpern AC, Guerry D, Elder DE et al. Dysplastic nevi as risk markers of sporadic (nonfamilial) melanoma. A case-control study. Arch Dermatol 1991;127:995–99.

Klein LJ, Barr RJ. Histologic atypia in clinically benign nevi: a prospective study. J Am Acad Dermatol 1990; 22:275–82.

Schneider JS, Moore DH, Sagebiel RW. Risk factors for melanoma incidence in prospective follow-up. The importance of atypical (dysplastic) nevi. Arch Dermatol 1994;130:1002–7.

Slade J, Maraghoob AA, Salopek TG et al. Atypical mole syndrome: risk factor for cutaneous malignant melanoma and implications for management. J Am Acad Dermatol 1995;32:479–94.

PIGMENTED BASAL CELL CARCINOMA
See Chapter 12.

SEBORRHEIC KERATOSIS
See Chapter 12.

SOLAR LENTIGO
Griffiths CE, Goldfarb MT, Finkel LJ et al. Topical tretinoin (retinoic acid) treatment of hyperpigmented lesions associated with photoaging in Chinese and Japanese patients: a vehicle-controlled trial. J Am Acad Dermatol 1994;30:76–84.

Rafal ES, Griffith CEM, Ditre CM et al. Topical tretinoin (retinoic acid) treatment for liver spots associated with photodamage. N Engl J Med 1992;326:368–74.

15
Benign Dermal Neoplasms

Other neoplasms
  Adnexal tumors
  Atypical fibrous xanthoma
  Hemangioma
  Histiocytic tumors (juvenile xanthogranuloma)
  Kaposi's sarcoma
  Keloid
  Other cysts (see text)
  Melanoma
  Metastatic carcinoma
  Nodular fasciitis

Tender tumors (ANGEL)
  Angiolipoma
  Neurilemmoma
  Glomus tumor
  Eccrine spiradenoma
  Leiomyoma

Vascular tumors

ALGORITHM FOR BENIGN DERMAL NEOPLASMS

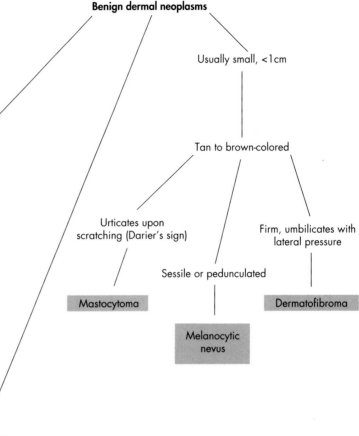

Benign dermal neoplasms

Usually small, <1cm

Tan to brown-colored

Urticates upon
scratching (Darier's sign)

Firm, umbilicates with
lateral pressure

Sessile or pedunculated

Mastocytoma

Dermatofibroma

Melanocytic
nevus

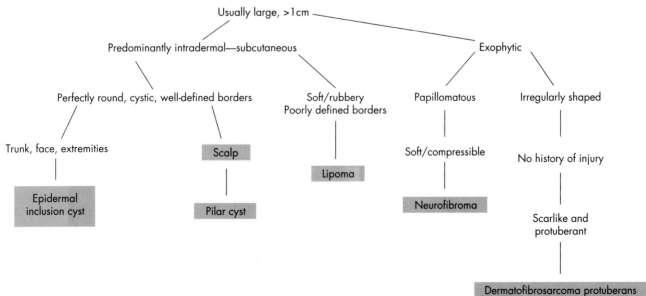

Usually large, >1cm

Predominantly intradermal—subcutaneous

Exophytic

Perfectly round, cystic, well-defined borders

Soft/rubbery
Poorly defined borders

Papillomatous

Irregularly shaped

Trunk, face, extremities

Scalp

Soft/compressible

No history of injury

Epidermal
inclusion cyst

Pilar cyst

Lipoma

Neurofibroma

Scarlike and
protuberant

Dermatofibrosarcoma protuberans

DIFFERENTIAL DIAGNOSIS

DISEASE DISCUSSION

Introduction

The dermis and subcutaneous tissue contain a wide variety of cell types from which neoplasms may develop. Fibroblasts, sebocytes, hair follicles, smooth muscle cells, and nerves all may give rise to a variety of both benign and malignant neoplasms. Despite this broad and complex spectrum of dermal tumors, the vast majority of neoplasms encountered in clinical practice are limited to a subset of common and readily identified growths. Recognition of the different types of neoplasms is often possible based on color, size, location, and tactile properties. The most common tan-brown growths are nevi and dermatofibromas. Dermatofibromas can be distinguished from nevi by their "center of gravity" in the mid to upper dermis and by the presence of puckering on lateral pressure. Mastocytomas are benign growths arising from mast cells, most commonly seen in children. Usually they are red-brown or tan, are larger than nevi, and develop a surrounding wheal when stroked. Neurofibromas typically present as large exophytic pedunculated growths that can be pushed back into the skin to produce a dimple. Cysts are mobile well-demarcated deep dermal nodules that sometimes have an overlying dilated pore. Lipomas are softer and less demarcated and often have lobulated borders. Despite clinical clues, biopsy needs to be performed for some dermal neoplasms to allow for accurate diagnosis. History of rapid growth, pain, or hemorrhage should prompt a close evaluation of any dermal neoplasm. This chapter helps clinicians develop a paradigm for deciding whether a neoplasm can simply be followed or whether it warrants biopsy or excision.

1. DERMATOFIBROMA
VERSUS
MELANOCYTIC NEVUS (INTRADERMAL)

Features in common: Tan to brown-colored dermal papules or nodules.

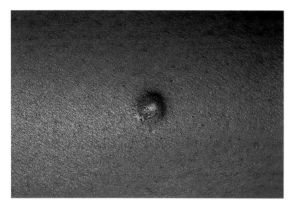

Figure 15.1.1 Dermatofibroma.

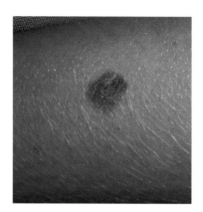

Figure 15.1.2 Melanocytic nevus.

Distinguishing features

	DERMATOFIBROMA	MELANOCYTIC NEVUS (INTRADERMAL)
Physical examination		
Morphology	Color: varies from yellow and reddish to dark brown	Color: less varied, various shades of brown to skin-colored
	Slight scale	No scale
	Not protuberant	Protuberant
Distribution	Dimples on lateral pressure (Fitzpatrick's dimple sign)	No dimple sign
	Most frequently on extremities	Anywhere
History		
Symptoms	Antecedent history of an insect bite, folliculitis, or cyst occasionally	No antecedent history of bite, folliculitis, or cyst
	Occasionally pruritic	Rarely pruritic
Exacerbating factors	None	None
Associated findings	None	Family history of multiple moles
Epidemiology	Adults	Children and adults
Biopsy	No	Sometimes
	Epidermal hyperplasia, within dermis increased number of haphazardly distributed fibroblasts surrounding and entrapping collagen bundles	Collection of melanocytes in nests; melanocytes "mature" and become more spindle-shaped in the deeper dermis

Continues

Distinguishing features (Continued)

	DERMATOFIBROMA	MELANOCYTIC NEVUS (INTRADERMAL)
Laboratory	None	None
Treatment	None necessary; excisional surgery if symptomatic	Complete excision if *asymmetry*, irregular *border*, variegated *color*, or change in *diameter* raise concerns about possible melanoma
Outcome	May involute over many years	May involute over many years

Differential diagnosis of brown lesions

Melanocytic nevus
Dermatofibroma
Lentigo: solar or simplex
Café au lait spot
Becker's nevus
Mongolian spot

Nevus of Ota
Nevus of Ito
Urticaria pigmentosa
Juvenile xanthogranuloma
Seborrheic keratosis
Pigmented basal cell carcinoma

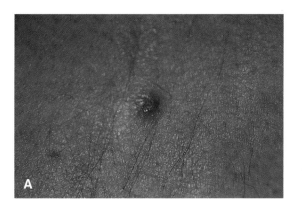 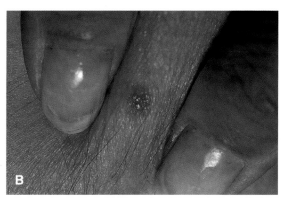

Figure 15.1.3 Dermatofibroma. *Clue to diagnosis:* Central pucker (A); upon pressure (B).

2. DERMATOFIBROMA
VERSUS
DERMATOFIBROSARCOMA PROTUBERANS

Features in common: Dermal plaques or papules.

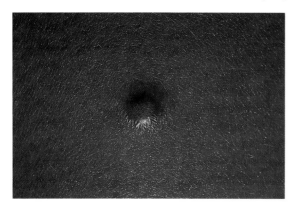

Figure 15.2.1 Dermatofibroma.

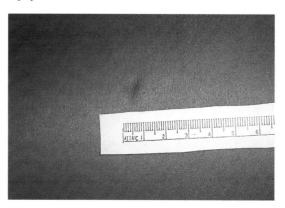

Figure 15.2.2 Dermatofibrosarcoma.

Distinguishing features

	DERMATOFIBROMA	DERMATOFIBROSARCOMA PROTUBERANS
Physical examination		
Morphology	Small, < 1 cm	Large, > 1 cm
	Symmetric	Asymmetric
	Dimples on lateral pressure (Fitzpatrick's, dimple sign)	No dimple sign
	Not protuberant	Protuberant tumor
	Epidermis acanthotic and does not ulcerate	Epidermis atrophic and shiny and may ulcerate
	Slight scale	No scale
Distribution	Most frequently on extremities	Most common on back
History	No growth	Slow growth
Symptoms	Occasionally antecedent history of an insect bite, "pimple," or antecedent cyst	No history of bite, "pimple," or antecedent cyst
	No history of recurrence	History of recurrence after prior removal in many cases
	Occasionally pruritic	Asymptomatic
Exacerbating factors	None	None
Associated findings	None	None
Epidemiology	Young adults	Adults
	Slightly more common in women	Male predominance

Continues

Distinguishing features (Continued)

	DERMATOFIBROMA	**DERMATOFIBROSARCOMA PROTUBERANS**
Biopsy	No Epidermal hyperplasia; increased number of haphazardly distributed fibroblasts surrounding and entrapping collagen bundles in dermis	Yes No epidermal hyperplasia; dense collection of fibroblast-like cells that form cartwheels and extend into subcutaneous tissue, forming fenestrated septae
Laboratory	None	None
Treatment	None necessary; excisional surgery if bothersome	Wide local excision with margin control
Outcome	May resolve or involute over many years	Continued growth: frequently recurrent; rarely metastatic

Synonyms for variants of dermatofibroma

Atrophic dermatofibroma
Dermatofibroma with monster giant cells
Epithelioid cell histiocytoma
Fibroma durum
Fibrous histiocytoma
Granular cell dermatofibroma
Nodular subepidermal fibrosis
Sclerosing hemangioma

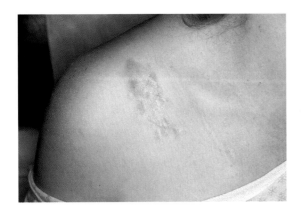

Figure 15.2.3 Dermatofibrosarcoma.
Clue to diagnosis: Irregular shape with protuberant nodules.

3. NEUROFIBROMA
VERSUS
MELANOCYTIC NEVUS (INTRADERMAL)

Features in common: Exophytic tumor.

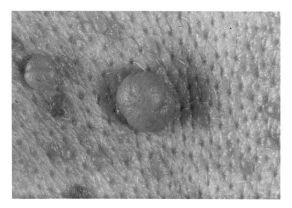

Figure 15.3.1 Neurofibroma.

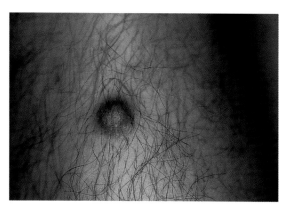

Figure 15.3.2 Melanocytic nevus.

Distinguishing features

	NEUROFIBROMA	MELANOCYTIC NEVUS (INTRADERMAL)
Physical examination Morphology	Skin colored	Various shades of brown to skin-colored
	Lesions polypoid or pedunculated "Button hole sign": invagination of lesion into skin with pressure	Lesions flat or sessile No invagination with pressure
Distribution	Any cutaneous surface	Any cutaneous surface
History Symptoms	None	None
Exacerbating factors	None	None
Associated findings	All ages No family history of multiple moles If multiple may be associated with neurofibromatosis: café au lait spots, axillary freckling, acoustic neuroma	All ages Family history of multiple moles No café au lait spots or axillary freckling
Epidemiology	Usually sporadic Neurofibromatosis: autosomal dominant inheritance	Young adults No sex predilection

Continues

Distinguishing features (Continued)

	NEUROFIBROMA	MELANOCYTIC NEVUS (INTRADERMAL)
Biopsy	No Small wavy spindle cells surrounded by a pale eosinophilic, slightly myxoid stroma containing mast cells	Sometimes Collection of melanocytes in nests Melanocytes "mature" and become more lymphoid and fibroblast-like in the deeper dermis
Laboratory	None	None
Treatment	None necessary except if changing	Complete excision if changing or worrisome
Outcome	Persists; rarely may evolve into neurofibrosarcoma in patients with neurofibromatosis	May involute over many years

Riccardi's classification of neurofibromatosis

Type A: Congenital onset with total body involvement; neurofibromas present
   1. Neurofibromatosis 1
      (NF-1, von Recklinghausen's neurofibromatosis): most common form
   2. Neurofibromatosis 2
      (NF-2, acoustic neurofibromatosis)
   3. Neurofibromatosis 3
      (NF-3, mixed neurofibromatosis)
   4. Neurofibromatosis 4
      (NF-4, variant neurofibromatosis)

Type B: Limited in distribution or late onset; neurofibromas not always found
   5. Neurofibromatosis 5
      (NF-5, segmental neurofibromatosis)
   6. Neurofibromatosis 6
      (NF-6, café au lait neurofibromatosis)
   7. Neurofibromatosis 7
      (NF-7, late-onset neurofibromatosis)
Type C: Neurofibromatosis 8
   (NF-8, unclassifiable)

Diagnostic criteria for von Recklinghausen's neurofibromatosis

Two of following seven criteria required
   1. Six or more café au lait spots over 5 mm in diameter in children or over 1.5 cm in diameter in adults
   2. Two or more neurofibromas or a single plexiform neurofibroma (histologic diagnosis)
   3. Crowe's sign: freckling in axillary or inguinal areas
   4. Optic glioma
   5. Lisch nodules on iris
   6. Osseous lesions: sphenoid dysplasia, thinning of long-bone cortex
   7. First-degree relative with neurofibromatosis

4. MASTOCYTOMA
VERSUS
MELANOCYTIC NEVUS (INTRADERMAL)

Features in common: Brown macules, papules, and nodules.

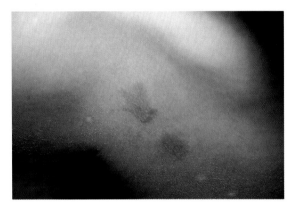

Figure 15.4.1 Mastocytoma.

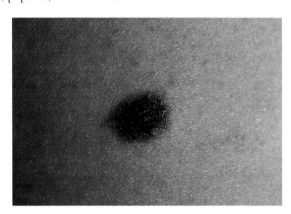

Figure 15.4.2 Melanocytic nevus.

Distinguishing features

	MASTOCYTOMA	MELANOCYTIC NEVUS (INTRADERMAL)
Physical examination		
Morphology	Brown to red	Various shades of brown to skin-colored
	Indistinct borders	Sharp borders
	Positive Darier's sign: production of a wheal upon rubbing the lesion	No Darier's sign
	Occasionally bullous lesions	No bullous lesions
Distribution	Predominantly truncal	Any cutaneous surface
History		
Symptoms	Intense pruritus	No pruritus
Exacerbating factors	Rubbing or scratching Medications: aspirin, codeine, morphine, alcohol, polymyxin B	None
Associated findings	Flushing attacks with headaches, dyspnea, wheezing, diarrhea, and syncope may be seen	Family history of multiple moles
Epidemiology	Predominantly babies, infants, and children	All ages

Continues

Distinguishing features (Continued)

	MASTOCYTOMA	MELANOCYTIC NEVUS (INTRADERMAL)
Biopsy	Yes Proliferation of mast cells in dermis	Sometimes Collection of melanocytes in nests Melanocytes "mature" and become more lymphoid and fibroblast-like in the deeper dermis
Laboratory	Usually none necessary Increased urine 5-hydroxyindoleacetic acid (5-HIAA) widespread and/or systemic lesions	None
Treatment	Topical steroids, excision psolaren plus ultraviolet A light (if many lesions, as in urticaria pigmentosa) Avoid mast-cell-degranulating agents	Complete excision if changing or worrisome
Outcome	Spontaneous resolution over several years	May involute over many years

Differential diagnosis of cutaneous dermal growths in infants and young children

Dermatofibroma

Dermoid cyst

Hemangioma

Infantile myofibroma

Juvenile xanthogranuloma or other histiocytic tumors

Leiomyoma and smooth muscle harmartoma

Mastocytoma (urticaria pigmentosa)

Melanocytic lesions

    Blue nevus

    Café au lait spot

    Congenital nevus

    Mongolian spot

    Nevi of Ito and Ota

    Spitz nevus

Molluscum contagiosum (mimicker of growth)

Neurofibroma

Pilomatrixoma

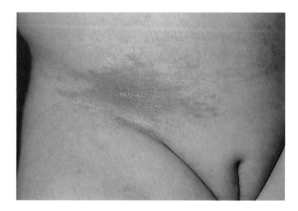

Figure 15.4.3 Mastocytoma. *Clue to diagnosis:* Darier's sign (i.e., an urticarial flare develops upon rubbing the lesion).

5. LIPOMA
VERSUS
EPIDERMAL INCLUSION CYST

Features in common: Mobile subcutaneous nodules.

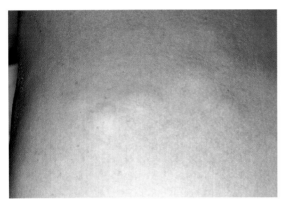

Figure 15.5.1 Lipoma.

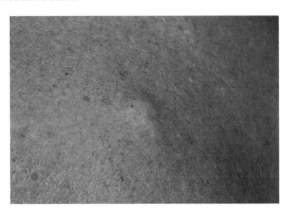

Figure 15.5.2 Epidermal inclusion cyst.

Distinguishing features

	LIPOMA	EPIDERMAL INCLUSION CYST
Physical examination		
Morphology	Lobulated subcutaneous nodule with indistinct borders	Smooth dermal and subcutaneous nodule
	Indistinct borders	Well-demarcated borders
	Soft, rubbery, and compressible	Firm but not soft
	No central punctum	Central punctum frequently present in overlying epidermis
	No surrounding erythema	Erythema if ruptured or secondarily infected
Distribution	Trunk, neck, and forearms	Trunk, face, and scalp
History		
Symptoms	None (angiolipomas may be painful)	None
	No history of drainage	Tender if ruptured or infected
		Drainage of yellow cheesy material occasionally
		Can form in hands after trauma
Exacerbating factors	None	Secondary infection
Associated findings	Obesity	Acne
	Rarely Gardner's syndrome	Rarely Gardner's syndrome
	Rarely inherited as autosomal dominant trait	
Epidemiology	Adults	Adults

Continues

Distinguishing features (Continued)

	LIPOMA	EPIDERMAL INCLUSION CYST
Biopsy	No Lobular aggregate of mature-appearing fat	No Keratin-filled cyst lined with epithelium resembling normal epidermis
Laboratory	None	None
Treatment	Excision if bothersome, or liposuction if biopsy-proven	Excision if bothersome
Outcome	Stable	Stable unless ruptures or becomes infected

Differential diagnosis of benign subcutaneous nodules

Adnexal tumors
Cysts
  Bronchogenic
  Cutaneous ciliated
  Dermoid
  Epidermal inclusion
  Hidrocystoma (apocrine and eccrine)
  Median raphae
  Mucous/ganglion
  Pilar
  Steatocystoma
  Thyroglossal duct
  Vellus
Lipomas
  Angiolipoma
  Hibernoma
  Spindle cell lipoma/pleomorphic lipoma

Painful tumors (ANGEL)
  Angiolipoma
  Neurilemmoma
  Glomus
  Eccrine spiradenoma
  Leiomyoma
Miscellaneous
  Dermatofibroma
  Foreign body granuloma
  Gouty tophus
  Osteoma/calcinosis cutis
  Pilomatrixoma
  Rheumatoid nodule
  Subcutaneous granuloma annulare
Vascular tumors
  Capillary hemangioma
  Cavernous hemangioma
  Lymphangioma

6. EPIDERMAL INCLUSION CYST

VERSUS

PILAR CYST

Features in common: Subcutaneous and dermal cysts.

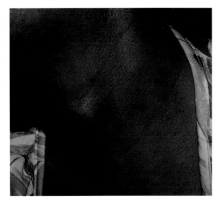

Figure 15.6.1 Epidermal inclusion cyst.

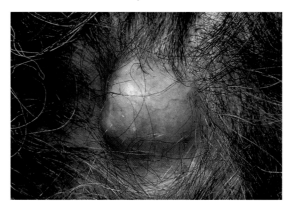

Figure 15.6.2 Pilar cyst.

Distinguishing features

	EPIDERMAL INCLUSION CYST	PILAR CYST
Physical examination		
Morphology	Compressible	Noncompressible
	Central punctum frequently in overlying epidermis	No central punctum
	Erythema if ruptured or infected	No erythema
Distribution	Trunk, face, and scalp	Scalp
History		
Symptoms	Tender if ruptures	None
	Drainage of yellow cheesy material occasionally	No history of drainage
	Can form in hands after trauma	
Exacerbating factors	Secondary infection	None
Associated findings	Acne	No acne
	Rarely Gardner's syndrome	Not associated with Gardner's syndrome
	Not inherited	Autosomal dominant inheritance occasionally
Epidemiology	Adults	Adults
Biopsy	No	No
	Loose keratin-filled cyst lined with epithelium resembling normal epidermis	Compact keratin-filled cyst lined with epithelium resembling follicular isthmus

Continues

Distinguishing features (Continued)

	EPIDERMAL INCLUSION CYST	PILAR CYST
Laboratory	None	None
Treatment	Excision if symptomatic	Excision if symptomatic
Outcome	Stable; only of cosmetic concern unless inflamed or infected	Stable; only of cosmetic concern

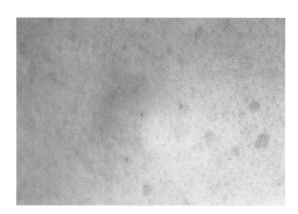

Figure 15.6.3 Epidermal inclusion cyst.
Clue to diagnosis: Central punctum.

Discussion

DERMATOFIBROMA

Definition and etiology: A dermatofibroma is a nodular benign proliferation of fibroblasts, histiocytes, blood vessels, and lymphocytes. Although historically classified as a neoplasm, a dermatofibroma is a reactive scar-like proliferation that may be caused by a wide variety of stimuli. Sometimes the lesions can be attributed to a ruptured cyst, an insect bite, folliculitis, or trauma.

Clinical features: Dermatofibromas are most commonly found on the lower extremities of young adults. Clinical examination reveals a firm, tan to light-brown dermal nodule. Slight epidermal lichenification due to rubbing and scaling may be present. Upon squeezing, the nodule puckers in from the side to the center; this phenomenon has been called Fitzpatrick's or dimple sign.

Dermatofibromas are frequently confused with intradermal nevi because of their brown color. Fitzpatrick's sign is not present in nevi, however. Nevi are usually more exophytic and soft and frequently are not round. If a dermatofibroma has a prominent vascular component, such as in the sclerosing hemangioma variant, it can also be confused with a hemangioma. Hemangiomas are bright red and have a lobular appearance. Early developing lesions of dermatofibrosarcoma protuberans may be mistaken for scars or

dermatofibromas. The clue to correct diagnosis of dermatofibrosarcoma protuberans is the typically larger size (greater than 1 cm), the irregular shape and borders, and the areas of protrusion from the skin. Dermatofibrosarcoma protuberans will also recur if not completely excised, and multiple recurrences are common because of subclinical extension of the tumor. Usually biopsies are not necessary to make a diagnosis of dermatofibroma. For worrisome or indeterminate lesions, biopsy results will reveal a nodular collection of haphazardly distributed fibroblasts that surround and entrap thick collagen bundles. A sparse inflammatory infiltrate, increased number of blood vessels, and lentiginous hyperplasia of the epidermis are also found.

Treatment: Since dermatofibromas are benign, no treatment is necessary; they gradually involute over many years. If they are bothersome, excision is the treatment of choice. Liquid nitrogen therapy can help flatten and soften the lesions.

DERMATOFIBROSARCOMA PROTUBERANS

Definition and etiology: Dermatofibrosarcoma protuberans (DFSP) is a low-grade sarcoma. Biopsy results reveal a spindle cell tumor arising within the dermis from fibroblast-like cells. DFSP recurs after incomplete removal and rarely metastasizes.

Clinical features: Dermatofibrosarcoma occurs most commonly on the upper back of adult men. A higher incidence is seen in blacks. Clinical examination reveals an irregularly shaped, asymmetric, firm, skin- to red-colored keloidal nodule or plaque on the skin that is several centimeters in size. The overlying epidermis is usually atrophic. Telangiectatic blood vessels are seen, and ulceration may be present. A characteristic feature of DFSP is single or multiple protuberant nodules.

The major diseases in the differential diagnosis are keloid and dermatofibroma. Dermatofibromas are smaller, symmetric, and brown and exhibit dimpling upon squeezing. Unlike in DFSP, keloids occur after an injury and are frequently multiple. They may also be symmetric exophytic masses. In all questionable cases or when dermatofibrosarcoma is suspected, the diagnosis should be confirmed with a biopsy.

Treatment: Since DFSP recurs very frequently and ultimately after numerous recurrences can metastasize, excision with wide margins is the treatment of choice. Mohs' surgery with microscopically controlled margins has been used successfully by a number of surgeons.

EPIDERMAL INCLUSION CYST

Definition and etiology: A cyst is a sac lined with epithelium. In an epidermal inclusion cyst, the lining epithelium resembles normal epidermis.

Clinical features: Cysts are easily recognized as mobile, well-circumscribed subcutaneous or dermal nodules. Accurate diagnosis of a cyst requires histologic confirmation because the majority of the neoplasm cannot be seen clinically. Epidermal inclusion cysts are the most common type of cyst seen in adults. They occur on the trunk, face, and sometimes the scalp. A central punctum in the overlying epidermis may be present. Associated diseases include acne and uncommon entities such as Gardner's syndrome. Epidermal inclusion cysts on the hands can be produced by traumatic inoculation of epidermis into dermis in a puncture wound. The major differential diagnostic considerations are other cysts. Pilar cysts are more firm and are commonly found on the scalp because they are derived from hair follicles. Dermoid cysts are a type of hamartoma and most commonly occur lateral to the eyebrows. They usually present in infancy or early childhood. Thyroglossal duct and bronchogenic duct cysts should be suspected with cystic lesions occurring in the midline area of the neck in babies and infants. Meningomyelocele should be suspected with centrally located cysts on the scalp in babies, infants, and young children. In adults, the sudden onset of multiple firm "cystic" nodules should raise the suspicion of metastatic tumor (see Ch. 16). If the lesions are firm and tender, the differ-

ential diagnosis includes so-called ANGEL tumors: angiolipoma, neurilemmoma, glomus tumor, eccrine spiradenoma, and leiomyoma.

Treatment: Since epidermal inclusion cysts are benign, no treatment is necessary. For larger or cosmetically bothersome lesions, complete removal of the cyst and epithelial lining is the treatment of choice. If cyst wall remains, the cyst is likely to recur. Other therapies include incision and drainage with curettage of the cyst wall or intralesional corticosteroids if the cyst is inflamed.

LIPOMA

Definition and etiology: A lipoma is a benign tumor composed of mature adipocytes.

Clinical features: Lipomas are well-circumscribed, mobile, subcutaneous nodules most commonly found on the trunk, neck, and proximal extremities. The tumors are usually asymptomatic, but if they contain a large number of blood vessels (e.g., angiolipoma), they can be painful. Upon palpation, tumors have a soft spongy texture. A higher incidence of lipoma occurs in obese people, and a female predominance has been reported.

The major differential diagnostic consideration is a cyst. Epidermal inclusion cysts are usually not quite as deep, are better circumscribed, and are firmer and often have a punctum in the overlying epidermis. Cysts may have surrounding erythema if they rupture or become secondarily infected. Drainage from epidermal inclusion cysts is often a cheesy material or pus. Other entities to be considered include metastatic carcinoma and adnexal tumors (ANGEL tumors). Metastatic tumors should be suspected when numerous subcutaneous lesions develop suddenly. The sudden development of numerous lipomas would be extremely unlikely. Metastases are firm and occur in elderly individuals who usually have a history of prior cancer (see Ch. 16). Adnexal tumors, like cysts, usually are firmer than lipomas.

Treatment: Since lipomas are benign, no therapy is necessary. Lipomas do not develop into liposarcomas. If they are bothersome clinically, the treatment of choice is resection. Liposuction can also be performed if numerous biopsy-proven lipomas are present.

MASTOCYTOMA

Definition and etiology: A mastocytoma is a benign tumor of mast cells.

Clinical features: Mastocytomas are tan to light brown macules, papules, and nodules most commonly found in children from birth to 2 years of age. A characteristic finding is Darier's sign (e.g., urtication upon rubbing). Usually the tumors are localized to the skin, but involvement of internal organs (bone, liver, and gastrointestinal tract) can produce flushing, headaches, diarrhea, dyspnea, and syncopal episodes.

Because of their brown color, mastocytomas can be mistaken for nevi. Small acquired nevi more commonly develop in older children, adolescents, and young adults. Congenital nevi are larger than mastocytomas and may contain hair. Nevi are also darker brown and do not exhibit Darier's sign. Other lesions to be considered in the differential diagnosis include non-X histiocytoses (such as juvenile xanthogranuloma) and adnexal tumors. Lesions of juvenile xanthogranuloma are usually more yellow. In clinically indeterminate lesions, a biopsy should readily lead to a correct diagnosis. The biopsy findings reveal a collection of uniform-appearing mast cells that stain blue on Giemsa staining, interspersed eosinophils, and slight hyperpigmentation of the basal cell epidermal layer.

Treatment: Lesions may spontaneously regress over 5 to 6 years. Mast-cell-degranulating agents such as aspirin, alcohol, polymyxin B, morphine, and codeine should be avoided. Parents of patients with multiple mastocytomas (urticaria pigmentosa) should be given a prescription for an epinephrine kit (e.g., Ana-kit, epi-pen) to prepare for the possibility of anaphylactic shock. Single lesions can be treated with a high-strength topical steroid under occlusion or with excision.

MELANOCYTIC NEVUS (INTRADERMAL)

Definition and etiology: A nevus or mole is a benign neoplasm of melanocytes. The major etiologic factors are sun exposure and familial inheritance.

Clinical features: The three most common types of nevi are the following.

1. Junctional, in which melanocytes are confined to the base of the epidermis. Junctional nevi are usually macules.
2. Intradermal, in which melanocytes are confined to the dermis. Intradermal nevi are usually papular.
3. Compound, in which the melanocytes are found in both the epidermis and the dermis. Compound nevi are usually papular or nodular.

Nevi vary in appearance and coloration but most often have a fairly symmetric configuration, regular border, uniform flesh to brown color, and relatively small diameter. Intradermal nevi are slightly raised soft papules or nodules and can be confused with dermatofibromas because of

their brown color and intradermal location. Dimpling upon squeezing (Fitzpatrick's sign) is not seen in nevi. Nevi also usually have a darker brown color. Juvenile xanthogranulomas, xanthomas, mastocytomas, and melanomas can be confused with intradermal nevi. Epiluminescent microscopy (dermatoscopy, skin-surface microscopy) can accentuate an underlying pigment network and aid in accurate diagnosis. If the diagnosis is in question, the lesion should undergo biopsy.

Treatment: For common nevi, no therapy is required unless there has been a change in color, shape, or size or if bleeding or symptoms have occurred. For clinically indeterminate lesions, an excisional biopsy is mandated, especially to exclude a diagnosis of malignant melanoma.

NEUROFIBROMA

Definition and etiology: A neurofibroma is a common tumor of nerve sheath origin. Solitary neurofibromas are idiopathic, but the tendency for multiple neurofibromas can be inherited as an autosomal dominant trait in von Recklinghausen's disease (neurofibromatosis).

Clinical features: Cutaneous neurofibromas are soft, sessile or pedunculated, skin-colored to light pink tumors most commonly found on the trunk. Tumors can be partially pushed back into the skin. This finding is known as the "buttonhole sign." Rarer uncommonly encountered variants of neurofibromas such as plexiform, diffuse, and nodular types present as deep subcutaneous nodules and masses. In patients with neurofibromatosis, other associated findings include café au lait spots, axillary freckling, and Lisch nodules on the iris of the eye. The major differential diagnostic considerations are intradermal nevi (which usually retain some brown color) and skin tags, which usually are smaller and occur around the neck or axilla. A biopsy is usually not required but reveals a collection of small wavy spindle cells surrounded by a loose myxoid-appearing stroma.

Treatment: Neurofibroma is a benign tumor, and therefore treatment is not necessary. Surgical excision is the treatment of choice for lesions that are irritated by clothing, cosmetically disfiguring, or painful or that require confirmation to make the diagnosis. Lesions in patients with von Recklinghausen's disease need to be followed closely because of the risk for sarcomatous change.

PILAR CYST

Definition and etiology: A pilar cyst (trichilemmal cyst) contains compact hair-type keratin with a cyst wall resembling the isthmus portion of a hair follicle.

Pilar cysts can be idiopathic or can be inherited as an autosomal dominant trait.

Clinical features: Pilar cysts are most commonly found on the scalp of middle-aged adults. Pilar cysts are slightly more predominant in women. Examination reveals a firm flesh-colored mobile dermal nodule. The major differential diagnostic consideration is an epidermal inclusion cyst. Epidermal inclusion cysts occur most commonly on the trunk, are not as firm, and contain a central umbilication in the overlying epidermis. Epidermal cysts more frequently rupture or become secondarily infected, producing surrounding erythema; they frequently may have a drainage of white cheesy material. The differential diagnosis also includes other cysts, metastatic tumors, and adnexal neoplasms. Dermoid cyst, a form of hamartoma, most commonly occurs lateral to the eyebrows in newborn babies. Thyroglossal duct and bronchogenic duct cysts should be suspected with cystic lesions in the midline area of the neck in babies and infants. In adults with the sudden onset of multiple firm "cystic" nodules, metastatic disease should be excluded (see Ch. 16). If the lesions are firm and tender, the differential diagnosis would also include ANGEL tumors (angiolipoma, neurilemmoma, glomus tumor, leiomyoma, and eccrine spiradenoma).

Treatment: Pilar cysts are benign and need only be excised for cosmetic reasons or if symptomatic.

Suggested Readings

DERMATOFIBROMA
Fish FS. Soft tissue sarcomas in dermatology. Dermatol Surg 1996;22:268–73.
Nestle FO, Nickoloff BJ, Burg G. Dermatofibroma: an abortive immunoreactive process mediated by dermal dendritic cells? Dermatology 1995;190:265–68.

DERMATOFIBROSARCOMA PROTUBERANS
Laskin WB. Dermatofibrosarcoma protuberans. CA Cancer J Clin 1992;42:116–25.
Mark RJ et al. Dermatofibrosarcoma protuberans of the head and neck. A report of 16 cases. Arch Otolaryngol Head Neck Surg 1993;119:891–96.

Norman RA et al. Dermatofibroma protuberans: report of a case. J Am Osteopath Assoc 1988;88:245–47.

EPIDERMAL INCLUSION CYST
Thaller SR, Bauer BS. Cysts and cyst-like lesions of the skin and subcutaneous tissue. Clin Plast Surg 1987; 14:327–40.

LIPOMAS
Osment LS, Cutaneous lipomas and lipomatosis. Surg Gynecol Obstet 1968;127:129–32.
Pinski KS, Roenigk HH Jr. Liposuction of lipomas. Dermatol Clin 1990;8:483–92.

MASTOCYTOMA
Kettelhut BV, Metcalfe DD. Pediatric mastocytosis. Ann Allergy 1994;73:197–202; quiz 202–7.
Soter NA. The skin in mastocytosis. J Invest Dermatol 1991;96:32S–38S; discussion 38S–39S.

MELANOCYTIC NEVUS
Bhawan J. Melanocytic nevi. A review. J Cutan Pathol 1979;6:153–69.
Sagebiel RW. "Doing things right": approach to the cutaneous pigmented lesion. Semin Dermatol 1989;8: 251–58.

NEUROFIBROMA
Mulvihill JJ, Parry DM, Sherman JL et al. NIH conference. Neurofibromatosis 1 (Recklinghausen disease) and neurofibromatosis 2 (bilateral acoustic neurofibromatosis). An update. Ann Intern Med 1990;113:39–52.
Reznik M. Cutaneous neuropathology: neurofibromas, schwannomas and other neural neoplasms with cutaneous and extracutaneous expressions. Clin Neuropathol 1991;10:225–31.
Riccardi VM. Neurofibromatosis update. Neurofibromatosis 1989;2:284–91.

PILAR CYST
Thaller SR, Bauer BS. Cysts and cyst-like lesions of the skin and subcutaneous tissue. Clin Plast Surg 1987; 14:327–40.

16

Malignant Dermal Neoplasms

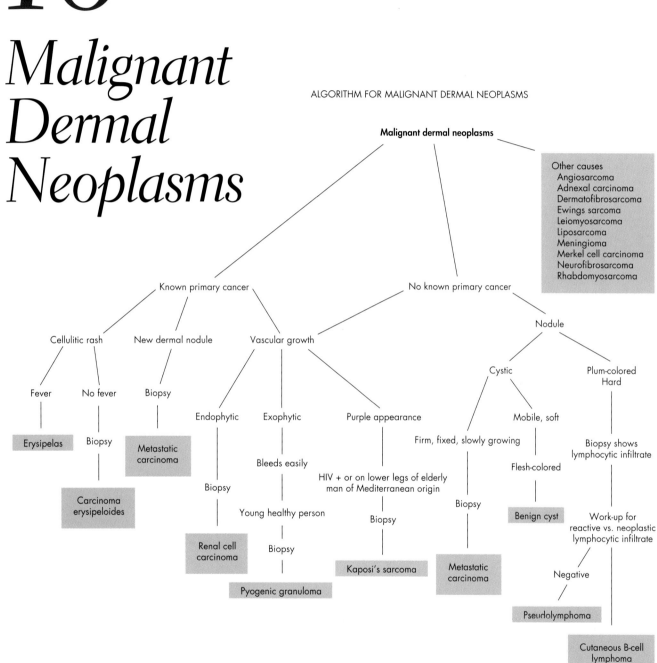

ALGORITHM FOR MALIGNANT DERMAL NEOPLASMS

Malignant dermal neoplasms

Other causes
  Angiosarcoma
  Adnexal carcinoma
  Dermatofibrosarcoma
  Ewings sarcoma
  Leiomyosarcoma
  Liposarcoma
  Meningioma
  Merkel cell carcinoma
  Neurofibrosarcoma
  Rhabdomyosarcoma

Known primary cancer

No known primary cancer

Nodule

Cellulitic rash

New dermal nodule

Vascular growth

Cystic

Plum-colored
Hard

Fever

No fever

Biopsy

Endophytic

Exophytic

Purple appearance

Firm, fixed, slowly growing

Mobile, soft

Biopsy shows
lymphocytic infiltrate

Erysipelas

Biopsy

Metastatic
carcinoma

Bleeds easily

HIV + or on lower legs of elderly
man of Mediterranean origin

Flesh-colored

Biopsy

Work-up for
reactive vs. neoplastic
lymphocytic infiltrate

Carcinoma
erysipeloides

Biopsy

Young healthy person

Biopsy

Biopsy

Benign cyst

Renal cell
carcinoma

Biopsy

Kaposi's sarcoma

Metastatic
carcinoma

Negative

Pyogenic granuloma

Pseudolymphoma

Cutaneous B-cell
lymphoma

Introduction

This chapter reviews the differential diagnosis of common malignant tumors and their benign simulators. Prompt recognition of malignant tumors is necessary to prevent morbidity and mortality. Cutaneous metastases are especially important to diagnose because they can assume a variety of different morphologies that can be mistaken for benign entities. Metastatic nodules are often misdiagnosed as cysts. Lesions of metastatic renal cell carcinoma are vascular and can be mistaken for hemangioma or pyogenic granuloma. Inflammatory metastases, so-called *carcinoma erysipeloides*, have a cellulitic or erysipelas-like appearance; it is inappropriate to treat them with intravenous antibiotics. Another malignant tumor that can be extremely difficult to diagnose is cutaneous B-cell lymphoma, especially since both the histologic and the clinical features of lymphomas and pseudolymphomas can be practically identical. Finally, with the onset of the acquired immunodeficiency syndrome (AIDS) epidemic, Kaposi's sarcoma is seen more frequently, and differentiation from its vascular simulators (such as hemangioma) is necessary.

1. NODULAR METASTATIC DISEASE
VERSUS
CUTANEOUS CYST

Features in common: Dermal nodules.

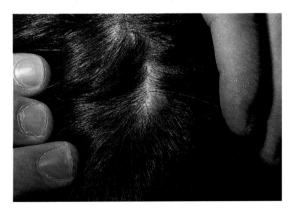

Figure 16.1.1 Epidermal inclusion cyst.

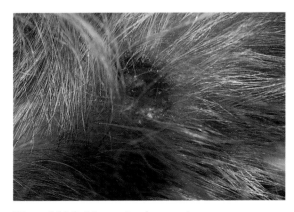

Figure 16.1.2 Metastatic adenocarcinoma.

Distinguishing features

	NODULAR METASTATIC DISEASE	CUTANEOUS CYST
Physical examination		
Morphology	Firm May be fixed to overlying skin No central punctum May ulcerate	Soft Not fixed to overlying skin Central punctum in epidermal inclusion cyst No ulceration
Distribution	Usually in vicinity of or body region near underlying cancer	Trunk, scalp, proximal extremities
History		
Symptoms	Sudden onset Often prior history of cancer Malaise, weight loss	Gradual onset No prior history of cancer No malaise or weight loss
Exacerbating factors	None	Secondary infection, rupture

Associated findings	Occasionally lymphadenopathy
	
	Hair loss if metastatic to scalp
	  (overlying metastasis)
		No lymphadenopathy
		  unless infected
		No hair loss with scalp cysts

Epidemiology	Elderly Familial history of cancer	Adults No familial history of cancer
Biopsy	Yes Malignant tumor cells Special stains can be performed	No, unless diagnosis is uncertain Cavity lined with epithelium
Laboratory	Depending on primary tumor	None

Treatment	Chemotherapy, radiation therapy,
	  surgical excision of primary tumor
	  and occasionally metastatic lesions
		Excision if symptomatic

Outcome	Poor	Excellent

Differential diagnosis of dermal nodules

Adnexal tumors
Calcinosis/osteoma cutis
Cysts
Dermatofibromas

If tender, consider ANGEL tumors:
  *a*ngiolipoma, *n*eurilemmoma,
  *g*lomus tumor, *e*ccrine spiradenoma,
  *l*eiomyoma

Lipomas
Metastatic tumors

2. CARCINOMA ERYSIPELOIDES
VERSUS
ERYSIPELAS

Features in common: Large erythematous macule.

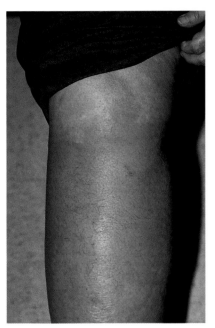

Figure 16.2.1 Erysipelas.

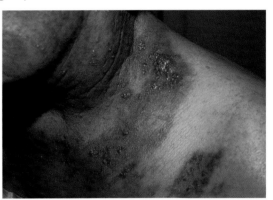

Figure 16.2.2 Carcinoma erysipeloides.

Distinguishing features

	CARCINOMA ERYSIPELOIDES	ERYSIPELAS
Physical examination		
Morphology	Dusky red-maroon color	Bright red color
	Skin is firm indurated	Skin not indurated
	Telangectasias may be present	No telangiectasia
	Gradual spread over days to weeks	Rapid spread over hours
	Nodular component may be present	Nodules rarely present
	On chest may be associated with nipple retraction, edema, and breast enlargement	No nipple retraction, edema, and breast enlargement
Distribution	Most common on chest	Usually on face or lower legs
History		
Symptoms	Prior history of cancer	No prior history of cancer
	No prior history of cellulitis	Sometimes prior history of cellulitis
	Weight loss, malaise	No weight loss or malaise
Exacerbating factors	Neglect or inappropriate treatment	Immunosuppression

Continues

Distinguishing features (*Continued*)

	CARCINOMA ERYSIPELOIDES	ERYSIPELAS
Associated findings	No fever Underlying malignancy No baseline lymphedema No prior history of thrombophlebitis	Fever No underlying malignancy Lymphedema: congenital, postsurgical, or stasis-related A prior history of thrombophlebitis or tinea pedis may be present with lesions on legs
Epidemiology	Adults Most often due to breast cancer	Adults Male and female
Biopsy	Yes Tumor cells within dilated lymphatic vessels	Not necessary Diffuse edema with neutrophilic infiltrate
Laboratory	Metastatic work-up	Leukocytosis, culture of skin biopsy or blood
Treatment	Chemotherapy, radiation therapy, surgery	IV or oral antibiotics that cover β-hemolytic streptococcus
Outcome	Poor	Resolves with treatment

3. METASTATIC RENAL CELL CARCINOMA
VERSUS
PYOGENIC GRANULOMA

Features in common: Red vascular-appearing nodules.

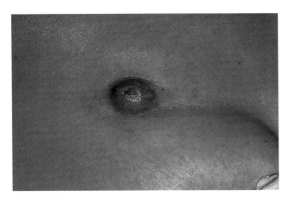

Figure 16.3.1 Metastatic renal cell carcinoma.

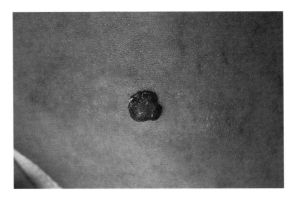

Figure 16.3.2 Pyogenic granuloma.

Distinguishing features

	METASTATIC RENAL CELL CARCINOMA	PYOGENIC GRANULOMA
Physical examination		
Morphology	Variable colored: flesh, red, blue, or black	Red-colored
	Dermal or subcutaneous nodules or plaques	Exophytic papules and nodules
	Ulceration and bleeding possible	Ulceration and bleeding common
	May be pulsatile	Not pulsatile
	Single or multiple lesions	Single lesion (rarely satellite lesions)
Distribution	Generalized	Generalized
History		
Symptoms	History of renal carcinoma	No history of carcinoma
	Weight loss, malaise	No weight loss or malaise
Exacerbating factors	None	Pregnancy
		Trauma
Associated findings	Hypertension, hypercalcemia, amyloidosis, and polycythemia are occasionally noted	No associated hypertension or hypercalcemia
	An associated bruit may be present	No associated bruit
Epidemiology	Adults	More common in children
Biopsy	Yes	Occasionally
	Neoplasm composed of lobules of clear-staining malignant cells with surrounding vascular stroma	Neoplasm composed of lobules of uniform round blood vessels surrounded by a collarette of epithelium and inflammatory cells
Laboratory	Work-up for metastatic disease	None
	Serum calcium	
Treatment	Chemotherapy	Excision, or curettage with electrodesiccation of base; occasionally lesions may recur
Outcome	Poor	Excellent

4. KAPOSI'S SARCOMA VERSUS HEMANGIOMA

Features in common: Red vascular-appearing papules, nodules, and plaques.

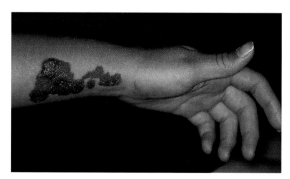

Figure 16.4.2 Hemangioma.

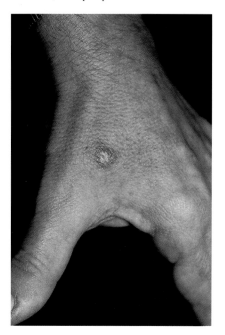

Figure 16.4.1 Kaposi's sarcoma.

Distinguishing features

	KAPOSI'S SARCOMA	HEMANGIOMA
Physical examination		
Morphology	Pink, purple, to brown colored	Red colored
	Patches, plaques, nodules	Papules, nodules
	Truncal lesions may follow skin lines	Does not follow skin lines
	May Koebnerize	Does not Koebnerize
Distribution	Classic: lower legs	
	HIV associated: face, trunk, extremities and mucosa	Trunk and extremities
History		
Symptoms	Asymptomatic	Bleeds with trauma
Exacerbating factors	Immunosuppression	Trauma
Associated findings	Occasionally pulmonary or gastrointestinal symptoms due to systemic involvement	Occasionally thrombocytopenia or disseminated intravascular coagulation

Continues

Distinguishing features (Continued)

	KAPOSI'S SARCOMA	HEMANGIOMA
Epidemiology	Classic: adult Mediterranean men HIV associated: homosexual men, human leukocyte antigen DR 25	Children

Biopsy	Yes
	Blood-filled slitlike spaces with
	  surrounding spindle cell proliferation
		No
		Uniform round-appearing
		  capillaries organized in lobules

Laboratory	Work-up for systemic disease as
	  indicated by symptoms
	Experimental: herpesvirus type 8 DNA
		Platelet, prothrombin and partial
		  thromboplastin times if clinical
		  symptoms of bleeding present

Treatment	Local: cryotherapy, excision, laser,
	  intralesional interferon, radiation
	Systemic: interferon, chemotherapy,
	  retinoids
		Surgical excision, laser ablation,
		  intralesional or systemic
		  corticosteroids in children

Outcome	Classic: chronic slowly progressive
	  disease
	HIV related: poor prognostic indicator
		Good: may spontaneously involute
		  during childhood

Abbreviation: HIV, human immunodeficiency virus.

Differential diagnosis of Kaposi's sarcoma

Common causes
  Dermatofibroma
  Hemangioma
    Angiokeratoma
    Capillary hemangioma
    Cavernous hemangioma
    Targetoid hemosiderotic
     hemangioma
  Hemorrhage trauma
  (talon noire)

Common causes (*continued*)
  Lichen planus
  Melanocytic nevus
  Postinflammatory
   hyperpigmentation
  Pyogenic granuloma
  Stasis dermatitis
   (acroangiodermatitis)

Rarer causes
  Angiosarcoma
  Bacillary angiomatosis
  Glomangioma
  Pityriasis rosea
  Psoriasis

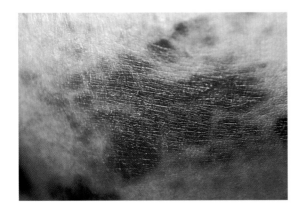

Figure 16.4.3 Kaposi's sarcoma. *Clue to diagnosis* Purple-colored plaques.

5. CUTANEOUS B-CELL LYMPHOMA
VERSUS
PSEUDOLYMPHOMA

Features in common: Red to plum-colored dermal nodules.

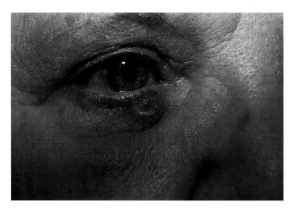

Figure 16.5.1 Lymphoma.

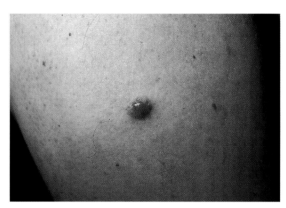

Figure 16.5.2 Pseudolymphoma.

Distinguishing features

	CUTANEOUS B-CELL LYMPHOMA	PSEUDOLYMPHOMA
Physical examination		
Morphology	*Identical appearance:* red to plum-colored nodules	*Identical appearance:* red to plum-colored nodules
	Lesions tend to be large (golf-ball-sized)	Lesions tend to be smaller than lymphoma
	Ulcerated nodules occasionally present	Ulcerated nodules rare
Distribution	More common on trunk but can occur on head and neck	Head and neck, rarely truncal
History		
Symptoms	Occasionally prior or concurrent history of systemic lymphoma	No history of systemic lymphoma
	Fever, weight loss, and night sweats if systemic involvement	No systemic symptoms
Exacerbating factors	Immunosuppression	Insect bites
		Lyme disease
		Medications
Associated findings	Lymphadenopathy or hepatosplenomegaly when systemic involvement is present	No lymphadenopathy or hepatosplenomegaly
Epidemiology	Adults	Any age

Continues

Distinguishing features (Continued)

	CUTANEOUS B-CELL LYMPHOMA	PSEUDOLYMPHOMA
Biopsy	Yes Nodular infiltrate is usually predominantly located in bottom of dermis or subcutaneous tissue with atypical cells	Yes Nodular infiltrate composed of benign lymphocytes predominantly located in middle to upper dermis; eosinophils are frequently numerous
Laboratory	Immunophenotypic and gene rearrangement studies clarify the diagnosis in histological indeterminate cases by demonstrating a clonal cell population Systemic work-up: computed tomography, chest x-ray	Immunophenotypic and gene rearrangement studies in histological indeterminate lesions; no clonal cell population
Treatment	Radiation and chemotherapy	Topical and intralesional steroids Cryosurgery and excision Radiation therapy for unresponsive lesions
Outcome	Curable if localized to skin Variable prognosis if systemic involvement	Excellent

Differential diagnosis of lymphocytic infiltrates in the skin

Benign lymphocytic infiltrate of Jessner

Cold panniculitis

Cutaneous lupus erythematosus

Drug eruption

Insect bite reaction

Lymphoma

Pernio (chilblains)

Polymorphous light eruption

Pseudolymphoma

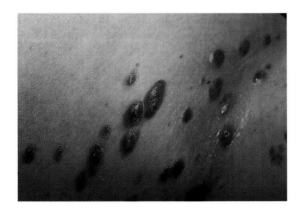

Figure 16.5.3 Lymphoma. *Clue to diagnosis*: Numerous nodules.

Discussion

CUTANEOUS B-CELL LYMPHOMA

Definition and etiology: Cutaneous B-cell lymphoma is non-Hodgkin's lymphoma of the skin. Although most patients with cutaneous B-cell lymphoma have systemic disease (secondary cutaneous B-cell lymphoma), some patients with lymphoma related to skin-associated lymphoid tissue (primary cutaneous B-cell lymphoma) have only cutaneous involvement.

Clinical features: Patients with cutaneous B-cell lymphoma present with either single or multiple dermal or subcutaneous nodules. Clinical findings are nondiagnostic, and the sudden onset of nodule(s) in a patient with non-Hodgkin's lymphoma requires a biopsy. The proximal lymph nodes frequently may be enlarged, and patients may also complain of fever, night sweats, and weight loss.

The lesions of cutaneous B-cell lymphoma are reddish-blue nodules that are most commonly found on the trunk, head, and neck. Surrounding papules or erythema and edema are present. Cutaneous B-cell lymphoma needs to be differentiated from a benign reactive lymphocytic infiltrate such as pseudolymphoma (lymphocytoma). Accurate diagnosis requires a skin biopsy. The biopsy results reveal a dense infiltrate composed of atypical lymphocytes. The infiltrate is denser in the deep dermis and subcutaneous tissue. Immunophenotypic and gene rearrangement studies demonstrate a clonal population of lymphocytes.

In some cases, in spite of having done a biopsy, the diagnosis may be uncertain, since there are reports of pseudolymphoma evolving into lymphoma. The development of nodules after an insect bite or after the start of a new medication provides evidence in favor of a benign reactive lymphocytic infiltrate rather than lymphoma. In all cases, work-up involves complete physical examination, screening laboratory tests, and radiologic studies in addition to biopsy.

Treatment: Patients with systemic involvement suffer significant morbidity and mortality. Aggressive treatment with radiation therapy or chemotherapy or both, is required. The prognosis for patients with cutaneous B-cell lymphoma limited to the skin is excellent, and lesions can be treated solely with radiation therapy.

CYST

Definition and etiology: A cyst is a sac lined by an epithelial layer. The two most common cysts are epidermal inclusion and pilar cysts (see Ch. 15).

Clinical features: Cysts are easily recognized as mobile, well-circumscribed, rubbery dermal and subcutaneous nodules. The ultimate classification of a cyst requires microscopic examination of its lining epithelium. Certain clinical clues may also help in differentiation. Epidermal inclusion cysts are by far the most common type of cyst encountered in clinical practice. They occur most frequently on the trunk, face, and scalp. Sometimes a central umbilication in the overlying epidermis is present. The second most common type of cyst is the pilar cyst. Pilar cysts (also known as isthmus-catagen cysts) are cysts with a lining epithelium resembling hair. They occur most commonly on the scalp. Dermoid cysts are a type of hamartoma. They occur most commonly lateral to the eyebrows and are most often detected at birth. Thyroglossal duct and bronchogenic duct cysts should be suspected with cystic lesions in the midline area of the neck and are usually first noted in infancy. In adults, the sudden onset of multiple firm "cystic" nodules should lead to the suspicion of metastatic disease. Metastatic nodular cutaneous lesions are easy to overlook or ignore. *If a patient with a history of a prior malignancy develops a new cutaneous nodule, a biopsy is mandatory.* The degree of suspicion is heightened if numerous "cysts" develop suddenly. Metastatic lesions are firmer than epidermal inclusion cysts. They are frequently irregularly shaped and fixed to the surrounding skin. Occasionally, metastatic nodules can be the presenting sign of an underlying malignancy. For any dermal or subcutaneous lesions for which the diagnosis is not certain, a biopsy should be done. If lesions are firm and tender, the differential diagnosis includes the so-called ANGEL tumors (benign tumors commonly associated with pain): angiolipoma, neurilemmoma, glomus tumor, eccrine spiradenoma, and leiomyoma.

Treatment: Since cysts are benign, no treatment is necessary. For larger or cosmetically bothersome lesions, the treatment of choice is surgery with removal of the entire lining epithelium to prevent recurrence. If the lining epithelium is not removed, the cyst is likely to recur. Incision and drainage with curettage to remove the cyst wall is done for ruptured or infected cysts.

ERYSIPELAS

Definition and etiology: Erysipelas is a cutaneous infection caused by *Streptococcus pyogenes.*

Clinical features: Patients present with fever, anorexia, headache, and even vomiting. There is a cellulitic rash. Erysipelas most commonly involves the face or lower extremities in older children or adults and the trunk in infants. The skin is bright red, hot, and painful and early on has a sharply defined and slightly raised margin. With time, edema, vesicles, and bullae may develop. The margin becomes less well demarcated.

The major differential diagnostic considerations are contact dermatitis, carcinoma erysipeloides, and an early lesion of herpes zoster. In contact dermatitis, fever is absent, pruritus is present, and history or patch testing will implicate a triggering antigen. The lesions of herpes zoster occur in a dermatomal distribution, and patients usually have prodromal hyperesthesia and complain of a prickly or lacerating pain. Eventually grouped vesicles will develop in areas of pain. The rash of carcinoma erysipeloides occurs in the vicinity of an underlying malignancy and does not spread as rapidly as erysipelas. Fever is not present, although the skin feels warm. Nodules and indurated areas are found on palpation. Blisters do not occur.

Treatment: The treatment of erysipelas includes oral or intravenous antibiotics like penicillin that cover streptococcal organisms.

HEMANGIOMA

Definition and etiology: A hemangioma is a benign neoplasm of blood vessels. Hemangiomas can be further classified into different subtypes, such as cherry angioma, targetoid hemosiderotic hemangioma, strawberry nevus, cavernous hemangioma, and arteriovenous hemangioma, based on clinical and histologic appearance. Rarer variants include epithelioid, verrucous, and tufted hemangiomas.

Clinical features: Cherry angioma and strawberry nevus derive their names from their clinical appearance: bright red papules and plaques resembling cherries and strawberries. Histologic examination reveals lobular proliferation of uniform round capillaries. Cavernous hemangiomas are larger, massive, deep-dermal red nodules and plaques that are several centimeters in size. Pathologic examination demonstrates large, dilated, thick-walled blood vessels. Targetoid hemosiderotic hemangiomas, primarily present in children and young adults, are small red angiomas with surrounding ecchymosis, which produces a targetoid appearance. Biopsy findings demonstrate irregularly shaped blood vessels that can be mistaken for Kaposi's sarcoma by unaware pathologists. Arteriovenous hemangiomas, collections of thick-walled arteries and veins, are red to skin-colored papules most commonly located on the face or on acral sites.

The major differential diagnostic considerations include pigmented nevi (see Ch. 14) and Kaposi's sarcoma. Usually, because of the bright red color, the diagnosis is relatively straightforward. Kaposi's sarcoma (discussed later) primarily occurs in adults and presents with violaceous, not red-colored, patches and plaques.

Treatment: Treatment of hemangioma is usually not necessary. Capillary hemangiomas in children usually involute over a period of 5 to 10 years. The treatment of choice for cosmetically unacceptable rapidly growing lesions or those that interfere with vision, eating, or breathing is laser surgery. Small lesions can also be destroyed with light electrodesiccation or can be removed with scalpel or scissors excision.

KAPOSI'S SARCOMA

Definition and etiology: Kaposi's sarcoma is a malignant neoplasm of blood vessels. Recently, Kaposi's sarcoma has been linked to herpesvirus-8 infection in some individuals.

Clinical features: A variety of different clinical forms of Kaposi's sarcoma exist. The classic adult form is found primarily in elderly Mediterranean, Jewish, or eastern European men. An endemic form is seen in Africa, and the immunosuppression-related form is most commonly seen in men with acquired immunodeficiency syndrome (AIDS). The cutaneous manifestations correlate with each of these clinical variants. In classic Kaposi's sarcoma, lesions are localized to the lower legs and can be confused with stasis dermatitis. The lack of pitting edema, the presence of violaceous-colored nodules, and the genetic and ethnic background of the patient will indicate the need for a skin biopsy, which confirms the diagnosis. The African endemic form commonly presents in children with generalized lymphadenopathy. The lesions in the immunosuppressed and AIDS-related forms are scattered and can involve the entire integument plus the oral mucosa. The tumor evolves through macule-patch, papule-plaque, and nodular stages. The macule patches are small, oval, round, nonscaly, and reddish-purple. Isolated lesions can be confused with dermatofibromas or hemangiomas. Dermatofibromas do not have purple color, however, are usually smaller, and umbilicate upon squeezing. Large hemangiomas are bright red (not purple) and are primarily seen in young infants and children. The smaller cherry angiomas in adults are red, small, and symmetric and only a few millimeters in size.

Lesions of Kaposi's sarcoma follow skin lines when present on the trunk and may be confused with pityriasis rosea. Unlike in pityriasis rosea, the lesions lack scale and there is no preceding herald patch. The lesions have a purple hue and last indefinitely. The papular lesions of Kaposi's sarcoma can be confused with pyogenic granuloma and bacillary angiomatosis. Pyogenic granulomas occur in young healthy children and adults, are isolated exophytic lesions, and bleed profusely when traumatized. Bacillary angiomatosis, an infection due to *Rochalimaea henselae*, occurs in immunocompromised patients, resembles pyogenic granuloma and Kaposi's sarcoma, and may be correctly diagnosed with a skin biopsy and a Warthin-Starry stain, which reveals the infectious organisms.

Plaquelike and nodular lesions of Kaposi's sarcoma can be confused with angiosarcoma. Angiosarcoma, however, develops most commonly on the scalp or in areas of chronic lymphedema. Ultimately, any lesion suspected to be Kaposi's sarcoma should undergo biopsy. Findings will reveal a proliferation of spindle cells, erythrocytes in slit-like spaces, and irregularly shaped blood vessels.

Treatment: Many treatment modalities exist for Kaposi's sarcoma. For a few isolated lesions, excision, laser therapy, sclerotherapy, intralesional chemotherapy, radiation therapy, cryosurgery, or intralesional interferon can be used. For widespread and systemic disease, chemotherapy, radiation therapy, retinoids, and interferon-α are of benefit. In patients with Kaposi's sarcoma who have other risk factors for AIDS, human immunodeficiency virus test should be done. The sarcoma may also improve with anti-retroviral therapy.

METASTATIC CARCINOMA

Definition and etiology: Metastasis is the spread of a malignant tumor beyond its primary site of origin to a discontinuous area. The spread can occur through vascular or lymphatic pathways. The majority of patients with cutaneous metastases have a known underlying primary malignancy, but cutaneous lesions may sometimes be the first sign of malignancy.

Clinical features: Cutaneous metastases can occur at any age. They are most common in elderly adults. Excluding melanoma, the majority of cutaneous metastases are from lung, breast (in females), or gastrointestinal tract tumors. Metastatic tumors can have a variety of different morphologies:

1. Nodules
2. Inflammatory metastases
   (carcinoma erysipeloides)
3. Cicatricial metastases
4. Carcinoma en cuirasse
5. Zosteriform metastases

Each of these different types can be confused with a variety of other diseases. Nodules of metastatic carcinoma are usually firm and vary in color from flesh-colored to red or purple. They can easily be confused with cysts, lipomas, or adnexal neoplasms. *Therefore, the sudden development of a new nodule in a patient with known malignancy mandates a skin biopsy.* A firm nodule that does not feel cystic and cannot be definitively classified should also undergo biopsy even if the patient does not have a history of underlying malignancy. Metastatic nodules in patients with renal cell carcinoma have a red vascular color and can easily be confused with hemangioma or pyogenic granuloma.

Pyogenic granulomas occur in young adults and children and are exophytic papules. A pyogenic-granuloma-like lesion in an adult should undergo biopsy. Similarly, because most hemangiomas (cherry angiomas) in adults are small papules, a large hemangioma-like lesion should undergo biopsy.

Inflammatory metastases appear as red plaques mimicking erysipelas and have been called *carcinoma erysipeloides.* Unlike erysipelas, fever is absent, the lesions progress at a slower rate, and an indurated and nodular component may be present. The lesions also most commonly occur in an area overlying a prior malignancy. Of note is that occasionally after surgical excision, some patients may also present with transient erythema lasting a few months to years in the site of surgery due to obstructed lymphatic vessels.

Cicatricial metastases appear as sclerotic plaques and can be mistaken for scars or sclerosing basal cell carcinoma. On the scalp, alopecia may be present (alopecia neoplastica). Therefore, cutaneous scar appearing without a prior history of injury or surgery should undergo biopsy, especially if the "scar" is enlarging.

Carcinoma en cuirasse refers to extensive metastatic involvement of the chest, which produces a circumferential fibrotic plaque. The tumor gives the patient the appearance of being encased in a breastplate of armor (en cuirasse).

Metastatic nodules that involve a dermatome are referred to as zosteriform metastases. This pattern may be confused with herpes zoster. The presence of nodules rather than vesicles leads to a correct diagnosis.

Treatment: The prognosis for patients with cutaneous metastases is poor but depends on the type of malignancy. Chemotherapy is the treatment of choice.

PSEUDOLYMPHOMA

Definition and etiology: Pseudolymphoma (also known as lymphocytoma) is a benign proliferation of lymphocytes that is often confused with lymphoma. The cause is unknown, but pseudolymphoma can be triggered by insect bites, medications, and *Borrelia burgdorferi* infection.

Clinical features: Pseudolymphoma primarily occurs in children and young adults. There is a slight predilection for females. The skin examination shows a single or occasionally multiple subcutaneous blue-red nodules on the earlobes, face, chest, and scrotum. The presence of large lesions that ulcerate and predominantly involve the trunk should, however, raise suspicion of the presence of an underlying lymphoma. A chest x-ray and complete blood count with differential should be ordered, and patients should be examined for lymphadenopathy and hepatosplenomegaly when the diagnosis is not certain.

Conversely, the history of occurrence of the lesions after an insect bite or onset of new medication would indicate a benign process. Phenytoin (Dilantin) has been associated with a pseudolymphoma-like reaction.

Clinically, the lesions cannot be differentiated from cutaneous lymphoma. If an etiologic agent cannot be ascertained with certainty, a biopsy is required for accurate diagnosis. Ultimately, all persistent lesions should undergo biopsy. Findings show a proliferation of lymphocytes in germinal centers mimicking a lymph node. Because of occasional histologic resemblance to lymphoma, ancillary tests such as gene rearrangement or phenotypic studies are necessary to confirm the reactive nature of the infiltrate. Lesions of lymphocytoma cutis can also be confused with benign lymphocytic infiltrate of Jessner-Kanof, which is another reactive lymphocytic infiltrate. Clinically, however, the lesions of lymphocytic infiltrate of Jessner-Kanof usually are annular, and histologically the infiltrate is less dense without germinal center formation.

Treatment: A variety of different treatment modalities have been used. None is entirely effective. Topical and intralesional steroid injections are most commonly used. Lesions associated with *Borrelia burgdorferi* respond to penicillin or doxycycline therapy. Any possibly associated medications should be discontinued. Cryotherapy and radiation therapy are also effective. Any lesion that does not respond to therapy should be followed carefully, since evolution of pseudolymphomas into true lymphomas has been reported.

PYOGENIC GRANULOMA

Definition and etiology: Pyogenic granuloma is a benign vascular proliferation. Whether the proliferation of blood vessels is reactive or neoplastic is yet to be determined.

Clinical features: Pyogenic granuloma can occur at any age but most commonly is found in young children. Pyogenic granuloma develops rapidly over a period of weeks with predilection for the head, neck, and arms. In pregnant women, mucosal lesions can occur. The skin examination reveals bright red, round, exophytic papules and nodules that bleed easily. Rarely, satellite lesions can occur after prior treatment or excision.

The differential diagnosis of pyogenic granuloma includes hemangioma, Kaposi's sarcoma, bacillary angiomatosis, primary cutaneous neoplasms such as Spitz nevus, atypical fibroxanthoma, amelanotic melanoma, and metastatic carcinoma. Hemangiomas usually start as macules and gradually grow into nodules in young children. They usually are larger, more lobulated masses as compared with the small, round, exophytic papules of pyogenic granulomas. A pyogenic-granuloma-like lesion in an immunocompromised patient, especially one with AIDS,

requires a biopsy to differentiate the lesion from both Kaposi's sarcoma and bacillary angiomatosis, since both tumors can be exophytic vascular papules. The additional presence of flat purple patches or plaques would be indicative of Kaposi's sarcoma. Some primary cutaneous malignancies such as amelanotic melanoma and atypical fibroxanthoma can appear as red papules or nodules. If the lesion is asymmetric and only parts of it bleed, and if it exhibits a dermal component on palpation, a malignancy rather then pyogenic granuloma should be suspected. Although a Spitz nevus can appear red, be perfectly symmetric, and develop rapidly, usually a Spitz nevus is more dome- or sessile-shaped, is nonulcerated, and has a more tan-colored appearance. Metastatic carcinoma, especially metastatic renal cell carcinoma, can also present as a red, rapidly growing dermal nodule. Asymmetry, a palpable dermal component, or occurrence in elderly adults should arouse suspicion. A biopsy of pyogenic granuloma should be done to confirm the diagnosis. It shows an exophytic lobular proliferation of uniform round-appearing blood vessels surrounded by edematous inflamed stroma and a collarette of epithelium.

Treatment: Pyogenic granuloma can be excised, removed with curettage and electrodesiccation, or treated with liquid nitrogen cryosurgery. Spontaneous resolution may also occur.

Suggested Readings

CUTANEOUS B-CELL LYMPHOMA
Burg G, Schmid MH, Kung E et al. Semimalignant ("pseudolymphomatous") cutaneous B-cell lymphomas. Dermatol Clin 1994;12:399–407.

Helm KF, Su WP, Muller SA et al. Malignant lymphoma and leukemia with prominent ulceration: clinicopathologic correlation of 33 cases. J Am Acad Dermatol 1992;27:553–59.

Landa NG, Zelickson BD, Peters MS et al. Lymphoma versus pseudolymphoma of the skin: gene rearrangement study of 21 cases with clinicopathologic correlation. J Am Acad Dermatol 1993; 29:945–53.

Patterson JW. Lymphomas (review). Dermatol Clini 1992; 10:235–51.

CYST
Thaller SR, Bauer BS. Cysts and cyst-like lesions of the skin and subcutaneous tissue. Clin Plast Surg 1987;14: 327–40.

ERYSIPELAS
Bratton RL, Nesse RE. St. Anthony's fire: diagnosis and management of erysipelas (see comments) (review). Am Fam Physician 1995; 51:401–4.

Chartier C, Grosshans E. Erysipelas (review). Int J Dermatol 1990;29:459–67.

Grosshans EM. The red face: erysipelas (review). Clin Dermatol 1993;11:307–13.

HEMANGIOMA
Bernstein EF, Kantor G, Howe N et al. Tufted angioma of the thigh. J Am Acad Dermatol 1994;31:307–11.

Fishman SJ, Mulliken JB. Hemangiomas and vascular malformations of infancy and childhood. Pediatr Clin North Am 1993;40:1177–200.

Lask GP, Glassberg E. 585-nm pulsed dye laser for the treatment of cutaneous lesions. Clin Dermatol 1995;13:63–67.

Low DW. Hemangiomas and vascular malformations. Semin Pediatr Surg 1994;3:40–61.

Morelli JG. Management of hemangiomas. Adv Dermatol 1993;8:327–44; discussion 345.

Upton J, Coombs C. Vascular tumors in children. Hand Clin 1995;11:307–37.

Wahrman JE, Honig PJ. Hemangiomas. Pediatr Rev 1994;15:266–71.

KAPOSI'S SARCOMA
Finesmith TH, Shrum JP. Kaposi's sarcoma (review). Int J Dermatol 1994;33:755–62.

Schwartz RA. Kaposi's sarcoma: advances and perspectives (review). J Am Acad Dermatol 1996;34:804–14.

Volm MD, von Roenn JH. Treatment strategies for epidemic Kaposi's sarcoma (review). Curr Opin Oncol 1995;7:429–36.

Zalla MJ. Kaposi's sarcoma. An update (review). Dermatol Surg 1996;22:274–87.

METASTATIC CARCINOMA
Kouroupakis D, Patsea E, Sofras F et al. Renal cell carcinoma metastases to the skin: a not so rare case? Br J of Urol 1995;75:583–85.

Lambert WC, Schwartz RA. Metastasis (editorial). J Am Acad Dermatol 1992;27:131–33.

Lookingbill DP, Spangler N, Helm KF. Cutaneous metastases in patients with metastatic carcinoma: a retrospective study of 4020 patients. J Am Acad Dermatol 1993;29:228–36.

Spencer PS, Helm TN. Skin metastases in cancer patients. Cutis 1987;39:119–21.

Williams JC, Heaney JA. Metastatic renal cell carcinoma presenting as a skin nodule: case report and review of the literature (review). J Urol 1994;152:2094–95.

PSEUDOLYMPHOMA
Helm KF, Muller SA. Benign lymphocytic infiltrate of the skin: correlation of clinical and pathologic findings. Mayo Clin Proc 1992;67:748–54.

Kuflik AS, Schwartz RA. Lymphocytoma cutis: a series of five patients successfully treated with cryosurgery. J Am Acad Dermatol 1992;26:449–52.

Magro CM, Crowson AN. Drugs with antihistaminic properties as a cause of atypical cutaneous lymphoid hyperplasia. J Am Acad Dermatol 1995;32:419–28.

Magro CM, Crowson AN. Drug-induced immune dysregulation as a cause of atypical cutaneous lymphoid infiltrates: a hypothesis. Hum Pathol 1996;27:125–32.

Rijlaarsdam JU, Willemze R. Cutaneous pseudolymphomas: classification and differential diagnosis (review). Semin Dermatol 1994;13:187–96.

Stein L, Lowe L, Fivenson D. Coalescing violaceous plaques forming leonine facies. Lymphocytoma cutis (pseudolymphoma). Arch Dermato 1994;130:1552–53.

Strle F, Pleterski-Rigler D, Stanek G et al. Solitary borrelial lymphocytoma: report of 36 cases. Infection 1992;20:201–6.

PYOGENIC GRANULOMA
Mooney MA, Janniger CK. Pyogenic granuloma. Cutis 1995;55:133–36.

Upton J, Coombs C. Vascular tumors in children. Hand Clin 1995;11:307–37.

Index

Page numbers followed by *f* indicate figures; those followed by *t* indicate tables.